Manual of Histological Techniques and their Diagnostic Application

For Churchill Livingstone:
Publisher: Geoffrey Nuttall
Project Editor: Lowri Daniels
Project Controller: Mark Sanderson
Copy Editor: Ruth Swan
Sales Promotion Executive: Duncan Jones

Manual of Histological Techniques and their Diagnostic Application

John D. Bancroft
Principal Medical Laboratory Scientific Officer,
Histopathology Department, Queen's Medical Centre, Nottingham,
University Hospital NHS Trust, UK

Harry C. Cook
Principal Medical Laboratory Scientific Officer,
Pathology Department, West Middlesex University Hospital NHS Trust,
Isleworth, Middlesex, UK

With a contribution by
Robert W. Stirling
Consultant Histopathologist, West Middlesex University Hospital NHS Trust, Isleworth,
Middlesex, UK

Foreword by
David R. Turner
Professor of Pathology, Medical School, Queen's Medical Centre, Nottingham,
University Hospital NHS Trust, UK

CHURCHILL LIVINGSTONE
EDINBURGH LONDON MADRID MELBOURNE NEW YORK AND TOKYO 1994

CHURCHILL LIVINGSTONE
An imprint of Harcourt Publishers Limited

© Longman Group UK Limited 1994
© Harcourt Publishers Limited 1999

First published 1984 as *Manual of Histological Techniques*
 Reprinted 1995
 Reprinted 1999

ISBN 0-443-04534-8

British Library of Cataloguing in Publication Data
A catalogue record for this book is available from the British
Library

Library of Congress Cataloging in Publication Data
Bancroft, John D.
 Manual of histological techniques and their diagnostic
applications/John D. Bancroft, Harry C. Cook; foreword by David R. Turner.
  p. cm.
 Includes index.
 ISBN 0-443-04534-8
 1. Histology, Pathological—Laboratory manauals. I. Cook, H. C. (Harry Charles)
II. Title.
 [DNLM: 1. Histological Techniques. QS 525 B213ma 1994]
RB30.B36 1994
616.07′583—dc20
DNLM/DLC   93-35533
for Library of Congress   CIP

The
publisher's
policy is to use
**paper manufactured
from sustainable forests**

Printed in China
CTPS/03

Contents

Foreword

This book is based on the earlier manual by Bancroft and Cook and shows extensive revision of that text, with the objective of including more scientific and medical background to the basic technical methodology. Increasingly, medical laboratory scientific officers are expected to have a deeper understanding of their subject. Indeed, better insight into the processes they are investigating means that they can collaborate in a true partnership with their medical colleagues for both diagnostic and research studies. We are seeing increasing evidence of this in our laboratory and it works to the benefit of laboratory staff, clinicians, patients and research studies.

Both authors are masters of their art, having long and detailed experience in the field of histotechnology. Between them they have seen and encouraged the revolution in demonstration techniques which play an increasing importance in diagnosis and research. The evolution from applying vegetable dyes to provide some colour contrast, through to specific identification of a wide range of organic and inorganic substances in tissues, has been a quiet but extraordinary development. The fascinating thing is that, with each improvement in specificity, we learn a little more about the interpretation of Haematoxylin–Eosin sections which remain the essential starting point of our investigations.

Diagnostic histopathology used to be concerned with the basic classification of disease processes present at autopsy and in major surgical resections provided interesting data but, perhaps, a little late. With increasing use of endoscopic and other biopsy techniques histopathological interpretation is now at the forefront of diagnosis in life and, in many cases, can assist the choice of appropriate therapy to modify the course of disease or even effect a complete cure. Even where therapy is still unavailable histopathologic diagnosis can contribute to assessing prognosis which is of major importance to the patient.

All these aspects of histopathological analysis are assisted by high quality histological preparations which are more readily achievable using the body of knowledge set out in this text, and which meets, in a comprehensive manner, the needs of today's histologists.

1994   D.R. Turner

Preface

The first book in this series was conceived as an integration of two previous books: Cook's *Manual of Histological Demonstration Techniques* and Bancroft's *Histochemical Techniques*. In the framework we endeavoured to meet three objectives. Firstly, to produce a textbook for courses in cellular pathology, both in the United Kingdom and elsewhere. Secondly, to produce a book as a practical companion of *Theory and Practice of Histological Techniques* (Bancroft and Stevens, Churchill Livingstone, now third edition, 1990) which is designed as a comprehensive reference book. Our third and major aim was to produce a laboratory manual containing a full repertoire of standard and non-standard, well-known and not-so-well-known histological techniques.

In continuing to meet these objectives we have tried to appeal to the laboratory scientist and pathologist by anticipating the techniques required in the busy laboratory situation. The book is still primarily designed to cover demonstration techniques; other specialized areas of cellular pathology are to be found in *Theory and Practice*.

In this book, which is an extension of our earlier *Manual of Histological Techniques* we have incorporated a number of new techniques and, where appropriate, different uses for existing ones. We have continued the overriding philosophy of discussion of the theoretical aspects of the various methods, and have given increased prominence to the associated pathology. We have sought to address the needs of today's laboratory in terms of new demonstration techniques. In particular, immunocytochemistry has assumed an important role since the first edition appeared. In view of its role in diagnosis, we have supplemented this chapter with the views of a diagnostician.

Nottingham and Isleworth, 1994

J.D.B
H.C.C.

Acknowledgments

It is a rare publication which is wholly and entirely the work of those persons whose names appear under the title. So it is with our 'Manual' and we are indebted to a number of people for their help. In particular the authors wish to acknowledge the assistance of the contributors to: *Theory and Practice of Histological Techniques* edited by Bancroft and Stevens, and other professional colleagues and friends.

Professor David Turner has provided useful advice in the revision of chapters one to four and we acknowledge, with gratitude, the implicit encouragement of our endeavours extended by both him and Dr Robert Stirling, the Clinical Directors of Pathology at the Queen's Medical Centre and the West Middlesex University Hospital, respectively. We would also like to express our appreciation for professional advice willingly extended to us by Dr Mark Wilkinson. The secretarial work was in the capable hands of Angela Prince whose patient, untiring assistance did much to alleviate the inevitable stress associated with the production of the final manuscript, and to her we extend our grateful thanks. We are also indebted to Dr Carol Bancroft for her patient proof reading and assistance with the Index.

Finally, we wish to place on record our appreciation of the support and help we both enjoyed from our senior staff. This support may not be easy to quantify but was, nonetheless, an important ingredient in the successful completion of this book.

Nottingham and Isleworth, 1994

J.D. Bancroft
H.C. Cook

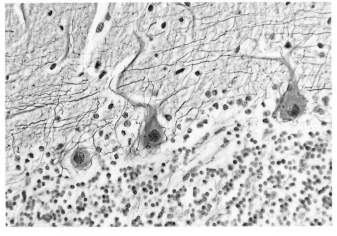

Plate 1
Cerebellum.
Purkinje cells and
nerve fibres.
Bielschowsky silver
technique. (medium
power)

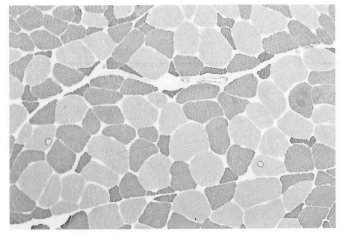

Plate 2
Voluntary muscle.
Type 1 fibres light
brown, type 2 fibres
dark brown. Myosin
ATP'ase (pH 9.4)
technique. (medium
power)

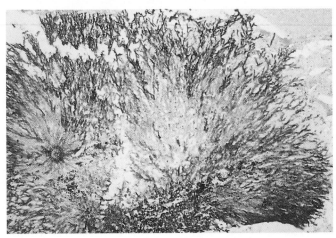

Plate 3
Lung. Aspergillus
hyphae. Grocott
hexamine silver
technique. (medium
power)

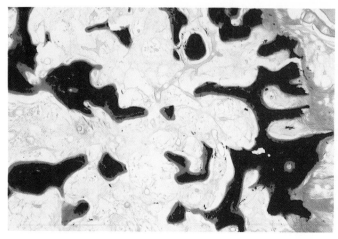

Plate 4
Bone. Enlarged osteoid seams in osteomalacia. Normal bone black, osteoid seams red. Tripp and Mackay — van Gieson technique (100)

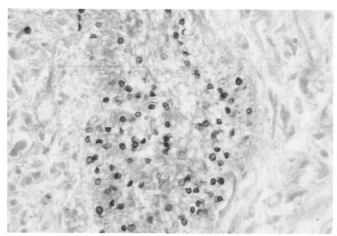

Plate 5
Lung. Pneumocystitis carinii. Grocott hexamine silver technique. (400)

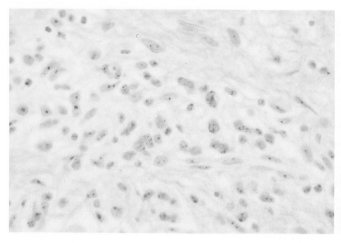

Plate 6
Carcinoma of stomach. Increased numbers of AgNORs (black intranuclear bodies). Silver technique. (400)

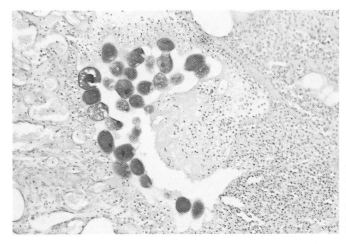

Plate 7
Colon. Cysts of
Balantidium coli in
abscess stained
magenta. PAS
technique. (100)

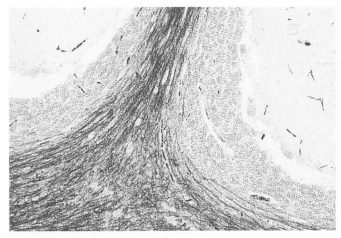

Plate 8
Cerebellum.
Myelinated
nerve fibres blue,
nuclei red. Luxol fast
blue — neutral red
technique. (100)

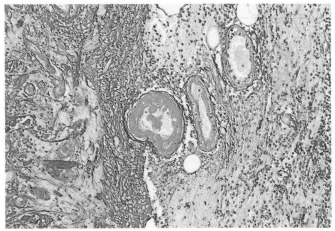

Plate 9
Stomach. Blood
vessels showing
fibrinoid degenera-
tion in vasculitis.
MSB technique.
(100)

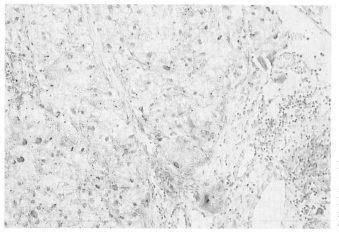

Plate 10
Carcinoma of adrenal cortex. Lipid deposits red, nuclei blue. Oil red O technique. (100)

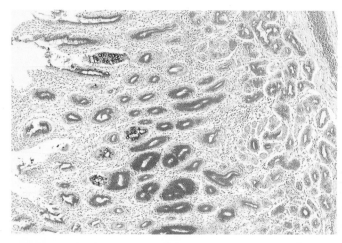

Plate 11
Stomach. Mucosal intestinal metaplasia. Normal gastric glands red, metaplastic glands blue. Alcian blue — PAS technique (41)

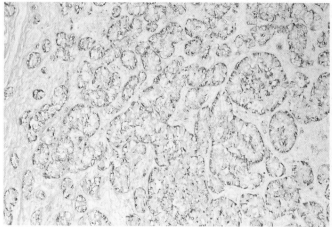

Plate 12
Carcinoid tumour. Diffuse Endocrine-type cells showing black granules. Grimelius silver technique. (250)

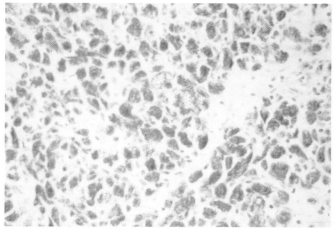

Plate 13
Lymph node.
Histiocytes
containing
Mycobacterium
avium intracellulare
organisms. Ziehl —
Neelsen technique.
(250)

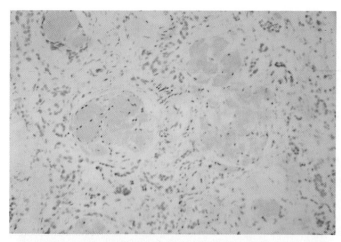

Plate 14
Kidney. Amyloid
deposits in
glomeruli stained
dull-orange. Congo
red technique.
(medium)

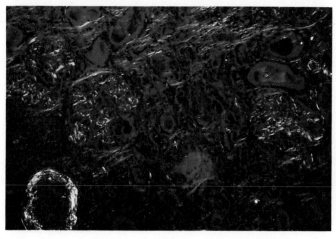

Plate 15
Kidney. Amyloid
deposits in
glomeruli showing
apple green
berefringence
effect. Polarising
microscopy-Congo
red technique.
(medium power)

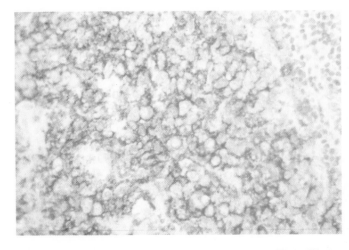

Plate 16
Lymph node. Non-Hodgkin's lymphoma B cell type showing cell surface reaction brown. Anti-L 26 immunoperoxidase technique. (250)

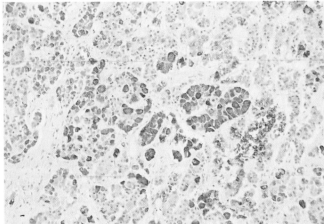

Plate 17
Anterior pituitary. ACTH secreting cells brown. Anti-ACTH immunoperoxidase technique. (128)

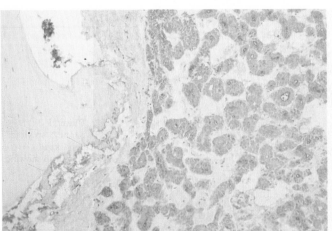

Plate 18
Bone. Thyroid carcinoma secondary deposits brown (a normal bone trabecula can be seen to the left of the field). Anti-thyroglobulin immunoperoxidase technique. (medium power)

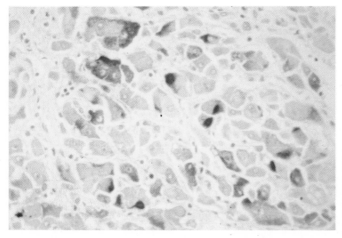

Plate 19
Liver. Hepatitis B
surface antigen
brown. Anti-
hepatitis B
immunoperoxidase
technique. (250)

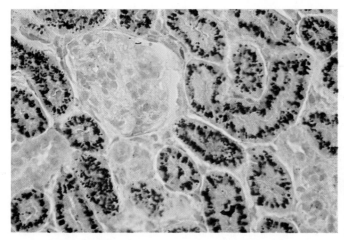

Plate 20
Kidney. Acid
phosphatase in renal
tubule cells. Gomori
metal precipitation
technique. (medium
power)

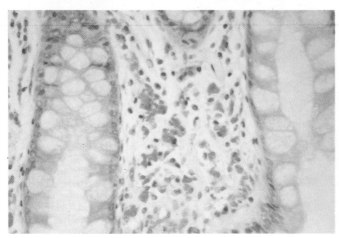

Plate 21
Colon.
Histiocytes
containing
melanosis coli
pigment stained
magenta. PAS
technique. (250)

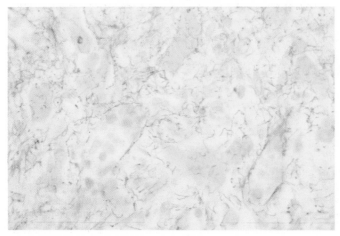

Plate 22
Liver. Spirochaetes.
Bertarelli silver
technique. (512)

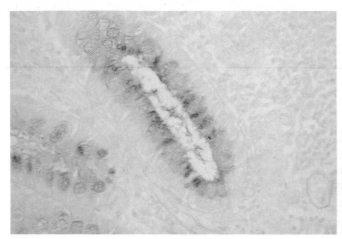

Plate 23
Colon. Mucosal
goblet cells
containing
sulphomucins
(brown) and
sialomucins (blue).
High iron diamine-
alcian blue
technique. (250)

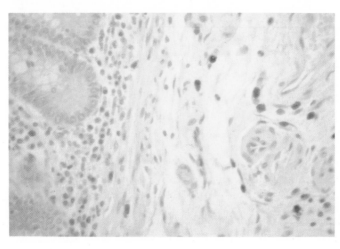

Plate 24
Small intestine.
Submucosal mast
cells bright red,
neutrophils paler
red. Chloroacetate
esterase technique.
(250)

1. Fundamentals of normal histology and histopathology

A basic knowledge of normal histology is a prerequisite for the successful practice and study of histological techniques. To achieve this it is necessary to have available the appropriate textbooks and, more importantly, stained histological sections. This chapter introduces the basic tissues that comprise the various organs and structures of the body and complements the demonstration techniques that are described subsequently. Complex organisms have evolved by specialization of different cell types to perform different functions. Nervous tissue is responsible for rapid conduction of information from one part of the organism to another and centrally coordinates sheets of cells from layers of epithelial tissue that line internal and external surfaces, and may also proliferate locally to form glandular tissue. The musculo-skeletal tissues provide the possibility of movement, connective tissue that is generally a loose fibrous and gelatinous system in which the blood vessels and nerves are distributed and the lymphoid system that is concerned with acquired immunity.

An elementary knowledge of pathological terms and lesions is of value in understanding how the various demonstration techniques can help in establishing a pathological diagnosis (see Table 1.2, p. 12). The following descriptions apply to formalin-fixed paraffin sections stained by haematoxylin and eosin. (H & E)

TYPES OF TISSUE SEEN IN NORMAL HISTOLOGY

EPITHELIUM

This type of tissue forms glands and lines surfaces (see Table 1.1). The cells are normally attached to a basement membrane at the interface with underlying connective tissues. There are three main subdivisions:

a. Simple (non-stratified)

Squamous (syn. pavement). This type of lining epithelium is specialized to facilitate diffusion. There is extensive flattened cytoplasm and in profile an elongated, central nucleus, as seen in a loop of Henle in the kidney, the lining of the alveoli of the lung and the endothelial and mesothelial cells found lining blood vessels and serous membranes respectively. This type of delicate lining could only survive deep within the body and is often formed from the middle or mesodermal layer of the embryo.

Cuboidal. These are small round cells having a central nucleus and are found forming the walls of small glandular intralobular ducts, and renal tubules.

1

Table 1.1   Epithelium: summary of types and location

Type	Location
Simple	
Squamous	Lung, kidney
Cuboidal	Kidney, glandular ducts
Columnar	Stomach, large and small intestine
Ciliated	Fallopian tubes, endocervix
Pseudo-stratified columnar	Bronchus, trachea
Stratified	
Squamous keratinized	Epidermis of skin
Squamous non-keratinized	Oesophagus, cervix
Transitional	Urinary bladder, ureters
Columnar	Large ducts, urethra
Mixed columnar-cuboidal	Epididymis
Glandular	
Exocrine {Tubular	Stomach, uterus
{Acinar	Pancreas, salivary glands
{Tubulo-acinar	Prostate
Endocrine	Pituitary
	Thyroid
	Parathyroids

Columnar. This takes the form of either 'low' or 'high' columnar and is an elongated cell having a basal nucleus. It may secrete mucin and is the lining epithelium for much of the alimentary tract (stomach onwards). In the small intestine the free border of the columnar cells has a so-called 'brush border'. This is a layer formed of microvilli to increase the surface area for absorption and can be seen as a darker staining line at the free surface.

Ciliated. Both cuboidal and columnar cells may carry on their free border fine hair-like motile processes termed cilia; they may also be found lining organs such as the Fallopian tubes, where they serve to transport ova to the uterine cavity.

Pseudo-stratified ciliated columnar. This type of epithelium is found in the upper respiratory tract and consists of apparently misshapen ciliated columnar cells that, although they appear to be arranged in layers, in reality extend from the basement membrane (basal lamina) to the free surface.

Goblet cells. A cell that is columnar in shape and includes a large mucin-filled secretory vacuole creating the impression of a wine glass or goblet. These cells are frequent in the respiratory and gastrointestinal tract.

b. Stratified (multilayered)

Squamous keratinized. This type of epithelium is specialized to withstand wear and tear. It forms the epidermis of the skin and consists of several layers, depending on the site. The skin on the inner aspect of the thigh is thinner than that on the sole of the foot.

The deepest or germinative layer is columnar in type compared to the middle layers (the so-called 'prickle cell' layers) that are polyhedral in shape. The 'prickle cells' have many desmosomal attachments on their surface that are artefactually exaggerated in conditions of epidermal oedema. The superficial layers become flatter or more squamous in shape with an uppermost granular layer, the cells of which contain many haematoxylophilic keratohyalin granules. Finally, there is a keratinous layer, the stratum corneum. (There is also a 'stratum lucidum'; we have yet to see a convincing example in routinely prepared skin.) Also to be found in normal epidermis are melanoblasts, melanocytes and melanophores, with Langerhans cells, which are related to the macrophage system.

Squamous non-keratinized. This is similar in structure to the foregoing but it lacks a keratinized layer and granular layer. It is found in the ectocervix and oesophagus.

Transitional is composed of cuboidal-like cells. It superficially resembles a stratified squamous epithelium, but careful examination reveals more uniform cells —the basal cells are only slightly more columnar than the most superficial cells; in addition, 'prickle', granular and keratinized layers are lacking. It is both stretchable and urine-proof and lines the urinary tract.

Columnar. True stratified columnar epithelium is only found in a few situations; these include the urethra and the major ducts of the salivary glands.

Mixed stratified. There are other variants of epithelial tissue that do not easily fit into one of the above categories. Such an epithelium occurs in the epididymis, where the tubules are lined by tall columnar cells, bearing stereocilia, with an underlying uniform layer of cuboidal-type cells.

c. Glandular

Local specialization of function within an epithelial tissue may occur as secretory glandular tissue. Essentially it represents a focus of epithelial downgrowth into the underlying connective tissue. Glandular tissue may be classified according to the shape of the glands, i.e. tubular, acinar, etc., but perhaps more importantly according to whether the glands retain a connecting channel or duct to the epithelial surface, i.e. an exocrine gland such as the salivary gland, or lose connection with the surface and secrete their product directly into the blood stream, i.e. an endocrine gland such as the anterior pituitary.

Tubular. These glands may be coiled or straight and have wide lumina lined by large columnar-type cells, with basal nuclei. This type of gland is found in the stomach and endometrium.

Acinar (syn. alveolar). The component cells have a broad base and narrow apex with the nucleus occupying a basal position. Each group of cells or acinus has an ill-defined central ductule that communicates with intra- and extralobular ducts. The pancreas and the salivary glands are good examples.

Mixed tubulo-acinar. As the name indicates, these are formed of mixtures of both of the above gland elements. The prostate shows this type of feature well.

MUSCLE

a. Skeletal muscle (syn. striated, voluntary)

This is a major component of the musculo-skeletal system and is under the direct control of the central nervous system. Examination of H & E-stained sections with the light microscope gives only limited information as to structure and composition of the muscle fibres, enzyme histochemistry and electron microscopy being necessary for systematic study. Skeletal muscle consists essentially of adjacent fibres varying in length from 1–40 mm, and in diameter from 10–100 μm. Each fibre is surrounded by a thin membrane, the sarcolemma, which encloses the cytoplasm or sarcoplasm. Nuclei are multiple and peripherally situated, a feature that is most easily seen when the fibres are in cross section. In volume a muscle fibre is much larger than other cells and this explains why its requirements cannot be served by a single nucleus.

Within the sarcoplasm are longitudinal myofibrils arranged in an ordered pattern to produce transverse (cross) striations. The latter cross striations consist of alternating light I discs with a narrow central darker Z band, and darker A discs having a lighter central H band. Skeletal muscle is rich in mitochondria and glycogen, and in H & E preparations usually stains a brighter red colour, compared with the other types of muscle.

b. Cardiac muscle

Under this heading are considered two different muscle fibres, the contractile heart muscle and the specialized conductor muscle that initiates and propagates heart contraction. The former type of muscle fibres are similar to skeletal in having longitudinal myofibrils and cross striations (although these are less evident in H & E preparations), but differ in that they branch and anastomose and are somewhat shorter (100–150 μm). Present in the sarcoplasm in the Z band region are intercalated discs which mark the cell boundaries. The nuclei are single and centrally placed. Mitochondria and glycogen are again abundant, and granules of lipofuscin are usually present in older age groups. The conducting system of the heart comprises the SA node, AV node and bundles of His, as well as the interventricular Purkinje fibres. These are not easily seen in human heart and indeed, careful dissection is needed to locate the various constituents (Hudson 1963).

The muscle cells of the nodes are somewhat smaller and more compact than the main cardiac muscle cells, whilst the Purkinje fibres are composed of larger somewhat ovoid muscle cells, which have a perinuclear centre rich in glycogen.

c. Smooth muscle (syn. involuntary, non-striated)

Muscle controlled by the autonomic nervous system has a wide distribution, being found in the walls of the alimentary, respiratory and genitourinary tracts. By comparison with skeletal and cardiac muscle it is more suited to slow, sustained and rhythmic contraction. As the name implies, there are no cross striations in the sarcoplasm of these cells, only longitudinal myofibrils. Typically, smooth muscle cells are 'cigar' shaped in that the poles are somewhat tapered. The nuclei are single and centrally placed, and the sarcoplasma contains fewer mitochondria and glycogen granules compared with the other muscle types. The overall size is significantly less, being about 20–10 μm in length, and in keeping with having only a single nucleus.

NERVOUS TISSUE

The microscopic study of both the central (CNS) and peripheral (PNS) nervous systems is carried out with the aid of special techniques, traditionally silver impregnation on frozen, paraffin- or celloidin-embedded material. A certain amount of detail can be visualized in H & E-stained paraffin sections and this is described below.

a. CNS (Central Nervous System)

This comprises the brain and spinal cord.

Neurones. The larger neurones such as the Betz cells of the cerebrum, Purkinje cells of the cerebellum and the anterior horn cells of the spinal cord have well-marked characteristics. There is a large cell body with discrete granules of ribonucleic acid (Nissl substance) and, as with cardiac muscle fibres, granules of lipofuscin pigment may be present in tissue from the older age groups. The nuclear membrane and chromatin are ill-defined but there is a prominent nucleolus. Small or medium-sized neurones have comparatively indistinct cell bodies and are often shown solely by their nuclei, which, compared to the large neurones, tend to have a more distinct chromatin pattern.

Neuroglia. There are several different types of glial cell having a variety of functions, varying from supportive astrocytes, to ventricular lining cells (ependymal) to myelin-forming oligodendrocytes. The microglial cell is embryologically not a true neuroglial element, being derived from mesenchyme, and is usually included for traditional reasons and for its possession of processes when appropriately stained; it is a reticulo-endothelial (RE) cell and has a marked phagocytic function.

Astrocytes. The two members of this group, the fibrous and protoplasmic, are indistinguishable in an H & E, and show virtually no cytoplasmic detail or evidence of processes. Their position is solely indicated by their round to ovoid moderately-sized nuclei, having a well-marked chromatin structure. Special stains reveal abundant and substantial processes.

Ependyma. These cells are found lining the ventricles of the brain and appear as ciliated cuboidal-like cells. Unlike the other neuroglial cells, special methods do not materially help in their identification.

Oligodendrocytes. These are the smallest cells of the neuroglial system and appear not unlike lymphocytes in an H & E-stained section, having a scanty cytoplasm and a small round pyknotic nucleus. Special methods reveal scanty, small processes.

Microglia. As with the astrocytes, H & E staining shows to advantage only the nuclei that are intermediate in size between astrocytes and oligodendrocytes. Unlike those cells, the microglial nucleus is more irregular in shape and usually more elongated. Special stains reveal a somewhat elongated cell body with short processes extending from each pole. As mentioned above, these cells are related to the reticulo-endothelial system rather than the nervous system in development terms.

Axons. These are the nerve fibres or elongated neuronal cell processes that comprise the main substance of both grey and white matter. They vary considerably in both length and diameter. Axons of white matter are surrounded by a dense fatty sheath termed *myelin*. By contrast, the fibres in the grey matter are largely nonmyelinated. Myelinated nerve fibres stain pink in H & E preparations, unlike the non-myelinated axons that may hardly stain at all. Fine fibrils, the *neurofibrils*, can be demonstrated within the axon by electron microscopy.

b. PNS (Peripheral Nervous System)

The appearance of the nerve fibres is similar to that in the CNS except that they may be formed into discrete nerve bundles with accompanying specialized connective tissue. The nerve cell bodies, or ganglion cells as they are termed in the PNS, tend to be modelled on the larger type of CNS neurone, although the Nissl substance is less pronounced. Lipofuscin is often a prominent feature. Posterior root ganglia of the spinal cord are formed of sensory neurones and their processes the nerve fibres, but in contrast to the CNS there is an abundant supporting framework of collagen fibres. Peripheral nerve fibres are lined externally by a thin layer of Schwann cells.

Nerve endings, either sensory or motor, are not usually distinguishable in H & E preparations. Exceptions to this rule are the Pacinian corpuscles. These are sensory end organs found prominently in the deeper layers of skin and neuromuscular spindles, another form of sensory nerve ending found in the skeletal muscle. The former is often quite large (up to 3 mm in diameter). It is fairly readily identified as it looks like an onion in appearance, consisting of concentric pale-staining layers of connective tissue surrounding a central nerve fibre. By contrast neuromuscular spindles are much less easily found. They appear as a pale-staining area in muscle, which on closer inspection is made up of thin muscle and nerve cells, invested and surrounded by fine connective tissue.

CONNECTIVE TISSUE

The connective tissue framework of the body is immensely variable and includes on the one hand the hard skeletal components of bone and cartilage connected by tough ligamentous tissues and the loose connective tissues in which the blood vessels and nerves are distributed to their destinations. The basic structure found in these situations is a fibrillar component lying within a muco-protein gel. The strength, elasticity and permeability of the connective tissue varies according to the density and nature of the fibrillar content and the firmness of the mucoprotein ground substance that is the case if bone becomes calcified.

The basic cell type of connective tissues is the fibroblast—that is an elongate spindle-shaped cell with a correspondingly shaped nucleus. Fibroblasts produce a protein, tropocollagen, that is the precursor substance for collagen fibres and secrete the associated muco-protein ground substance.

Types of connective tissue

Collagen fibres are inelastic non-branching fibres with an average diameter of about 64 μm and usually arranged in bundles lying within a muco-protein ground substance. The individual fibrils can only be recognized with the electron microscope since they are too narrow to be visualized with the light microscope, but bundles of fibres will be visible using conventional stains such as eosin.

Biochemical analysis has shown that there are several chemical variants of collagen: the most important of these are type I collagen, described above, and type III collagen that is the variant that forms reticulin fibres.

Reticulin fibres. As stated above, these fine fibres are formed from type III collagen and can be visualized with the light microscope using silver impregnation techniques. They tend to be found in situations where free diffusion of fluids and cells are important, as for example within the internal structure of lymphoid tissues and lining the sinusoids of the liver.

Elastic fibres. These are branching fibres of variable diameter (1–10 μm). They are truly elastic and are found in sites where this function could be anticipated, i.e. in the walls of large blood vessels to withstand the pulsatile effect of cardiac contraction, and in the lung that is stretched by every inspiration and then recoils on expiration. It is assumed that elastic fibres are synthesized by modified fibroblasts.

Loose connective tissue (syn. areolar tissue). This could easily be dismissed as a loose packing tissue around and between the other tissues of the body. It is composed of a composite mixture of fine collagen fibres, elastic fibres and reticulin associated with fibroblasts, lying in muco-protein that allows ready diffusion. The blood vessels and nerves are embedded within this loose connective tissue, and an occasional mast cell may be encountered. Mast cells are densely granulated cells capable of releasing histamine and serotonin. Other blood cells will normally only enter this zone when an inflammatory reaction is in progress although there may be some resident histiocytes remaining from previous inflammatory episodes. Histiocytes are large phagocytic cells with pale bean-shaped nuclei.

Adipose tissue. This is the fat depot of the body, containing the major proportion of adipose tissue as in the mesentery and omentum of the abdominal cavity and the subcutaneous layer of the skin. Individual fat cells have a distended and vacuolated cytoplasm in paraffin sections with a thin nucleus compressed to one side. Fine collagen or reticulin fibres surround the cells, which are grouped into lobules. Small blood vessels run in the more compact collagen fibres of the interlobular tissue.

Lymphoid tissue. It is convenient to describe lymphoid tissue in this context, although its function is far removed from that of being supportive. Many cellular elements of lymphoid tissue and the supportive connective tissue have a common origin and remain closely associated. Lymphoid tissue is primarily found in lymph nodes, tonsil, spleen and large and small intestine.

The following simplified description of this complex and controversial tissue is an attempt to highlight the more important constituents. It must be appreciated that many of these constituents are not readily identified with conventional H & E preparations. A typical lymph node exhibits the following structure:

Gross structure. The efferent lymph flow is from the medullary sinuses. The afferent lymphatics enter via channels in the fibroreticular membrane that covers the lymph node, and thence into subcapsular sinuses. A dense reticulin pattern can be demonstrated throughout most of the lymph node and this supports a system of cortical and medullary sinuses with the latter leading into the efferent lymphatic at the hilum of the organ.

Cortex. An unstimulated node contains primary follicles consisting largely of small lymphocytes (B type) and dendritic reticulum cells; the former cells have compact nuclei and the latter have larger irregular pale-staining nuclei. An active node will show secondary follicles or germinal centres. These are paler-staining zones compared with the primary follicles. They contain tingible body macrophages and different forms of B lymphocytes such as the cleaved (centrocyte) and non-cleaved forms (centroblast); this description refers to the nuclear conformations.

Immunoblasts and plasma cells may also be present, plus occasional T lymphocytes. Reticulin fibres are scanty.

Paracortex. This occupies a position internal to the cortex, but external to the medullary cords, and is primarily the domain of the T lymphocyte series. Both cortex and paracortex are drained by a system of cortical sinuses, having a reticulin fibre framework, that lead into the medullary region.

Medullary cords. The cortical sinuses drain into a system of medullary sinuses. These run between medullary cords that are formed of various lymphocytic cells, plasma cells and histiocytes.

Blood cells. In non-haemopoietic tissue these comprise neutrophils, lymphocytes and eosinophils, and have the classic normal features of the circulating blood cells. They may be seen to greatest advantage in loose connective tissue such as the lamina propria of the alimentary tract.

Mast cells. These occur in loose connective tissue and in the wall of the large and small intestines. Where they are known as 'mucosal' mast cells, these cells are small with a large central nucleus and prominent cytoplasmic basophilic granules. The human mast cell granules are not easily seen in H & E-stained sections. They proliferate in hypersensitivity reactions, when they produce the IgE immunoglobulin and histamine. They are related to the basophils in the blood.

Plasma cells. These are found in many situations such as lymphoid tissue, spleen, bone marrow and the loose connective tissue of the alimentary tract. They have an ovoid cytoplasm and eccentric nucleus with prominent radial chromatin. They are derived from B lymphocytes and produce immunoglobulins. Although termed plasma cells, they are only rarely seen in the blood in occasional cases of plasma cell leukaemia.

Histiocytes. Found in similar situations to fibroblasts, these are round to oval cells intermediate in size between a fibroblast and a mast cell. The cytoplasm and nucleus stain weakly and are typically oval or indented (kidney-shaped). These cells have an important phagocytic role in removing larger items of debris such as dead cells and nuclei. They are the equivalent of monocytes in the blood.

Cartilage. This forms the precursor of the adult skeleton and consists of a hard glassy ground substance that is secreted by specialized cells or chondrocytes that remain in spaces within the dense muco-protein matrix. The fibre content of cartilage modifies its function. Thus hyaline cartilage is glassy in appearance, covers joint surfaces and has a low collagen fibre content.

Fibro-cartilage has a high collagen fibre content which increases its strength but reduces the opportunity for diffusion of materials through its substance. The best example of fibro-cartilage is an intervertebral disc. Elastic cartilage has a high elastic fibre content and is the type of cartilage found in the pinna of the ear and epiglottis where both firmness and elasticity are required.

Bone. Structurally, bone develops either as dense compact material, as is found forming the cortex of long bones, or as the cancellous (spongy) tissue of the medulla of the long bones. The latter encloses the cells of the bone marrow. In either case, bone is composed of collagen and a ground substance termed osteoid impregnated by various calcium salts.

The mature bone cells are termed osteocytes, and have small dense round to elongated nuclei with an ill-defined cytoplasm. These cells lie in bone spaces called lacunae, which interconnect by means of fine channels—the canaliculi—to permit diffusion of nutrients. Active or growing bone is evidenced by the presence of bone-forming cells, the osteoblasts, and multinucleated bone-remodelling cells — the osteoclasts, Both cells are found principally at sites of new bone formation and sites of remodelling.

GENERAL NOTES

Having set out the various tissue types and subtypes, it may be helpful to note the following points. The structure of a tissue often mirrors its mechanical or physiological function. For example, epithelial cells lining an intralobular duct in an acinar gland are usually cuboidal in type, whereas those cells lining the extralobular, i.e. larger, ducts will tend to be more columnar. The main duct for the gland may be lined by stratified (layered) columnar cells. Stratified squamous epithelium forming external skin surfaces is keratinized to varying degrees, whereas the internal 'skin' surfaces such as the oesophagus in man lack a protective layer of keratin. Both examples demonstrate the arrangement of cells according to their role: for the ducts the degree of secretion required and resistance to the flow-stress of the duct contents, and for the skin layers the degree of surface protection required against trauma. When comparing sections of tissues with descriptions or pictures in textbooks, remember that 'normal' is a relative word and that, of necessity, textbook illustrations show tissue under ideal conditions of fixation, preservation and demonstration. It is logical to expect appearances to be modified when there are variations in these ideal conditions.

In the authors' experience the most useful microscope objectives for studying the histology of stained slides are the low-power scanning lens, e.g. × 2.5, and the high-power × 40. The low-power should be initially employed to afford a general idea of the cellular arrangement, followed by examination at a higher power to confirm or resolve important fine structural details. The × 100 oil-immersion objective is rarely called for in histology, apart from identifying acid-fast bacilli in Ziehl-Neelsen preparations.

BASIC HISTOPATHOLOGY

The pathological changes to be discussed in this section are those that are likely to be encountered routinely in a diagnostic laboratory. They will be described in relation to the type of material handled by such a laboratory.

NON-TUMOUR PATHOLOGY

A wide spectrum of disorders is included in this category and often includes some degree of inflammatory change that may be the primary lesion, or a secondary reaction to other disease processes. The following explanation of some common terms may be found useful:

Aneurysm. A localized dilatation of an artery due to either a congenital or acquired defect in the structural components of the vessel wall. It may involve vessels of various sizes, from congenital berry aneurysms to those affecting the aorta (atheromatous and dissecting).

Diverticulum. A pouch-like dilatation of the bowel wall, in which the mucosa protrudes through an attenuated muscle coat. The condition known as diverticulosis commonly affects the sigmoid colon and, if inflammation is present, is termed diverticulitis.

Embolism. There are various forms of embolism, caused by a detached mass of material which is transported from one part of the blood circulation to another. Examples of emboli are pieces of thrombus, fat or tumour.

Endometriosis. Endometrium may develop in abnormal anatomical sites causing the condition of endometriosis where nodular lesions occur in abnormal or 'ectopic' sites including the ovary, umbilicus and gut. The wall of the uterus frequently shows this condition—known in this site as 'adenomyosis'.

Granuloma. Inflammatory reactions may develop a variety of patterns. A granulomatous reaction is one where there is a marked proliferation of abnormal histiocyctes called 'epithelioid' cells with giant cells, which represent fused epithelioid cells. Examples of this type of reaction are found in tuberculosis and sarcoidosis.

Infarct. Infarction is a localized area of tissue necrosis caused by a partial or complete interruption to the blood supply (resulting in leakage of red blood cells into the area). Whilst this can occur in almost any situation, it is seen particularly in the heart (myocardial infarction), brain, lung, kidney, spleen and placenta.

Inflammation. In histological terms an acute inflammatory reaction involves, to varying degrees, hyperaemia, oedema, fibrin deposition and neutrophil proliferation. This initial reaction is followed by an influx of monocytes and macrophages that remove the debris. If substantial tissue damage has occurred there will be either regeneration of the original tissue or repair by granulation tissue to produce a collagenous scar.

Ischaemia. Sometimes the blood supply to a given tissue is decreased due to partial obstruction or narrowing of a blood vessel. This partial occlusion may affect the heart muscle in coronary artery disease, and results over a period in patchy fibrosis of the myocardium or even infarction. A similar diminution of blood supply can affect the large intestine, a condition termed 'ischaemic colitis'.

Necrosis. Implied in this term is death of cells or tissues from any cause, with a loss of normal cellular detail and architecture. Nuclear changes are evident including pyknosis (condensation of chromatin) and karyorrhexis (nuclear breakdown). Calcification is often present, so this type of tissue change is less than popular with the microtomist! There are some specific types of necrotic change: infarction (see above) is one and caseation necrosis associated with tuberculous lesions is another.

Disturbances of growth

Anaplasia. The term 'anaplastic' implies a lack of differentiation with associated immaturity; tumours showing anaplasia often present as highly malignant neoplasms.

Atrophy. 'Atrophic change' is applied to the macroscopic appearance of shrinkage of a structure and can be due to a decrease in number or size of the component cells. Examples are disuse atrophy of muscle, and renal atrophy due to ureteric blockage.

Dysplasia. This denotes an abnormal growth pattern and rather confusingly has been used for a variety of abnormalities including cystic renal dysplasia and premalignant change in epithelial tissues.

Hyperplasia/hypoplasia. An increase or decrease in the number of component cells. Endocrine glands such as the thyroid or adrenal may exhibit these features; also haemopoietic bone marrow in a variety of diseases.

Hypertrophy. This is the converse of atrophy and denotes an increase in cell volume. An example is ventricular hypertrophy of heart muscle in hypertension.

Metaplasia. Denotes a change in differentiation of tissue from one mature type to another. This is thought to be due to the proliferation and differentiation of stem cells. Metaplastic change can be non-specific or result from inflammation. Examples are squamous metaplasia of bronchial mucosa in chronic bronchitis, bony areas in scar tissue, and intestinal metaplasia of the stomach. The term 'tumour metaplasia' is used to describe the corresponding change in a neoplasm. Squamous metaplasia is a common example, particularly in adenocarcinoma of the uterus and transitional cell carcinoma of the bladder.

Neoplasm. An abnormal mass of tissue, the growth of which exceeds and remains uncoordinated with the tissues that surround it.

Tumour. Common term for neoplasm, benign or malignant.

TUMOUR PATHOLOGY

A benign tumour usually differs in a number of significant respects from a malignant tumour. This is true not only clinically but histologically, and the following guidelines may be found useful. It is important to remember that there is frequently a degree of overlap of the histological parameters of benign and malignant tumours; this situation calls for greater interpretative skills and is assisted by high quality technical preparations.

Benign tumours. These may be small or large, but the component cells tend to have a relatively uniform appearance with little variation in size and shape of either nucleus or cytoplasm. Growth is by expansion. These tumours do not spread to distant sites. Examples are lipomas and uterine leiomyomata ('fibroids').

Malignant tumours. Most malignant tumours arise from epithelium and are termed 'carcinoma'. They develop from both glandular and surface epithelia. Microscopically the cells exhibit some or all of the following features:

1. Pleomorphism (variation in size and shape of nuclei and cytoplasm)
2. Invasion of deeper structures
3. Nuclear immaturity (abnormal chromatin clumping, prominent nucleoli)
4. Mitotic activity
5. Spread to distant sites or metastasis—this is the ultimate test of whether a tumour is malignant.

The other, less common, type of malignant tumour is the sarcoma, which consists of tissue elements of mesenchymal origin. This is a complex group and tends to present the pathologist with greater diagnostic problems. The names of the individual sarcomata reflect the type of tissue from which they spring, e.g. fibrosarcoma, myosarcoma, osteosarcoma, liposarcoma, etc. The sarcomas affect all age groups, unlike the carcinomas which have a predilection for the older age groups.

The following explanations of some commonly employed terms may be found useful:

Adenoma. A benign tumour of glandular or secretory tissue. Common examples are to be found in rectum, skin appendages and thyroid. The malignant variant is known as an adenocarcinoma and is the commonest type of tumour in the gastrointestinal tract.

Papilloma. A papillomatous growth consists of finger-like projections of epithelium overlying a series of connective tissue cones. Originally intended to describe a form of benign tumours the 'papillary pattern' may also be seen in some well-differentiated carcinomas.

Polyp. 'Polyps' or 'polypi' are rounded, usually benign growths with a connecting stalk and are often 'pedunculated'; a non-pedunculated polyp is termed 'sessile'. Certain types of polyps are prone to malignant change, particularly the adenomatous polyps arising in the gastrointestinal tract. The nose and cervix uteri are common sites for polyps.

Tumour differentiation. When a given malignant tumour is termed histologically *well* or *poorly differentiated*, it denotes the degree to which the malignant tissue resembles the normal parent tissue. A '*well-differentiated*' adenocarcinoma of the colon will show a well-marked glandular structure, often with mucin secretion. A '*poorly-differentiated*' adenocarcinoma may consist of cell masses with little or no glandular structure or mucin secretion, and the cells themselves will possess the stigmata of immaturity, particularly about the nuclear configuration. Analogous to the mucin production of the *well-differentiated* adenocarcinoma is the keratin formation of *well-differentiated* squamous cell carcinomas. In a similar way, a fibrosarcoma if *well-differentiated* will show a greater *fibrillar* content of the intervening connective tissue stroma and a lessened *cellularity* compared to a poorly-differentiated sarcoma, which will be more cellular and less fibrillar. However, the behaviour of a given tumour is only loosely related to its morphological characteristics.

The more important organs and structures in the body and their relationship to the more important histopathological conditions are shown in Table 1.2. It is not an exhaustive list, merely an attempt to highlight the location of the more common lesions that are likely to be presented to the average histology laboratory.

Table 1.2   Some commonly received specimens in the surgical laboratory and their more common pathologies

Tissue	Non-tumour pathology	Tumour pathology
Appendix	Appendicitis Mucocele	Carcinoid tumour Carcinoma, primary (rare) Carcinoma, secondary (uncommon)
Artery	Arteritis Atheroma Aneurysm	
Bladder (biopsy or cystectomy)	Cystitis Diverticula Fistulae Tuberculosis (uncommon) Schistosomiasis (uncommon)	Transitional cell carcinoma Squamous cell carcinoma (uncommon) Adenocarcinoma (uncommon)
Bone and bone marrow	Osteoporosis Osteomalacia Osteomyelitis Paget's disease	Osteochondroma Myeloma Metastatic tumour (e.g. breast, bronchus, thyroid, prostate, kidney)

Table 1.2   *(continued)*

Tissue	Non-tumour pathology	Tumour pathology
Bone and bone marrow (contd)		Leukaemia Osteosarcoma
Breast (biopsy or mastectomy)	Cysts Fibrocystic disease Abscess Fat necrosis	Adenoma Fibroadenoma Adenocarcinoma Paget's disease of nipple
Bronchial biopsy	Inflammation Squamous metaplasia	Squamous carcinoma Small cell carcinoma Carcinoid tumour
Cervix (cone or punch biopsy)	Inflammation	Squamous carcinoma (in-situ [CIN] or invasive)
Colon and rectum (biopsy or colectomy)	Ulcerative colitis Crohn's disease Amyloidosis Fistulae Amoebiasis (uncommon) Diverticular disease	Adenocarcinoma Carcinoid tumour Lymphoma (uncommon) Polyps (various types)
Endometrium (curettings)	Endometritis Abnormalities of cycle Hyperplasia	Adenocarcinoma Sarcomas (uncommon) Polyps
Epididymis	Cysts Inflammation Tuberculosis	Adenocarcinoma (rare)
Fallopian tubes	Salpingitis Ectopic pregnancy Endometriosis	Adenocarcinoma (rare)
Gall bladder	Cholecystitis Calculi	Adenocarcinoma (uncommon)
Joints/tendons	Osteoarthritis Rheumatoid arthritis Crystal synovitis (e.g. gout)	Sarcoma (rare)
Kidney (biopsy or nephrectomy)	Amyloidosis Glomerulonephritis Pyelonephritis Cysts/calculi Tuberculosis	Adenocarcinoma Renal tubular cell carcinoma Transitional cell carcinoma of pelvis
Larynx and vocal cords	Laryngeal nodules Inflammation	Squamous cell carcinoma Polyps
Liver (biopsy)	Hepatitis Cirrhosis Obstructive jaundice Sarcoidosis Amyloidosis Storage disorders (rare)	Hepatocellular carcinoma Secondary tumour, e.g. colon, stomach, breast and pancreas Lymphoma (rare) Cholangiocarcinoma (uncommon)
Lung (biopsy)	Pneumonia Alveolar fibrosis Infections, e.g. AIDS-related	Squamous carcinoma Small cell carcinoma

Table 1.2   *(continued)*

Tissue	Non-tumour pathology	Tumour pathology
Lung (biopsy) (contd)		Adenocarcinoma Secondary tumours
Lymph node	Reaction to inflammation Tuberculosis Sarcoidosis	Hodgkin's and non-Hodgkin's lymphoma Secondary tumours, e.g. lung, breast, colon, testis
Muscle, voluntary (biopsy)	Myopathies Neuropathic atrophy	Rhabdomyosarcoma (rare)
Nasal mucosa	Inflammation	Muco-epidermoid carcinoma Squamous cell carcinoma Polyps
Oral cavity	Cysts (dental) Inflammation	Squamous cell carcinoma Salivary gland tumours Polyps
Oesophagus (biopsy)	Oesophagitis Strictures Ulceration (peptic)	Squamous cell carcinoma
Ovary	Cysts Endometriosis	Both benign and malignant tumours of: epithelium, e.g. mucinous/serous cystadenoma; stroma, e.g. thecoma; germ cells, e.g. dysgerminoma.
Pancreas	Cysts Pancreatitis	Adenocarcinoma (exocrine elements) Endocrine tumours
Parathyroid glands	Hyperplasia	Adenomas
Placenta and umbilical cord	Malformations Infarction	Hydatidiform mole Choriocarcinoma (uncommon)
Pleural biopsy	Inflammations Tuberculosis	Mesothelioma Secondary tumour, e.g. lungs, breast Adenocarcinoma
Prostate gland	Hyperplasia Prostatitis	Adenocarcinoma
Salivary glands	Calculi Sialoadenitis	Pleomorphic adenoma Adenolymphoma (Warthin's) Muco-epidermoid tumour
Skin (biopsy)	Cysts Dermatitis Reactive changes	Naevi Warts Skin appendage tumours Squamous cell carcinoma Basal cell carcinoma Malignant melanoma Carcinoma-in-situ (Bowen's disease)
Small intestine	Infarction Diverticula	Carcinoid tumour Lymphoma

Table 1.2   *(continued)*

Tissue	Non-tumour pathology	Tumour pathology
Small intestine (contd)	Crohn's disease Coeliac disease	Adenocarcinoma (uncommon)
Spleen	Traumatic rupture Thrombocytopenic purpura Hypersplenism syndromes Amyloidosis	Lymphoma Leukaemia
Stomach	Gastritis Peptic ulceration	Adenocarcinoma Lymphoma Leiomyoma Carcinoid tumour
Testis	Infertility Orchitis Hydrocele	Seminoma Teratoma Lymphoma (uncommon)
Thyroid	Nodular goitre Thyrotoxic hyperplasia Hashimoto's thyroiditis	Adenoma Follicular carcinoma Papillary carcinoma Medullary carcinoma (amyloid associated)
Uterus (hysterectomy)	Abnormal cyclical bleeding Endometritis Adenomyosis	Leiomyoma (fibroid) Adenocarcinoma of endometrium Choriocarcinoma (uncommon)
Vulva (biopsy or excision)	Leukoplakia Inflammation Lichen sclerosis	Squamous carcinoma (in-situ or invasive)

REFERENCE

Hudson R C B 1963 The human conduction-system and its examination. Journal of Clinical Pathology 16: 49

2. Principles of tissue demonstration and routine morphological staining

To visualize detail and tissue structure at the light microscope level it is usually necessary to impart colour to the element to be studied. When Zernicke, in 1932, and Kohler and Loos, in 1941, introduced the phase contrast microscope it was hailed as the means of examining tissue that, it was confidently forecast by many workers, would soon render conventional histological demonstration techniques obsolete. Phase contrast microscopy has taken its place in our repertoire, particularly for studying fine detail in living material. It is the colouring of cells and tissues that remains fundamental to the science of histology with the light microscope.

When tissues are studied by electron microscopy colour definition is not involved, and 'staining' of cells is by application of salts of heavy metals such as lead and uranium. These build up a detailed image by varying the electron lucency or opacity, depending on the way they are bound to the tissue. There are three ways to impart colour to tissue: staining with dyes, impregnation with metallic salts and the formation of coloured compounds in situ by chemical reactions. It is a complex subject and only the outline of the principles of tissue demonstration can be given. For more detailed information see Horobin (1982, 1990).

STAINING WITH DYES

Fixed protein has approximately the same refractive index as glass, so, when looking at a stained section under the microscope that has been cleared and mounted in one standard medium, it is not the tissue that is seen but dye particles attached to the protein molecules. The way in which we do this profoundly affects the tissue image. The basic principle used when applying a staining method to tissue sections is to choose a dye that has a particular affinity for the element to be studied; this is the *primary* stain. To highlight the stained *primary* element it is common practice to counterstain the background; this *secondary* staining is applied using dyes of a contrasting colour that have an affinity for the background tissues.

DYES AND THEIR DEVELOPMENT

Dyes of natural origin (animal and vegetable) have been in use for the study of tissue for a considerable period, possibly starting with Grew in 1682, who stained plant tissue with cochineal, and Leeuwenhoek who, in 1714, stained muscle fibres with saffron. These dyes were of animal (cochineal beetle) and plant (crocus) origin respectively. Not until Perkin successfully synthesized the dye aniline violet in 1856 did a viable dye industry emerge, from which dyes for histological and bacteriological purposes were developed. The impetus for a flourishing and successful dye industry came largely from German workers, as did the staining of tissue sections in the laboratory. Prominent among these workers are the well-known names of Ehrlich, Weigert and Koch. Today, most dyes used in histology and cytology are synthetic but it is interesting to reflect that probably the most important early dye still in widespread use today is a naturally derived one—namely haematoxylin that is extracted from a tropical logwood.

When dyes were first introduced their mode of action was ill-understood, and up to the early 1950s many tissue–dye reactions remained empirical. These reactions are now better understood generally; the dyes themselves have been classified and to some extent standardized. There is little room for complacency; even today there are staining reactions for which there is no accepted rationale. The histologist is still too often plagued by differences in the quality and content of dye batches. Not infrequently there is variation in the proportion of chemicals, such as dextrin or sodium chloride, combined with the dye during manufacture. These are added to improve the solubility or flow properties of the dye, but it is the amount of dye present that is important to the laboratory user. Most dyes were developed for use in the textile industry and histologists' needs have been secondary to those of the industrial users when considering the enormous disparity in the quantities used. One means of establishing the uniformity of dye samples is paper chromatography. This shows whether there are secondary dye fractions present, and gives some indication of dye particle size by the extent of travel in the paper in a given solvent and developing solution. A number 1 Whatman filter paper can be used for this exercise; the procedure is set out in an article by Rosenthal et al (1965).

Reference has been made to the importance of the natural dye haematoxylin in histology and cytology; it was introduced in 1863 by Waldeyer and is still used extensively. Other natural dyes include carmine from the cochineal beetle, and orcein that is derived from a species of lichens; both dyes continue to have a significant, if small role in current histological practice. In latter years comparatively few 'new' dyes have entered the repertoire and remained there. Examples are luxol fast blue, solochrome cyanine, Sirius red, brilliant crystal scarlet, amido black, alcian blue and fluorescent dyes such as thioflavine T and fluorescein isothiocyanate (FITC). Dye nomenclature is often descriptive and reflects either the colour of the product, e.g. *light green*, or occasionally an association with a particular use, e.g. *wool green*, or even a particular event, e.g. *Congo red*, whose introduction to the dye market coincided with the founding of the Congo Free State in 1885. Occasionally the dye name is followed by various letters or numbers, e.g. alcian blue GX, allotted by the manufacturer to designate slight modifications in production.

THE CHEMISTRY OF DYES AND THEIR MODE OF ATTACHMENT TO TISSUE

Dyes. These are essentially aromatic benzene ring compounds or derivatives that possess the twin properties of colour and ability to bind to tissues. At one time most dyes were coal tar derivatives but an increasing number are now by-products of oil distillation.

Chromophores. The group on the benzene ring that confers colour is known as a chromophore and alters the light resonance properties of the compound, so that unequal absorption occurs when white light is passed through. The colour *emission* of a given object depends on the colour spectrum *absorbed* when white light falls on it. A red rose is red because the arrangement of the rose fibre molecules is such that the blue-green component is absorbed out.

An important chromophore is the quinoid ring where two of the hydrogen atoms on the benzene ring have been replaced by oxygen atoms. The quinoid chromophore may occur alone, as in the triphenyl methane dyes (e.g. basic fuchsin), or with other chromophores such as the azo group (Congo red). Other important chromophoric groups are xanthene (eosin) and the quinone-imine group. The latter group is subdivided according to the element present in the inter-benzene bonds. These include the *oxazins* where an oxygen atom is incorporated (cresyl fast violet), and the thiazins where a sulphur atom is incorporated (toluidine blue). Possession of colour alone does not itself constitute a dye; an auxochromic or binding group is necessary (a substance possessing a chromophore is known as a chromogen), therefore;

chromogen + auxochrome = a dye

Auxochromes. In order for tissue to bind firmly it is necessary for the dye to possess auxochromic groups. These are groups on the benzene ring that can impart a net charge to the molecule by conferring the property of electrolytic dissociation. This electrical charge is an important mechanism in the attachment of dyes to tissues. The amino group is an important cationic auxochrome and the hydroxyl and carboxyl groups important anionic auxochromes. Other forms of binding are described below under the heading 'Tissue–dye reactions'.

DYE MODIFIERS

The possession of a chromophore and auxochrome is integral to the formation of a dye, but there are other radicles that affect either the colour or properties of that dye; they literally 'modify' the dye. Ethyl and methyl groups on the benzene ring have this effect, e.g. increased methylation of methyl violet produces a bluer shade of dye, namely crystal violet. Another type of dye modifier is the sulphonic acid radical that can increase the water solubility of a dye and confer anionic properties, even in the presence of a cationic auxochrome. Acid fuchsin is virtually sulphonated basic fuchsin and, as their names imply, they have quite different staining properties.

Leuco dyes. Dyes that lose their colour by a process of reduction are termed 'leuco' dyes. A good example of this is the dye patent blue which becomes colour-less on hydrogenation, but may be restored to its original colour by a suitably catal-ysed oxidation process. Schiff's reagent is sometimes incorrectly called a 'leucofuchsin', a term that is best avoided as strictly speaking it is a sulphurated fuchsin, rather than a reduced fuchsin. The use of Schiff's reagent is fundamental to the practice of histochemistry: it is essentially a sulphurated pararosanilin dye capable of forming a magenta compound with tissue di-aldehydes. The precise nature of the magenta compound is still in some doubt and is discussed in greater detail in Chapter 7.

Fluorescent dyes. Fluorescence is emitted by certain substances when high energy, i.e. low wavelength, light is used to raise them to a higher energy level.

Subsequently there is a fall to a lower energy level and because there is an energy loss, the energy they emit is of a longer wavelength. This is the basis of fluorescence microscopy, which is used for identifying or visualizing certain tissue entities. These fluorescent substances can be shown to increase the wavelength of the exciting light from the invisible (e.g. ultraviolet) to visible, or alternatively to increase the wavelength of visible exciting light and change the colour from blue to yellow. Structures such as elastic fibres possess an inherent fluorescence property that is known as auto or primary fluorescence (more properly the latter). In addition there are compounds known as fluorochromes or fluorescent dyes that bind to non-fluorescent tissue entities and demonstrate them by indirect fluorescence properties; this is termed secondary fluorescence. Examples of commonly employed fluorescent dyes are acridine orange, thioflavine T and fluorescein isothiocyanate (FITC). One useful advantage of fluorescent over conventional dyes is that they are more sensitive and can aid the visualization of minute structures, but they are usually less selective.

TISSUE – DYE REACTIONS

Tissue will bind dyes by one of the following mechanisms:

Electrostatic. Most tissue–dye reactions involve some form of electrostatic mechanism, so that a cationic dye (neutral red) will bond to anionic compounds (nucleic acids). Conversely, anionic dyes (light green) will bond to cationic substances (basic protein as in red blood cell envelopes). Amphoteric reactions also apply, an example being muscle protein that will behave as a base in the presence of an acid dye and bind that dye or vice versa. Dyes too, may be amphoteric and behave as an acid or base when suitably buffered to below or above their isoelectric point.

Hydrogen bonding. Although relatively few staining effects are based on this type of reaction, it is important because some of the most useful and diagnostically significant techniques in the histological repertoire are involved; Congo red for amyloid, carmine for glycogen and the Weigert-type resorcinol dye methods for elastic fibres are examples.

van der Waals forces and covalent bonding. There has been, in recent years, an increased awareness of the role played by van der Waals Forces in dye binding. It has been shown that large dye–mordant complexes may bind to tissue by van der Waals forces; an example of this binding is the staining of cell nuclei by alum haematoxylin solutions. Covalent bonding is also thought to be involved in dye–mordant–tissue reactions, but the precise nature of the binding is less clear.

Physical staining. The staining of lipids by dyes known collectively as Sudan dyes is the only noteworthy histological reaction where a purely physical mechanism pertains. These dyes of the azo chromophoric group possess the unique property of being more soluble in certain types of lipid than in their solvent, so that diffusion, which is reversible, takes place from one medium to the other. The Sudan dyes, with one exception, lack an auxochromic group so they are not dyes in the true sense of the word. The exception is Sudan black, which possesses an amino group auxochrome; because of this, it has enhanced staining properties compared to others of the Sudan group and a wide range of lipids can be stained.

Natural affinity. There are a few examples where living material has an affinity for a particular dye, the most noteworthy being that of Janus green for mitochondria in vital dyeing.

FACTORS INFLUENCING DYE UPTAKE

These include *spatial relationships*, where the stereochemistry of the dye molecule and tissue results in a specific staining reaction, and the *dye particle size related to tissue pore size* in controlled sequential staining by different coloured dyes having a similar electrical charge. Both factors will be further discussed in the chapters dealing with the demonstration of nucleic acids and connective tissue respectively, but these merely *influence* the way in which dyes are bound to tissue by *conventional* (electrostatic) forces.

The third influencing factor in some staining reactions is the use of *mordants*. These are double salts of metals such as lead, aluminium, copper, iron, molybdenum and tungsten, and serve to enhance or make possible the binding of a particular dye to a particular tissue moiety. In a sense they act as a bridge between tissue and dye. Mordants can be incorporated into the stain solution, e.g. aluminium potassium sulphate in haematoxylin solutions, or as a separate step usually preceding the staining solution, as in the Loyez technique for myelin.

EFFECTS OF FIXATION ON STAINING OF TISSUES

To discuss this topic in detail is beyond the scope of this chapter. Certain fixatives either enhance or inhibit dye uptake by modifying the tissue proteins, which means that dye diffusion is affected, or reactive radicals either exposed or masked by protein rearrangement (denaturation). For example, formalin forms cross-links with protein and tends to mask cationic tissue binding sites for anionic dyes so that acid dye uptake, e.g. eosin, is suppressed. Conversely, anionic binding sites are exposed, so that basophilia of nuclei are enhanced.

IMPREGNATION WITH METALLIC SALTS

Only two metallic salts are used for demonstrating tissue morphology; silver nitrate has a wide use. The other salt, gold chloride, was employed to a limited extent in an empirical manner by early workers in the field of nerve fibre and nerve ending demonstration. The only technique employing a gold salt that is still used is that of Cajal, that incorporates an impregnating solution of gold chloride and mercuric chloride to demonstrate neuroglial astrocytes. The use of silver nitrate in histological demonstration techniques is not new—von Recklinghausen used it as long ago as 1862. It has many applications and these can be divided into three forms.

ARGYROPHIL REACTIONS

There are many techniques to be found under this broad umbrella, quite often differing only in the length of the various steps or in the composition of the silver solutions employed. Essentially the reactions are those employed in black and white photography, although the precise rationale for many of these closely related methods is poorly understood. Certain tissue elements have a natural affinity (argyrophilia) for silver nitrate. This bound colourless silver salt (various complex silver oxide solutions are employed), if subsequently reduced by substances such as hydroquinone or formalin, will form a black reduced silver compound and show the particular elements demonstrated as black structures against a colourless or pale yellow background. Examples of tissue elements demonstrated by an argyrophil technique are reticulin and nerve fibres and calcium salts, although this involves a different type of argyrophil reaction (q.v.).

ARGENTAFFIN REACTIONS

In this type of technique, use is made of the presence in structures of an appropriate reducing agent such as a phenolic group. These reducing agents are capable of reducing silver salts and other metallic salts, i.e. they do not need an extraneous reducer as in the argyrophil method. One of the earliest applications of this principle was to demonstrate carcinoid tumours. Tissue granules, such as melanin, and certain forms of enterochromaffin cells are good examples of argentaffin material.

ALDEHYDE REDUCTION

Certain carbohydrate-containing tissues when treated with suitable oxidants form aldehydes, and are then able to reduce a compound formed of hexamine (methenamine) and silver nitrate, under appropriate conditions of temperature and pH (q.v.). Fungi, glycogen and basement membranes (basal laminae) can be demonstrated by this means.

FORMATION OF COLOURED COMPOUNDS BY A CHEMICAL REACTION

Like the silver techniques described above, the use of colour formation methods has a firm place in the routine histological repertoire. In this type of technique sections are treated with organic or inorganic salts that react with the moiety to be demonstrated and will either directly form a coloured reaction product in situ, or a colourless intermediate product capable of forming a coloured end-product when suitably treated in its turn. This principle is not new. As far back as 1849, Millon devised a histochemical technique for tyrosine, and in 1867 Perls introduced his now classic method for the demonstration of iron. Other techniques still in common use, and based upon colour formation by a chemical reaction, include the Schmorl method for melanin and the Fouchet technique for bile that was adapted from its original use in biochemistry. These methods are discussed in detail in the relevant chapters.

Another significant group of histochemical techniques is the demonstration of enzymes that received its impetus from Gomori in 1939. He, with Takamatsu, described the technique for the demonstration of alkaline phosphatase, using a metallic substitution principle to produce a brown-black reaction product. Another later enzyme demonstration milestone, by Menton and co-workers in 1944, was the use of diazonium salts which react with enzyme-substrate reaction products to form an azo dye in situ. It is interesting that the field of enzyme histochemistry took on a new lease of life with the development of immunocytochemistry, one important technique in this context being the DAB technique, introduced in 1966 by Graham and Karnovsky for the demonstration of the enzyme peroxidase in blood cells. How little could they have anticipated its eventual worldwide use in the immunoperoxidase method, which was become a standard immunocytochemistry technique, and for which new applications are constantly being sought and found.

SUMMARY OF COMMON TERMS USED IN TISSUE DEMONSTRATION

Argentaffin. Affinity of substances for silver salts and capability of reducing them to a black metallic silver without the need for an extraneous reducer, e.g. melanin pigment.

Argyrophil. Affinity of substances for silver salts that are subsequently reduced to black metallic silver and demonstrated, e.g. nerve fibres, using a reducing agent.

Auxochrome. A charged group present on dye molecules responsible for electrochemical binding of charged tissue molecules, e.g. OH, NH_2.

Chromophore. An organic group, the presence of which confers colour to benzene ring compounds, e.g. quinoid group.

Diazonium salt. Organic compounds that have been nitrogenated ('diazotized') and combine with certain organic groups, such as naphthol, to form azo dyes. Used commonly in methods for tissue enzymes.

Fluorochrome. When tissues are stained with a fluorochrome, e.g. acridine orange, this confers the property of secondary fluorescence. A fluorochrome can increase the wavelength of high energy light passed through it and so can be used to confer secondary fluorescence.

Metachromasia. A metachromatic dye is one capable of staining certain negatively charged tissue moieties a colour that is not inherent in the dye itself, e.g. toluidine blue will stain cartilage metachromatically purple-red and the surrounding tissue blue. *Polychromasia*, by contrast, is when tissues are stained varying colours by a compound containing more than one dye fraction, e.g. Giemsa stain.

Mordant. Some dye–tissue reactions require the presence of an intermediate binding agent. This agent is termed a mordant and consists of the salts of various metals, e.g. aluminium potassium sulphate that facilitates the binding of haematoxylin to cell nuclei.

ROUTINE MORPHOLOGICAL STAINING

HAEMATOXYLIN AND EOSIN (H&E)

H&E staining usually means staining of nuclei by oxidized haematoxylin (haematein) through mordant (chelate) bonds of metals such as aluminium, followed by counterstaining by the xanthene dye eosin, which colours in varying shades the different tissue fibres and cytoplasms. A general tissue demonstration picture is produced and serves as the main diagnostic technique for the histopathologist.

Haematoxylin is extracted from a tropical logwood but is not strictly a dye as it possesses neither tissue binding properties, nor colour to any marked degree. For nuclear staining it is necessary to oxidize haematoxylin to haematein—a weakly anionic purple dye. This oxidation or 'ripening' may be accomplished by a natural process of exposure to light and air over a long period, or by the addition of oxidizing agents. Examples of the latter are sodium iodate in Mayer's, Gill's and Carazzi's solutions, iodine in Cole's and mercuric oxide in Harris's haematoxylin. Haematein is anionic, having no particular affinity for the nucleic acids of cell nuclei. It is necessary to combine a metallic salt or 'mordant' with haematoxylin to confer a net positive charge to the dye compound. The cationic dye-metal complex will bind to the anionic nuclear chromatin. Haematoxylin solutions containing 'alums' formed of aluminium sulphate with either potassium or ammonium sulphate are known as 'alum haematoxylins', and are suitable for routine nuclear staining with eosin as a counterstain. An alternative nuclear stain is provided by the 'iron haematoxylins'. These use mordants that combine ferric sulphate with ammonium sulphate and form a much stronger nucleic acid–dye bond. Consequently, these iron haematoxylins are employed when a particularly vigorous counterstain such as van Gieson is to be used, which might decolourize the weaker nuclear staining obtained with the alum haematoxylins.

Some haematoxylin solutions, such as Harris's, stain background tissue as well as nuclei, although to a lesser degree, and subsequent acid-alcohol differentiation will be required so that only the nuclei are stained. This *regressive* staining is the standard technique employed in routine morphological staining. Other haematoxylins stain the background tissue to a much lesser extent, so differentiation may not be necessary or need only be minimal. This *progressive* staining is used with haematoxylins of Mayer and Carazzi. The haematoxylin solutions are complex and contain one or more of the following substances forming a composite solution bearing the originator's name:

An alum. This is the mordant, of which the aluminium cation is the main reactant and is obtained as a combined salt with either potassium or ammonium sulphate.

An acid. Aims at making staining more precise—what is termed an 'accelerator'.

An oxidizing agent. Gives speedy conversion of haematoxylin to haematein.

Glycerol. Slows the oxidation of naturally oxidizing haematoxylin and improves the keeping properties.

The choice of a haematoxylin solution is a personal decision, as all the popular ones are capable of giving good results. There are minor attributes to be borne in mind. Mayer's and Carazzi's haematoxylin solutions have a shorter staining time and can be used progressively. Harris's haematoxylin solution needs filtering before use and careful differentiation, but is regarded by many as giving the most intense and precise staining. Gill's haematoxylin is popular, particularly amongst cytologists, for its avid staining allied to a short staining time, and may be used in the Papanicolaou technique for cervical smears. Ehrlich's haematoxylin solution, on the other hand, keeps well and stains certain of the mucins blue, but requires a longer staining time. Differentiation of haematoxylin is done by using an alcoholic solution of hydrochloric acid. It is thought that the differentiation is achieved by the acid attacking and breaking the tissue–mordant bond, rather than the mordant–dye bond (Baker 1962).

Eosin was first used in 1875 as 'Eosine' for the dyeing of silk and wool. There are various forms available commercially but the most commonly used is the water-soluble (ws) yellowish. Other variants are eosin B (a bluish form) and eosin ethyl, an alcohol–soluble form. Eosin is an anionic dye and combines electrostatically with tissue such as collagen and muscle, the latter in an amphoteric manner. Raising the pH of the solution causes eosin to stain more intensely. This can be achieved either by the use of a suitable buffer or by dissolving the dye in tap water (the latter treatment will vary in its efficacy in different areas).

In the following procedures, dogmatic times of haematoxylin treatment will be omitted as these will depend on the preparation of the solutions and sections. The staining time of Ehrlich's haematoxylin will vary according to the degree of oxidation obtained. Paraffin sections from tissue fixed for a long time in formalin will stain more heavily with haematoxylin and more weakly with eosin, than sections of tissue fixed for a short time in Helly's solution for example. Frozen sections stain more quickly than paraffin.

STAINING SOLUTIONS

Ehrlich's haematoxylin solution (Ehrlich 1886)

Haematoxylin	16 g
Ethyl alcohol	480 ml
Potassium or ammonium alum	48 g
Distilled water	240 ml
Glycerol	240 ml
Glacial acetic acid	24 ml

Dissolve the haematoxylin in the alcohol with the aid of gentle heat (56°C oven or water bath). Dissolve the alum in the distilled water using heat (bunsen) and whilst warm add the glycerol. Allow to cool. Add the alcoholic haematoxylin solution in small volumes to the alum-glycerol solution, mixing well. Add the acetic acid and mix, plug the container with cotton wool and allow to oxidize by exposure to light. This will take at least 6 weeks, but ripening may be allowed to continue indefinitely. Filter prior to use. Immediate oxidation may be achieved by adding 0.1 g sodium iodate per 100 ml volume of prepared solution, then mixing and allowing to stand for at least 1 hour before use.

Mayer's haematoxylin solution (Mayer 1903)

Haematoxylin	1 g
Distilled water	1000 ml
Potassium or ammonium alum	50 g
Sodium iodate	0.2 g
Citric acid	1 g
Chloral hydrate	50 g

Dissolve the haematoxylin, alum and sodium iodate in distilled water, standing the mixture overnight at room temperature. Add the chloral hydrate and citric acid, mix and boil for 5 min. Cool and filter. The solution is ready for use and should not need re-filtering.

Harris's haematoxylin solution (Harris 1900)

Haematoxylin	5 g
Ethyl alcohol	50 ml
Potassium or ammonium alum	100 g
Distilled water	950 ml
Sodium iodate	1 g
Glacial acetic acid	40 ml

Dissolve the haematoxylin in the alcohol using gentle heat (56°C oven or water bath) and dissolve the alum in the distilled water using heat (bunsen) with frequent stirring. While the aqueous alum solution is still hot, add the alcoholic haematoxylin solution and bring to the boil stirring frequently. (Turn off the bunsen just before adding the mercuric oxide as the resultant effervescence may cause spillage.) Cool quickly by plunging the container into cold water, then add the acetic acid and filter. The solution is ready for immediate use but will need re-filtering.

Cole's haematoxylin solution (Cole 1943)

Haematoxylin	1.5 g
Saturated aqueous potassium or ammonium alum	700 ml
1% iodine in 95% alcohol	50 ml
Distilled water	250 ml

Dissolve the haematoxylin in the distilled water using gentle heat (56°C oven or water bath). Add to this the iodine solution and bring to the boil, then cool quickly. The solution is ready for immediate use but will need re-filtering.

Carazzi's haematoxylin solution (Carazzi 1911)

Haematoxylin	10 g
Glycerol	200 ml
Potassium or ammonium alum	50 g
Distilled water	800 ml
Potassium iodate	0.2 g

Dissolve the haematoxylin in the glycerol, and the alum in 750 ml of distilled water. The alum solution should be prepared at room temperature and left overnight for the alum crystals to dissolve. Mix the alum and haematoxylin solutions in small volumes, shaking well, dissolve the iodate salt in the remaining volume of distilled water and add to the main solution with thorough mixing. Filter and the solution is ready for use.

Gill's haematoxylin solution (Gill et al 1974)

Haematoxylin	2 g
Sodium iodate	0.2 g
Aluminium sulphate	17.6 g
Distilled water	750 ml
Ethylene glycol	250 ml
Glacial acetic acid	20 ml

Mix the distilled water and ethylene glycol and add the haematoxylin. Next add the sodium iodate followed by the aluminium sulphate and mix. Finally add the acetic acid and stir for 1 hour at room temperature using a magnetic stirrer. The solution is ready for immediate use and should be filtered when required.

Eosin 1% aqueous ws yellowish

Add a crystal of phenol or thymol to the prepared solution to inhibit mould formation. Filter prior to use.

Differentiator
1% hydrochloric acid in 70% alcohol.

Blueing agent
2% aqueous sodium bicarbonate.

HAEMATOXYLIN AND EOSIN (H & E)

Technique

1. Sections to water.
2. Stain with haematoxylin solution for the requisite time, e.g. Carazzi's, Mayer's and Harris's 5 min; Cole and Gill's up to 10 min (smears 2 min); Ehrlich's up to 25 min.
3. Wash briefly in water and differentiate in acid-alcohol.
4. Wash well in water and blue for 10–30s. Check microscopically—the nuclei should be a deep blue colour with the vesicular nuclei showing a well-marked chromatin pattern. The background should show only weak residual haematoxylin colouration.
5. Wash in water and stain with eosin solution for 5 min.
6. Wash quickly in water, differentiate and dehydrate in alcohol. Clear and mount as desired.

Results

Keratohyalin, nuclei, cytoplasmic RNA, some calcium salts, urates, bacteria (weakly)	blue
Muscle, keratin, coarse elastic fibres, fibrin, fibrinoid	bright red
Collagen, reticulin, myelinated nerve fibres, amyloid	pink
Red blood cells	orange

Besides the haematoxylin solutions detailed above there are others having a more specialized role (see Table 2.1) including: Celestine blue-haematoxylin, Heidenhain, Weigert, Verhoeff, Loyez, PTAH, Solcia lead and Thomas molybdenum haematoxylins.

Table 2.1   Specialized (non-nuclear) uses of haematoxylin-haematein

Technique	Mordant	Demonstration
Baker	Potassium dichromate	Phospholipids
Heidenhain	Iron alum	Mitochondria, striated muscle
Kultschitsky	Potassium dichromate, chromic fluoride	Normal myelin
Loyez	Iron alum	Normal myelin
Mallory	Phosphotungstic acid	Fibrin, glial fibres, striated muscle
Mallory	None	Lead, copper
Mayer	Aluminium chloride	Mucins
Solcia	Lead nitrate	Diffuse endocrine cells
Thomas	Molybdenum	Diffuse endocrine cells, collagen
Verhoeff	Ferric chloride	Elastic fibres
Weigert	Ferric chloride	Normal myelin
Weil	Iron alum	Normal myelin

CARMALUM STAIN FOR NUCLEI (Mayer 1892)

This can be used as a red nuclear stain. Unlike neutral red it is stable even if the section is mounted in an aqueous mountant. It is valuable as a nuclear counterstain to the Sudan black stain for lipid but is not a particularly avid stain and a lengthy (30 min) staining time is required. Formalin-fixed material gives poor results; mercuric chloride-containing solutions are preferred.

Carmalum staining solution

Carminic acid	2 g
5% aqueous ammonium alum	100 ml
Salicylic acid or thymol	0.2 g

Add the carminic acid to the ammonium alum solution and dissolve by boiling for 1 hour. Cool and restore to original volume with distilled water. Add the fungicidal agent and mix thoroughly. Filter and use. The solution keeps quite well if stored at 4°C.

RAPID STAINING FOR URGENT FROZEN SECTIONS

H&E TECHNIQUE FOR FRESH CRYOSTAT SECTIONS

Notes

Whilst fixation prior to staining is not essential, brief (1–2 min) immersion of the slide in 10% formalin will enhance the nuclear basophilia. Sections of certain material, e.g. mucoid tumours, may lift off the slides when placed in the formalin and this step should, therefore, be avoided and a dry section celloidinized instead.

Solutions

Harris's haematoxylin (pre-filtered) (see p. 25)
1% acid-alcohol (see p. 27)
2% aqueous sodium bicarbonate (see p. 27)
1% aqueous ws yellowish eosin (see p. 26)

Technique

1. Wash sections in water for 10–20 s.
2. Stain with haematoxylin for 1 min.
3. Wash briefly in water, differentiate in acid-alcohol for 1–2 s.
4. Wash briefly in water and 'blue' in sodium bicarbonate for 10 s or so.
5. Wash in water 10–20 s and, if time permits, check nuclear staining microscopically.
6. Stain with eosin for 30 s.
7. Wash briefly, dehydrate, clear and mount as desired.

Results

Nuclei	blue
Background	shades of pink to red

H&E TECHNIQUE FOR FORMALIN-FIXED FROZEN SECTIONS

Notes

The essential differences in technique when staining fixed, as opposed to unfixed, frozen sections are based upon the former's tendency to lift from the slide more easily during staining, and that eosin staining is depressed and nuclear staining enhanced. Providing a celloidin film is applied that is reasonably thin and even, there should be no need to remove it at the conclusion of staining.

Solutions

As for the previous technique except for the eosin solution.
2% eosin ws yellowish in tap water, see notes on page 24.

Technique

1. Mount the frozen sections on a slide and blot dry.
2. Rinse in equal parts ether-alcohol and then cover with 0.5% celloidin in ether-alcohol.
3. Drain slide, allow to air dry, before washing in water for $\frac{1}{2}$–1 min to complete the process of hardening the celloidin film.
4. Stain with haematoxylin for 40–50 s.
5. Wash briefly in water and differentiate in acid-alcohol for up to 5 s.
6. Wash briefly in water and 'blue' in sodium bicarbonate solution 10 s or so.
7. Wash in water and, if time permits, check nuclear staining microscopically.
8. Stain with eosin for 1 min.
9. Wash briefly in water, dehydrate thoroughly because of the celloidin film; clear and mount as desired.

Results

Nuclei	blue
Background	shades of pink to red

POLYCHROME METHYLENE BLUE TECHNIQUE (Morris 1947)

Notes

The use of polychrome methylene blue for rapid frozen sections was popular at one time, either for the H&E stain, or as a preceding stain so that the pathologist could study the methylene blue-stained section whilst the comparatively slower H&E-stained section was completed. Touch or imprint smears of unfixed tumours, breast lumps or lymph nodes may also be stained to advantage with polychrome methylene blue. Polychroming of methylene blue is achieved by mixing with potassium carbonate, when various azures are formed. This process is accentuated by ageing of the solution.

Staining solution

Methylene blue	1 g
Potassium carbonate	1 g

Glacial acetic acid	3 ml
Distilled water	300 ml

Place the distilled water in a 1 litre flask and add, with mixing, methylene blue and potassium carbonate. Boil for 10–15 min. While still hot add glacial acetic acid drop by drop, shaking vigorously until the formed precipitate is dissolved. Boil until the volume of fluid is reduced to 100 ml. Cool and filter. Allow to stand 4 weeks prior to use.

Technique

1. Rinse frozen sections and imprint smears in water.
2. Filter on the polychrome methylene blue for $\frac{1}{2}$–1 min.
3. Wash in water and blot dry.
4. Dehydrate in tertiary butyl alcohol, clear in xylene and mount in a DPX-type mountant (conventional ethanol dehydration will diminish the polychromasia).

Results

Nuclei	blue
Background	various shades of red-purple

ROUTINE STAINING FOR THIN PLASTIC RESIN SECTIONS

Staining resin sections for light microscopy presents problems that are absent when dealing with paraffin or frozen material. This is the result of the inability of dye molecules to penetrate certain plastic resins, and it is necessary to dissolve the resin from the section prior to staining. The acrylic resins permit staining without the need for resin extraction, but epoxy resin sections require treatment. Whether or not section resin extraction is required, it may be necessary to modify the normal staining times or precede staining by permanganate oxidation to intensify the reaction. In the H&E technique haematoxylin stains nuclei effectively in thin resin sections, but eosin does not stain the cytoplasm to the same degree. It is common practice to use a related dye, phloxine, instead. Described below is toluidine blue staining, which is the standard morphological technique for general overnight staining of resin-embedded tissue. It gives nuclear detail not obtained in staining of paraffin or frozen sections.

Resin extraction of sections prior to staining (sodium ethoxide)

1. Dissolve 2 g sodium hydroxide in 100 ml absolute ethanol and allow to stand overnight.
2. Place sections in the solution for 1 h at room temperature. Wash well in water (at least 15 min).

TOLUIDINE BLUE TECHNIQUE FOR THIN RESIN SECTIONS

Notes

Epoxy resins are difficult to stain, even after sodium ethoxide extraction, and require a heated toluidine blue solution. Other resins such as LR White and glycol methacrylate are adequately stained using the solution at room temperature. At the conclusion of staining it is better to air dry and mount, as the usual alcohol-xylene treatment may cause cracking or lifting of the section.

Staining solution

1% toluidine blue in 1% aqueous borax (sodium tetraborate). Filter. The solution has a pH of approximately 11.0.

Technique

1. Rinse sections in distilled water.
2. Stain with re-filtered toluidine blue, either (see Notes) at room temperature for 15 s or for $1\frac{1}{2}$–2 min on a hot plate (temperature in the region 60–65°C).
3. Blot and allow to thoroughly air dry.
4. Mount as desired.

Results

Nuclei	deep blue
Background	pale blue

HAEMATOXYLIN-PHLOXINE TECHNIQUE FOR THIN RESIN SECTIONS

Notes

The nuclei of resin sections will usually stain perfectly well but less readily than non-plastic resin sections, so that it is important to use an avid alum haematoxylin. Harris's haematoxylin is commonly used. It will be noted that longer times of staining are necessary with fairly brief subsequent acid-alcohol differentiation.

Solutions

Harris's haematoxylin (see p. 25)
1% acid-alcohol (see p. 25)
2% aqueous sodium bicarbonate (see p. 27)
1% aqueous phloxine
Add a few crystals of thymol after filtering to prevent fungal growth.

Technique

1. Rinse sections in water.
2. Stain with haematoxylin for 10 min.
3. Rinse in water.
4. Differentiate in acid-alcohol for 1–2 s.
5. Wash in water and blue in sodium bicarbonate 10 s or so.
6. Wash in water.

7. Stain with phloxine for 5 min.
8. Blot and allow to thoroughly air dry. Mount as desired.

Results

Nuclei	blue
Background	pale pink

SECTION ADHESION AND TRANSFERENCE

Having considered general staining techniques it would be profitable to consider two practical aspects of staining sections on slides. These concern keeping the section on the slide during treatment with reagents, and the measures to be adopted when a slide is broken that carries an all-important section and for a variety of reasons is impossible to replace. Most *well-processed, well-cut* paraffin sections, if adequately dried on the slide, present few problems during staining. Badly prepared and dried sections are likely to become detached, as are sections of tissues such as brain, bone, keratinous skin lesions and material containing tuberculous caseation. Besides the above, techniques involving high temperatures or exposure to strongly alkaline solutions will produce conditions where sections will float off the slide. Immunocytochemistry and in-situ hybridization techniques present problems of section adhesion, and popularly employed slide adhesives are poly-L-lysine and 3-aminopropyltriethoxy-silane respectively.

Recommended procedures in cases of difficulty

1. Mount the section on a microscope slide pre-washed in 1% acid-alcohol (as used for the standard H&E technique) for 10 min then wash in water and wipe dry. When the section has been mounted on the slide it is worthwhile drying at a lower than usual temperature but for a longer period, e.g. 3–4 h at 56°C or overnight at 37°C.

2. Should the above procedures fail, it will be necessary to coat the slide with a section adhesive. For an occasional section it is effective to smear the slide with a thin layer of *normal* plasma (Cook 1965). The mounted section is then heat dried in the usual way. Note that too thick a layer of plasma will take up a counterstain such as eosin. From a health and safety aspect it is important to check that the plasma has been obtained from patients in whom there is no risk of serum hepatitis. For a larger numbers of sections we would recommend the following procedure in which slides are prepared en masse in advance. Prepare a 0.2% aqueous solution of gelatin to which a few crystals of thymol have been added to discourage bacterial growth. Allow to dissolve at 56°C (30 min will suffice). Dip clean microscope slides into the gelatin solution *when cool*, agitating for several seconds. Take out the slides, drain thoroughly and allow to dry on edge (for maximum drainage) at room temperature. It is useful if slide racks are used; place these on clean cloth to obviate the collection of gelatin solution at the bottom edge of the slides. Dry the coated slides for 1 h at 56°C. Allow to cool and store until required in suitable containers. Sections may be subsequently mounted in the usual way from the floating-out bath, followed by conventional drying treatment.

TRANSFERENCE OF SECTIONS (Clayden 1955, slightly modified)

Notes

The transfer of a section from one glass slide to another is effectively achieved by covering the section with a plastic resin film, which when hardened can be soaked off with the section. For a successful result, it is important that the solution be of the right consistency and that hardening of the film be complete. If the film is too thin it will fail to attach to the section, conversely if the film is too thick problems will be encountered when coverslipping.

Solution

DPX mountant	1 part
Butyl acetate	6 parts

This is conveniently done in a glass test-tube and requires thorough mixing by repeated inversion.

Technique

1. Remove the coverslip from the section to be transferred and completely remove the existing mountant in xylene.
2. Cover the whole slide with the resin solution and leave for up to 30 min at 56°C until a hard film is formed. (This is conveniently done by resting the slide on glass rods in a Petri dish.)
3. Using a sharp scalpel blade, make a firm cut in the resin film around the section.
4. Place the slide in distilled water until film plus section starts to lift. This may take several minutes and can be expedited by levering one corner of the film with a scalpel blade. When the section has completely floated off, take up on a clean slide, wipe off the excess water and place in a rack in the 56°C incubator until completely dry.
5. Wash carefully with several changes of butyl acetate, then in xylene, and finally mount as desired.

REFERENCES

Baker J R 1962 Experiments on the action of mordants: 2, aluminium-haematin. Quarterly Journal of Microscopic Science 103: 493
Carazzi D 1911 Eine neue Hamatoxylinosung. Zeitschrift für wissenschaftliche Mikroskopie und für mikroskopische Technik 28: 275
Clayden E C 1955 Practical section cutting and staining. Churchill, London
Cole E C 1943 Studies in haematoxylin stains. Stain Technology 18: 125
Cook H C 1965 A comparative survey of section adhesives and of factors affecting adhesion. Stain Technology 40: 321–328
Ehrlich P 1886 Frageskasten. Zeitschrift für wissenschaftliche Mikroskipie und für mikroskipische Technik 3: 150
Gill G W, Frost J K, Miller K A 1974 A new formula for a half-oxidised haematoxylin solution that neither overstains or requires differentiation. Acta Cytologica 18: 300–311
Harris H F 1900 On the rapid conversion of haematoxylin to haematein in staining reactions. Journal of Applied Microscopic Laboratory Methods 3: 777

Horobin R 1982 Histochemistry. Butterworth, London

Horobin R 1990 Theory of staining. In: Bancroft J D, Stevens A (eds) Theory and practice of histological techniques, 3rd edn. Churchill Livingstone, Edinburgh

Mayer P 1892 Uber das Farben mit Carmin, Cochenille und Hamatein-Tonerde. Mitt. Zool. Stat. Neapel 10: 480

Mayer P 1903 Notiz über Haematein und Hamalaum. Zeitschrift für wissenschaftliche Mickroskopie und für mikroskopische Technik 20: 409

Morris A A 1947 The histological use of the smear technique in the rapid histological diagnosis of tumour of the central nervous system. Journal of Neurosurgery 4: 497

Rosenthal S I, Puchtler H, Sweat F 1965 Paper chromatography of dyes. Archives of Pathology 80: 190–196

3. Connective tissues

The term connective tissue is used here in a broad sense to include fibrillar connective tissue, and tissues that are histologically associated, including basement membranes (basal lamina) and muscle. The types of staining technique falling within this group are those involving the more colourful dyes, the origins of which are set in the early empirical years of histological staining. Their role has changed little over the decades as has their value to the histologist, for these methods include some of the most frequently requested in the repertoire of the routine diagnostic laboratory. The chief components of connective tissue are dealt with in this chapter; other entities, because of their specialized chemical constituents, are dealt with elsewhere. Cartilage, with its high mucin content, is dealt with under *Carbohydrates*, adipose tissue under *Lipids*, and *bone* is dealt with as a biopsy.

MUSCLE

In an H&E stain muscle fibres react strongly with eosin. This is particularly true for voluntary muscle, and the demonstration of different types of muscle can be emphasized by using a trichrome technique. The latter clearly distinguishes muscle from connective tissue in a tinctorial manner, although the different types of striated muscle fibre (types 1, 2a, 2b, 2c) can only be reliably separated by enzyme histochemistry (see Ch. 13). Voluntary muscle striations are birefringent, those in cardiac muscle less obviously so.

COLLAGEN FIBRES

These fibres are formed by fibroblasts and may be arranged in either fine or coarse bundles. They are compact in dermis of skin and in tendon, and form a much more open meshwork in lymphoid tissue and liver where they are called reticulin fibres. They are birefringent and stain weakly with eosin compared with muscle. Collagen is present in loose areolar tissue together with reticulin and elastin fibres. A variety of different cell types are found in loose connective (areolar) tissue and include histiocytes, mast cells, fibroblasts, neutrophils and lymphocytes. van Gieson's technique (which follows) with the methyl blue variant, is the most widely used technique with the trichromes for the demonstration of collagen. Collagen stains are of particular value in identifying the increase in collagenous tissues that occurs in chronic inflammatory processes. In neoplastic processes collagen deposition is more usually a reactive process of the stroma than a product of the tumour cells. It may nevertheless be a characteristic feature of a particular tumour type and thereby may assist diagnosis.

VAN GIESON'S TECHNIQUE (van Gieson 1889)

Notes

van Gieson's technique is probably the most successful single histological technique devised; over a hundred years after its inception it is still in regular use in histological laboratories. Its success is due to the specific staining of collagen with clear colour distinction from other tissues. A potential flaw however is the non-staining of young collagen fibres; for their demonstration use a trichrome stain (see p. 39). Apart from its role as a specific collagen stain, van Gieson's stain makes a useful counterstain in many techniques, e.g. Fouchet for bile (see p. 201) and von Kossa for calcium (see p. 410). In the latter the van Gieson stain contrasts effectively the osteoid material in bone (red) with the mineralized bone (black). The rationale of the method is that when combined solutions of picric acid and acid fuchsin are used the small molecules of picric acid penetrate all tissues rapidly, but are only retained in the close-textured red blood cells and muscle. The larger molecules of the acid fuchsin are able to enter the larger pores of the collagen fibres where they displace the picric acid (Seki 1932). Hydrochloric or nitric acid can be added to the van Gieson's solution (0.25 ml per 100 ml of stain) resulting in brighter staining. The acid tends to cause further differentiation of haematoxylin and elastin stains and must be used cautiously.

Other dyes can be used in combination with picric acid in place of acid fuchsin and will give similar results: these include methyl blue, aniline blue, amido black 10B and violamine. Due to the tendency for the picric acid moiety to differentiate haematoxylin it is customary to stain the nuclei with iron salt-mordant haematoxylin solutions such as Weigert's iron haematoxylin, or a celestine blue-Mayer's haematoxylin sequence. If using the latter it should be borne in mind that celloidin strongly retains celestine blue, therefore avoid celloidinization of sections prior to staining; Weigert's stain is to be preferred. A ferrous sulphate iron haematoxylin is included and will give an intense, dark nuclear stain suitable for use with the van Gieson and trichrome techniques. For the brightest staining results avoid tap water rinsing before and after van Gieson staining; use distilled water instead or blot dry. Dehydrate quickly at the conclusion of the technique as the highly alcohol-soluble picric acid will be extracted. Differentiation of the haematoxylin with the acid-alcohol should be minimal because further differentiation will occur during staining with van Gieson's solution.

Staining solutions

Weigert's iron haematoxylin (Weigert 1904). This is stored as two solutions and mixed in equal proportions immediately prior to use. It has been shown (Ibeachum 1971) that the working solution retains its staining avidity for up to 60 days if stored at 4°C. The alcoholic haematoxylin solution gives better results when young. In older solutions over-oxidation results when the ferric chloride is added. The hydrochloric acid probably acts as an accentuator.

Solution A:

| Haematoxylin | 1 g |
| Ethyl alcohol | 100 ml |

Dissolve with gentle heat.
Solution B:

30% aqueous ferric chloride	4 ml
Conc. hydrochloric acid	1 ml
Distilled water	100 ml

Add equal volumes of A and B prior to use.

Celestine blue (Gray et al 1958):

Celestine blue B or R	1 g
Conc.sulphuric acid	0.5 ml
2.5% aqueous ferric ammonium sulphate	86 ml
Glycerol	14 ml

Grind the celestine blue to a paste with sulphuric acid and gradually add the iron alum solution with frequent mixing. Add the glycerol, mix and place in the 56°C oven to dissolve. Cool and filter. It is advisable to filter again prior to use. We find this variant gives particularly intense staining.

Ferrous sulphate iron haematoxylin (Slidders 1968). In the following solution the ferrous salt is used for a ferric salt mordant. This gives a more stable vigorous solution as it does not over-oxidize the haematoxylin. Aluminium chloride is incorporated as a stabilizing salt. A staining time of 5–10 min is recommended and may be followed by a counterstain, i.e. van Gieson. Nuclei are stained almost black.

Iron haematoxylin:

Haematoxylin	1 g
Aluminium chloride	10 g
Ferrous sulphate	10 g
Conc.hydrochloric acid	2 ml
95% ethanol	100 ml
Saturated (9%) aqueous sodium iodate	2 ml
Distilled water	100 ml

Dissolve the haematoxylin in the 95% ethanol. Add the aluminium chloride and ferrous sulphate to the distilled water. Mix the two solutions together, add hydrochloric acid and sodium iodate solutions. Mix, stand for 48 h and filter before use.

van Gieson stain:

| Saturated aqueous picric acid | 100 ml |
| 1% aqueous acid fuchsin | 10 ml |

Boil for 3 min, cool and filter.

Curtis's stain. This modification of van Gieson's stain gives brighter results and is claimed to fade less than the conventional stain.

| Saturated aqueous picric acid | 100 ml |

| 1% aqueous Ponceau S | 10 ml |
| Glacial acetic acid | 1 ml |

Technique

1. Take sections to water.
2. Stain nuclei with either Weigert's haematoxylin solution for 15–30 min, or with celestine blue for 5 min, wash in water then stain in Mayer's haematoxylin solution for 5 min.
3. Wash in water, differentiate with acid-alcohol. Wash and blue.
4. Check microscopically; the nuclei should be a dark blue-black and the background a paler blue-black colour.
5. Rinse well in distilled water.
6. Stain with van Gieson's solution for 5 min.
7. Rinse in distilled water or drain, rinse in alcohol. Dehydrate, clear and mount in DPX.

Results

Nuclei	brown-black
Mature collagen	red
Other tissue, e.g. muscle and red blood cells	yellow
Some bile pigments	green

METHYL BLUE-VAN GIESON TECHNIQUE FOR YOUNG AND MATURE COLLAGEN (Herovici 1963)

Notes

The method depends on the affinity of young collagen and reticulin for methyl blue and mature fibres for acid fuchsin. It may be used in the demonstration of recent fibrosis in healing processes in tissue. The variable affinity of the two dyes is due to variation in particle size and in the structure of the fibres, the mature collagen having larger intermicellar spaces and the younger fibres smaller spaces. Formal-acetic-alcohol (10:5:85) is the recommended fixative. On occasion the method may be capricious and we have noticed that fibrin may also stain blue. The original method used a final metanil yellow step to stain cytoplasm but we usually omit this.

Staining solution

0.5% aqueous methyl blue	50 ml
0.1% acid fuchsin in saturated aqueous picric acid	10 ml
Mix, then add glycerol	10 ml
Saturated aqueous lithium carbonate	0.5 ml

Technique

1. Sections to water.
2. Stain nuclei with an iron haematoxylin solution. Differentiate and blue.

3. Stain with modified van Gieson's solution for 2 min.
4. Wash in 1% acetic acid solution for 2 min.
5. Dehydrate, clear and mount as for the conventional van Gieson technique.

Results

Nulcei	brown-black
Reticulin, young collagen and (?) fibrin	blue
Mature collagen	red
Red blood cells, muscle, etc.	yellow

TRICHROME METHODS

Under this heading are grouped most multi-stage techniques that are capable of distinguishing between tissue structures such as collagen and muscle in contrasting colours. The rationale underlying these methods is the firm attachment of one dye to a specific tissue that is probably electrostatic in nature. The means by which sequential staining with a series of anionic dyes is achieved relates to the physical structure of the dyes and the tissues. For example, red blood cells may be stained first with a dye of small particle size such as orange G. This is more firmly retained in the small intermicellar spaces of the red cell than in the looser texture of structures such as collagen or muscle. If this is followed by acid fuchsin staining, which has a larger particle size, the dye molecules are unable to enter the red cell pores, but can enter those of muscle and collagen. If the tissue is then treated with phosphomolybdic or phosphotungstic acid solutions there is a displacement of acid fuchsin particles from collagen, where they are insecurely held in the large intermicellar spaces. Finally, a dye of large particle size, such as aniline blue, is used that is able to enter collagen.

The trichrome stains are of particular value for demonstrating fibrin or young collagen fibres and for differentiating muscle from connective tissue. They may also be valuable in the interpretation of partly autolysed post-mortem tissues where conventional H & E staining can be relatively poor. The precise method used is a matter of choice; good results are possible with all. Mercuric chloride, potassium dichromate and picric acid fixation give best results. Formalin fixation can lead to indifferent results that may be partly overcome by pre-mordanting sections in Helly's fixative (see Appendix 1) for at least 5 h. A useful tip, when dealing with a section in which there are few normal tissue structures to act as a guide to staining, is to select a reasonably sized artery to act as a control, relying on the fact that the tunica media should be red and the tunica adventitia blue or green. When staining voluntary (striated) muscle it will be found that type 1 fibres stain a deeper red colour than type 2. This effect is heightened if formalin fixation only was used and is less easily seen if the normally recommended fixation was carried out. It appears the formaldehyde cross-linking masking effect on amino group acidophilia is less pronounced with type 1 muscle protein, probably due to the higher mitochondria content of these fibres. In mitochondrial myopathy this phenomenon is sufficiently enhanced that the term 'ragged red fibres' has been used to describe muscle fibres containing large aggregates of abnormal mitochondria.

MALLORY'S TECHNIQUE (Mallory 1905)

Notes

One of the earliest trichrome methods, it is now no longer widely used in Britain. Mallory slightly modified the method in later years; the following technique is the original. We see no reason why nuclei may not be stained first with haematoxylin.

Solutions

0.5% aqueous acid fuchsin
Orange G-aniline blue stain:

Orange G	2 g
Aniline blue	0.5 g
Phosphomolybdic acid	1 g
Distilled water	100 ml

Dissolve the phosphomolybdic acid in water, add the two dyes and mix. Filter before use.

Technique

1. Take sections to water.
2. Stain with the acid fuchsin solution for 5 min.
3. Drain and stain with the orange G-aniline blue solution for 20 min.
4. Differentiate in 95% alcohol, dehydrate, clear and mount as desired.

Results

Nuclei	blue or red, depending on whether or not a haematoxylin step was introduced
Muscle, fibrin	red
Collagen, reticulin	blue
Red blood cells	yellow
Elastin	weak red colour

PICRO-MALLORY TECHNIQUE (McFarlane 1944)

Notes

When differentiating the picro-orange solution leave a little in the background as it will be masked by the subsequent dyes. Differentiation of acid fuchsin is more prolonged than the collagen staining so treat as long as necessary to obtain the desired effect—a maxim that can be applied to all histological methods. The optional alcian green step is repeated following haematoxylin staining, giving a more intense colouration of any acid mucins present.

Solutions

1% alcian green 2GX in 3% acetic acid (optional)
0.2% orange G in saturated alcoholic picric acid

Ponceau-acid fuchsin solution

Equal volumes of 0.5% ponceau 2R and 0.5% acid fuchsin in 1% acetic acid.

Aniline blue solution

Boil 97.5 ml of distilled water and add 2 g aniline blue ws. While still hot, add 2.5 ml glacial acetic acid. Cool and filter.

Stock solution:

Phosphotungstic acid	25 g
Picric acid	2.5 g
95% alcohol	100 ml

Red differentiator:

Stock solution	40 ml
95% alcohol	40 ml
Distilled water	20 ml

Blue differentiator:

Stock solution	20 ml
Distilled water	80 ml

Technique

1. Sections to water.
2. Stain with the alcian green solution for 3 min (optional).
3. Wash in water and stain the nuclei with an iron haematoxylin solution. Differentiate well and blue.
4. Wash, then stain with the alcian green solution for 3 min (optional).
5. Wash in water and stain with the picro-orange solution for 7 min.
6. Differentiate in water for approximately 5 s until red blood cells are yellow and background is faint yellow.
7. Treat with the ponceau-acid fuchsin solution for 2–3 min.
8. Rinse in 2% acetic acid then differentiate in red differentiator until the muscle is red and connective tissues are almost colourless; this may take several minutes. To check microscopically, rinse in 2% acetic acid — this will stop further differentiation.
9. Finally, rinse in 2% acetic acid then in tap water for 10 s or so to remove the acetic acid.
10. Stain with the aniline blue solution for 10 min.
11. Rinse in 2% acetic acid and differentiate in the blue differentiator until excess blue staining is removed (usually 10–20 s).
12. Rinse in 2% acetic acid. Dehydrate, clear and mount as desired.

Results

Nuclei	blue-black (may be red)
Acid mucins	green (optional step)
Fibrin, muscle	red
Reticulin, collagen	blue
Red blood cells, colloid	yellow

HEIDENHAIN'S 'AZAN' (Heidenhain 1915)

Notes

This is a less-used trichrome method. To obtain good results, stain strongly with the azocarmine and slightly under-differentiate with the aniline-alcohol, otherwise the counterstain will mask the staining of muscle. Although orange G is incorporated into the counterstain, little yellow colouration is imparted to such structures as red blood cells. We have found the technique useful when examining renal tissue.

Staining solutions

Azocarmine
    Add 0.1 g azocarmine GX or 1 g azocarmine B to 100 ml distilled water and bring to the boil. Cool and add 1 ml acetic acid. Filter.
Orange G-aniline blue
    Dissolve 0.5 g aniline blue ws and 2 g orange G in 100 ml of 8% aqueous acetic acid solution. Dissolve with the aid of gentle heat (56°C oven). Cool and filter. Dilute 1:3 with distilled water prior to use.

Technique

1. Sections to water.
2. Stain with the azocarmine solution for 45–60 min at 56°C in a Coplin jar.
3. Cool to room temperature for approximately 10 min before removing the slide and washing in water.
4. Differentiate in 0.1% aniline in 95% alcohol so that the muscle is red and the collagen a paler red colour (usually 10–30 s).
5. Rinse in 2% acetic acid to stop differentiation. Wash.
6. Complete differentiation in 5% phosphotungstic acid in 25% methanol (30–60 min).
7. Wash in water, and counterstain in the orange G-aniline blue solution for 15 min.
8. Wash, dehydrate and differentiate in alcohol; clear and mount as desired.

Results

Nuclei, red blood cells, fibrin	red
Muscle	orange-red
Collagen	blue

MASSON'S TECHNIQUE (Masson 1929)

Notes

The success of this method depends on the degree of differentiation of the ponceau-acid fuchsin by phosphomolybdic acid. It is important to prolong differentiation until the connective tissue is almost unstained. This may be expedited at 56°C. (Phosphotungstic acid may be used.) Aniline blue or light green can be used for the fibre stain but we prefer the latter for photomicrographs.

Solutions

Ponceau-acid fuchsin solution (see p. 41)
1% aqueous phosphomolybdic acid
Aniline blue solution (see p. 41) or 2% light green in 2% acetic acid; dilute 1:10 with distilled water prior to use.

Technique

1. Sections to water.
2. Stain nuclei with an iron haematoxylin solution. Differentiate and blue. Wash in water.
3. Treat with the ponceau-acid fuchsin solution for 2–3 min.
4. Wash in water and differentiate in the phosphomolybdic acid solution (usually for between 5 and 15 min at room temperature).
5. Wash well in water.
6. Counterstain either with aniline blue for 5 min, or the light green solution for 1 min.
7. Wash, dehydrate, clear and mount as desired.

Results

Nuclei	blue-black
Muscle, red blood cells, fibrin	red
Connective tissue	blue or green according to the counterstain used

GOMORI RAPID ONE STEP TRICHROME (Gomori 1950a)

Notes

This method is simple and the inexperienced worker can obtain good results. A variant of the method is used to demonstrate nemaline rods in nemaline rod myopathy, the traditional formula being used but at a slightly higher pH and with frozen not paraffin sections (Francis 1982).

Solutions

Staining solution:

Chromotrope 2 R	0.6 g
Fast green FCF	0.3 g
Phosphotungstic acid	0.6 g
Glacial acetic acid	1 ml
Distilled water	100 ml

The solution keeps well. For demonstrating nemaline rods adjust the pH of the solution to 3.4 using 1 M sodium hydroxide (Dubowitz 1985).

0.2% glacial acetic acid

Technique

1. Sections to water.
2. Stain nuclei with an alum haematoxylin.
3. Differentiate in acid-alcohol and blue as in the standard technique.
4. Wash well in tap water, then in distilled water.
5. Stain in the Gomori solution 5–20 min.
6. Rinse well in the acetic acid solution.
7. Blot dry, dehydrate, clear and mount as desired.

Results

Nuclei	grey-blue
Collagen	green
Muscle, cytoplasm, red blood cells, fibrin	red

Using the higher pH solution:

Nemaline rods	red
Background	blue-green

MALLORY'S PHOSPHOTUNGSTIC ACID-HAEMATOXYLIN

Notes

This is an example of a 'standard' method, which is anything but standard in its application, as no two laboratories seem to use it in an identical manner. It is a popular method, demonstrating a wide range of fibrillar elements clearly and in a progressive manner. The results are less subjective than in the more usual regressive type of technique. The mechanism by which two-colour staining is achieved from a mixture of haematein and phosphotungstic acid is obscure. Terner et al (1964) concluded that the blue colour produced was a metachromatic-type staining effect. The technique can be capricious, probably as a result of variation in batches of dye. Fixation in a mercuric chloride-containing solution gives the brightest staining, although satisfactory results may be obtained with most routine fixatives, providing fixation times are not prolonged. An effective means of improving staining is by immersing sections in Helly's fluid for several hours prior to staining.

The important modifications of the PTAH technique are those of Mallory (1900), Lieb (1948) and Bohacek (1966). We prefer the method of Shum & Hon (1969) who say that the proportion of phosphotungstic acid to haematein is important (0.9%: 0.08%), that pre-mordanting is unnecessary, and that long room-temperature staining gives more precise results than shorter staining at 56°C. We concur with the last statement. The solution may be used repeatedly but requires filtering after use. The potassium permanganate (oxidation) step promotes staining and is employed as a pre-staining stage in many different tinctorial methods.

Staining solution

Take 0.08 g haematein and grind to a chocolate-brown paste with 1 ml distilled water (an unsatisfactory batch of haematein will appear lighter, more straw-coloured and should be discarded). Dissolve 0.9 g phosphotungstic acid in 99 ml distilled water and mix with the ground haematein solution. Bring to the boil, cool and filter.

Technique

1. Sections to water.
2. Treat with 0.25% aqueous potassium permanganate solution for 5 min.
3. Wash, then bleach with 5% aqueous oxalic acid solution.
4. Wash well, then stain in the PTAH solution for 12–24 h at room temperature.
5. Wash in distilled water. Dehydrate, clear and mount in a DPX-type mountant.

Results

The following have variously been reported as staining blue; keratin, red blood cells, nuclei, some fibrin, intercellular bridges of squamous cells, muscle, bile canaliculi, cilia, Paneth cells, neuroglia fibres, coarse elastin, α pancreatic cells, myelin, oncocytes and alcoholic hyaline.

    Collagen, reticulin, mucins   brick red

LISSAMINE FAST RED TECHNIQUE (Lendrum, 1947)

Notes

Not strictly a trichrome, this method gives clear-cut differentiation of smooth muscle from collagen. Its main attribute is the striking demonstration of myofibrils; cross-striations of voluntary muscle are not well-shown. It is used to advantage in the demonstration of smooth muscle tumours if they are reasonably well differentiated. Differentiation of the lissamine fast red by phosphomolybdic acid should be stopped when there is still a little excess dye in the collagen. The final tartrazine counterstain tends to remove some of the red dye. Should differentiation be too rapid at 56°C, try the procedure at room temperature. The lissamine fast red solution does not keep and should be discarded after 3 weeks. As in all trichrome-type techniques mercuric chloride, potassium dichromate fixation gives improved results. This is achieved by secondary fixation in Helly's solution of either tissue or sections of formalin-fixed material.

Solutions

1% lissamine fast red in 1% acetic acid
1.5% tartrazine in 1.5% acetic acid
1% aqueous phosphomolybdic acid

Technique

1. Sections to water.
2. Stain nuclei with an iron haematoxylin solution. Differentiate well and blue.

3. Stain with the lissamine fast red solution for 5 min.
4. Wash briefly in water then differentiate in the phosphomolybdic acid solution at 56°C until the connective tissue is destained (5 min will usually suffice).
5. Wash briefly in water.
6. Counterstain with the tartrazine solution for 5 min.
7. Wash briefly in 90% alcohol.
8. Dehydrate, clear and mount as desired.

Results

Nuclei	blue-black
Smooth muscle and red blood cells	deep red
Connective tissue, etc.	yellow

ACID FUCHSIN TECHNIQUE FOR EARLY MYOCARDIAL INFARCTION
(Poley et al 1964)

Notes

This method for detecting ischaemic and degenerating myocardium before changes are evident in conventional H&E sections is based on the affinity of degenerating myocardium for acid fuchsin, compared with normal myocardium that is counter-stained a contrasting blue-green. The practical utilization of the idea was introduced by Selye (1958) and modified by Poley et al (1964). The rationale is not fully under-stood, but it has been suggested that a pH change or electrolyte shift is responsible for the increased affinity of acid stains for damaged myocardium (Lie 1968). Lie examined the usefulness of acid fuchsin for detecting early myocardial infarction, and found it a sensitive technique. It is important to take through a set of control slides: a normal myocardium, one showing minimal infarction and one showing well-marked infarction changes. The staining times are variable and are altered according to the results with the control material. In our limited experience with this technique, we have found that practice is necessary to achieve consistent results, for like most trichrome-type techniques, the results are subjective. According to Berry (1967) mechanical mixing during acid fuchsin staining increases reproducibility.

An alternative method is that of Carle (1981), utilizing the enhanced acidophilia of necrotic myocardium when examining conventional H&E preparations under a fluorescence microscope. Necrotic muscle fibres give a bright yellow secondary fluorescence compared to the dull green of normal myocardium.

Solutions

Stain A:
  Stock solution:

Cresyl fast violet	0.2 g
Distilled water	100 ml

Allow to stand 1 h and filter.

  Working solution (prepare on day of use):

Stock solution	10 ml

| Distilled water | 40 ml |
| 1% aqueous oxalic acid | 0.2 ml |

Stain B:

0.01% aqueous acid fuchsin	20 ml
0.01% aqueous orange G	15 ml
0.01% methyl green	0.1 ml
1% aqueous oxalic acid	0.2 ml

1% aqueous phosphotungstic acid
0.05% glacial acetic acid

Technique

1. Sections to water.
2. Place in stain A for 15 min.
3. Wash in running water for 10 min.
4. Mordant in the phosphotungstic acid for 15 min.
5. Wash in running water for 3 min.
6. Place in stain B for 30 min at 60°C (if possible using a mechanical stirrer).
7. Rinse in the weak acetic acid.
8. Dehydrate, clear and mount as desired.

Results

Myocardial fibres are stained progressively red in proportion to the degree of infarction.

    Normal myocardium   blue-green

COLLAGENASE DIGESTION

Notes

Collagenase, derived from the Clostridia group of organisms, was recommended by Green (1960) as an enzyme that could be used for the digestion of collagen and reticulin fibres in tissue sections. This, used with the appropriate connective tissue method, enables presumptive identification of these fibres. Another variant (Vice 1968) gives better results, we think, and is described below. The rationale is similar in that collagen and reticulin are depolymerized into their constituent peptides. Fixation should be in Carnoy's fluid or alcohol and, after thorough washing in water, frozen sections should be prepared. We have found it necessary on occasion to extend digestion times but, even so, complete digestion of collagen and reticulin fibres may not be achieved.

Solution

1 mg high-purity collagenase, 800–1600 units/mg, dissolved in 1 ml pH 7.0 buffer (see Buffer Tables, Appendix 3).

Technique

1. Take two test and two positive control sections to distilled water.
2. Treat one test and one control section with collagenase for at least 5 h, and if necessary up to 24 h at 37°C. Duplicate sections are treated with buffer only for a similar period.
3. Wash all sections well in running tap water. Carry out a suitable demonstration technique, e.g. trichrome or van Gieson for collagen, and a silver method for reticulin.

Results

Collagen and reticulin fibres will fail to stain and will be absent or substantially reduced when the digested sections are compared with the undigested control sections. Young collagen is reported to be more susceptible to digestion than mature fibres (Montford & Perez-Tanyayo 1975). When silver techniques for reticulin are carried out following collagenase digestion, an increase in background argyrophilia will be seen and consequently should not be regarded as the result of faulty technique.

RETICULIN

Reticulin fibres (collagen type III) are fine branching fibres that are difficult to see in H&E preparations and need other techniques to be properly visualized. The fibres are normally seen to best advantage in lymphoid tissue and liver. They result from the interaction of at least three proteins: fibronectin, collagen type III and a non-collagenous reticulin component (Scott et al 1984). A trichrome-type technique may be used to demonstrate these fibres, which appear blue or green. They also stain positively with the PAS technique.

The most successful way to identify reticulin fibres is to use their argyrophilia. There are many silver techniques in use, the more important of which will be described below. We prefer the Gordon and Sweets' technique but all the methods described are capable of good results when the necessary expertise is available. The various silver methods for reticulin are modifications of the Bielschowsky techniques for nerve fibres in which, by means of various metallic sensitizers, silver is selectively deposited on the fibres. This is subsequently converted to reduced (black) silver by suitable reducing agents, allowing visualization of the fibres. Most silver techniques for reticulin are preceded by a permanganate oxidation step; this prevents the normal argyrophilia of structures like nerve fibres. Toning in gold chloride is optional and if used will give a clearer background and render collagen a purple-grey colour instead of a yellow-brown. We prefer not to tone, retaining the colour distinction between collagen and reticulin fibres (brown and black respectively). The final step in silver methods is to remove any remaining un-reduced silver by treating with sodium thiosulphate ('hypo'). This prevents subsequent background precipitation due to light reduction, but does not appear to be strictly necessary in reticulin methods. Formalin is probably the best fixative, but most are satisfactory except for Helly's. Decalcified material often gives poor results with reticulin methods but this can be circumvented if EDTA at 48°C is used. Needle biopsies of bone may exhibit argyrophilia of the red blood cells in the marrow.

An obliteration of the normal reticulin framework of a lymph node may be an important piece of evidence in the diagnosis of malignant lymphoma. Similarly, a reticulin stain is valuable in recognizing when liver architecture is sufficiently disturbed to warrant a diagnosis of cirrhosis.

GORDON AND SWEETS' TECHNIQUE (Gordon & Sweets 1936)

Notes

This is a popular and reliable method. The ammoniacal silver solution may be kept without deterioration for many weeks, even when stored at room temperature in a clear container. The formalin is best diluted with tap water, maintaining a better and more even reduction of the silver solution. This is partly a result of the dissolved chlorides, which give a more intense reduction, and partly the higher pH of tap water.

Solutions

5% aqueous oxalic acid
2% aqueous ferric ammonium sulphate (iron alum)
Acidified potassium permanganate solution:

0.25% aqueous potassium permanganate	47.5 ml
3% aqueous sulphuric acid	2.5 ml

These may conveniently be kept as stock solutions; the composite solution will keep for several weeks.
Ammoniacal silver solution:

10% aqueous silver nitrate	5 ml

Add concentrated ammonia drop by drop with frequent mixing until the formed precipitate just re-dissolves. Add 5 ml of 3.1% aqueous sodium hydroxide and mix. A precipitate will form that gradually dissolves upon the addition of ammonia, drop by drop as before. Stop when there are only a few precipitate granules remaining. Make up the final volume to 50 ml with distilled water.
5% aqueous sodium thiosulphate (hypo)

Technique

1. Sections to water.
2. Treat with acidified potassium permanganate solution for 5 min.
3. Wash off in water and bleach with oxalic acid solution for approximately 1 min. Wash well in water.
4. Rinse in distilled water then treat with the iron alum solution for 5 min.
5. Wash well in several changes of distilled water.
6. Treat with ammoniacal silver solution for 4–5 s with agitation of the slide.
7. Wash well in several changes of distilled water.

8. Reduce in 10% formalin in tap water for $\frac{1}{2}$–1 min with agitation of the slide.
9. Wash and tone if desired in 0.1% aqueous yellow gold chloride for 2 min.
10. Wash in water, treat with 5% hypo for 5 min.
11. Wash in water, counterstain if desired in 1% aqueous neutral red for 5 min.
12. Dehydrate, clear and mount as desired.

Results

Reticulin	black (some pigments such as lipofuscins and melanin are also weakly impregnated)
Collagen	yellow-brown if untoned
Background	clear if not counterstained, red if counter stained

WILDER'S TECHNIQUE (Wilder 1935)

Notes

This rapid method tends to give background silver deposition.

Solutions

0.25% aqueous potassium permanganate
5% aqueous oxalic acid
1% aqueous uranyl nitrate
Ammoniacal silver solution (as for Gordon & Sweets' method)
Reducer:

1.5% aqueous uranyl nitrate	1.5 ml
Formalin	0.5 ml
Distilled water	50 ml

5% aqueous sodium thiosulphate (hypo)

Technique

1. Sections to water.
2. Treat with the potassium permanganate solution for 1 min.
3. Wash in water and bleach with the oxalic acid solution for approximately 1 min.
4. Wash well in water, then in distilled water.
5. Treat with the 1% uranyl nitrate solution for 3–5 s.
6. Wash well in distilled water.
7. Treat with the ammoniacal silver solution for 1 min.
8. Dip quickly into 95% alcohol.
9. Reduce for 1 min. Wash in water and tone if desired in 0.2% aqueous gold chloride.
10. Wash in water and treat with 5% hypo for 5 min.
11. Wash and counterstain in 1% aqueous neutral red if desired.
12. Wash, dehydrate, clear and mount as desired.

Results

Reticulin (and some pigments)	black
Collagen	yellow-brown if untoned
Background	light brown if not counterstained, red if counterstained

LAIDLAW'S TECHNIQUE (Laidlaw 1929)

Notes

This is a more time-consuming method but gives good results.

Solutions

1% iodine in 95% alcohol
0.25% aqueous potassium permanganate
5% aqueous oxalic acid
Ammoniacal lithium-silver solution

To 230 ml saturated aqueous lithium carbonate add 20 ml 60% aqueous silver nitrate, in a 250 ml measuring cylinder. Mix and allow the formed precipitate to settle to a 70 ml volume. Decant the supernatant and replace with distilled water. Mix well, repeat the washing of the precipitate twice more. Finally, decant the supernatant for a third time, add concentrated ammonia, with mixing, until the precipitate is almost dissolved. Make up the final volume to 120 ml with distilled water and filter.

5% aqueous sodium thiosulphate (hypo)

Technique

1. Sections to water.
2. Treat with the alcoholic-iodine solution for 5 min.
3. Wash in water and treat with 5% hypo to bleach the iodine colouration.
4. Wash in water then treat with the potassium permanganate solution for 4 min.
5. Wash in water, bleach with the oxalic acid solution for approximately 1 min.
6. Wash well in water, then in several changes of distilled water.
7. Treat with the ammoniacal lithium-silver solution for 5 min at 56°C (pre-heated).
8. Rinse well in distilled water.
9. Reduce in 1% formalin in a Coplin jar until satisfactory reduction is obtained; this may take from 3–60 min.
10. Wash in water, tone if desired, treat with 5% hypo. Counterstain in 1% aqueous neutral red.
11. Dehydrate, clear and mount as desired.

Results

Reticulin (and some pigments)	black
Collagen	yellow-brown if untoned

Background   light brown if not counterstained, red if
                                              counterstained

ROBB-SMITH'S TECHNIQUE (Robb-Smith 1937)

Notes

This is a laborious flotation method that gives a crisp reticulin picture. A convenient
method is to float the paraffin sections onto the reagent in a glass Petri dish. After
the treatment time, take off the solution using a suction pump. Pour in the new
solution with care; with practice it is fairly easy to take off the solution in the dish
without losing or damaging the section.

Solutions

10% aqueous ammonia (conc. ammonia diluted 1:10)
0.25% aqueous potassium permanganate
5% aqueous oxalic acid
1.5% aqueous silver nitrate
Ammoniacal silver

Add 6 drops of 10% aqueous sodium hydroxide to 8 ml 10% aqueous
silver nitrate. Mix, and add conc. ammonia with mixing until the resulting
precipitate is almost re-dissolved. Make up to 28 ml volume with distilled water.

30% formalin
5% aqueous sodium thiosulphate (hypo)

Technique

1. Cut loose paraffin sections and float them onto distilled water at room
   temperature.
2. Transfer to the ammonia solution for 5 min.
3. Wash in three changes of distilled water.
4. Treat with the potassium permanganate solution for 10 min.
5. Wash with one change of distilled water, then bleach in the oxalic acid
   solution for 1–2 min.
6. Give four changes of distilled water then treat with aqueous silver nitrate
   solution for 1 h.
7. Give three changes of distilled water.
8. Treat with the ammoniacal silver solution for 15 min.
9. Wash with three changes of distilled water.
10. Reduce in 30% formalin for 3 min.
11. Wash in water, tone if desired in 0.2% aqueous gold chloride and fix in
    5% hypo. Wash in water.
12. Float onto warm water to flatten the section, pick up on a clean slide and
    dry in a 56°C oven for 30 min.
13. De-wax in xylene, rinse in clean xylene and mount as desired.

Results

Reticulin (and some pigments)   black

Collagen	yellow-brown if untoned
Background	pale yellow

GOMORI'S TECHNIQUE (Gomori 1937)

Notes

This is comparable with Gordon and Sweets' method in technique and consistency of result. Gomori indicated a second reducing step following toning.

Solutions

1% aqueous potassium permanganate
3% aqueous potassium metabisulphite
2% aqueous ferric ammonium sulphate (iron alum)
Ammoniacal silver

To 20 ml of 10% aqueous silver nitrate add 4 ml of 10% aqueous potassium hydroxide. Add conc. ammonia with repeated mixing until the formed precipitate is just dissolved. Then add 10% aqueous silver nitrate slowly with frequent mixing, until only a faint opalescence remains. Dilute with an equal volume of distilled water.

5% aqueous sodium thiosulphate (hypo)

Technique

1. Sections to water.
2. Treat with the potassium permanganate solution for 1–2 min.
3. Wash in water, bleach with the potassium metabisulphite solution. Wash well in water.
4. Treat with the iron alum solution for 1 min. Wash well in tap and then distilled water.
5. Treat with ammoniacal silver solution for 1 min.
6. Wash briefly in distilled water and reduce in 10% formalin for 3 min.
7. Wash, then tone in 0.2% gold chloride for up to 10 min.
8. Rinse in distilled water, then treat with the potassium metabisulphite solution for 1 min.
9. Rinse with distilled water and fix with 5% hypo for 1–2 min.
10. Wash, dehydrate, clear and mount as desired.

Results

Reticulin (and some pigments)	black
Nuclei	grey
Collagen	grey-purple

JAMES' TECHNIQUE (James 1967)

Notes

Good results may be obtained with this technique that has the added advantage of a standard treatment time for each step.

Solutions

Acidified potassium permanganate:

> 0.3% aqueous potassium permanganate
> 3% sulphuric acid

Mix equal parts immediately prior to use.

5% aqueous oxalic acid
5% aqueous silver nitrate
Ammoniacal silver solution

> To 20 ml of 10% aqueous silver nitrate add concentrated ammonia drop by drop with frequent mixing until the formed precipitate just re-dissolves. Add one drop of 10% aqueous silver nitrate and 20 ml distilled water. Filter and store in the dark.

5% formalin
5% aqueous sodium thiosulphate (hypo)

Technique

1. Sections to water.
2. Treat with the acidified permanganate for 5 min.
3. Rinse three times in distilled water.
4. Treat with the oxalic acid for 5 min.
5. Rinse three times in distilled water.
6. Treat with the 5% silver nitrate for 5 min.
7. Rinse three times in distilled water.
8. Treat with the ammoniacal silver for 5 min.
9. Rinse three times in distilled water.
10. Reduce in formalin for 5 min.
11. Rinse three times in distilled water.
12. Fix in hypo for 5 min.
13. Wash well in water.
14. Dehydrate, clear and mount as desired.

Results

Reticulin fibres	black
Collagen	yellow to brown

ELASTIC FIBRES

Elastic fibres are branching fibres of varying size and diameter that consist of the protein elastin and glycoprotein microfibrils. They are easily seen in tissue sites such as dermis of skin, lung, heart and blood vessel walls. Elastic fibres may be increased because of a stromal reaction to the presence of tumour cells, as in breast cancer, or secretion by tumour cells, as in the rare elastoma dorsi. More usually, however, specific staining is required to identify changes in the elastic laminae of blood vessel walls that may be increased due to hypertension or lost because of a degenerative process. The finer elastic fibres are not easily delineated in an H&E preparation unless special stains are used. The fibres are monofringent and weakly PAS-positive, they exhibit a primary fluorescence and stain with Congo red and related dyes. Prior methylation will block the reactivity of elastin (Fullmer 1958). Fixation is not critical although Heidenhain's 'Susa' appears inferior. Celloidinization of sections prior to staining, particularly of skin and blood vessels, is desirable as they may detach from the slide. This slide detachment is more likely to occur if the method (such as the Weigert group) incorporates a preliminary treatment with a potassium permanganate-oxalic acid sequence.

WIEGERT-TYPE TECHNIQUES

Notes

There are several variations of the Weigert technique, resulting in a choice of final colour product. The rationale of these methods is obscure. Baker (1966) thought resorcinol fuchsin stained elastin by a hydrogen bonding mechanism; the same mechanism probably underlies the staining of elastin by Congo red. Most of the Weigert-type methods show a remarkable selectivity for elastic fibres and give, we think, the best demonstration of fine fibres. The techniques tend to be slow and the solutions are time-consuming to prepare. If the solutions fail to stain satisfactorily the likely cause is a poor batch of either the dye or ferric chloride. An avid staining solution may be used repeatedly, it is merely necessary to filter the solution after use. The main variants are Weigert's resorcinol fuchsin (1898) and Hart's modification (1908) that stain elastic fibres dark blue-black, French's modification (1929) dark blue-green and Sheridan's modification (1929), green.

These solutions stain well at room temperature and may be used repeatedly. Some variation in staining avidity will be found with different dye batches so a variation in staining times will occur. Staining at room temperature for longer periods gives better results than a shorter time at 56°C. Pre-treatment with an acidified permanganate-oxalic acid solution sequence gives a clearer background.

Solutions

Weigert's resorcinol fuchsin solution

Basic fuchsin	2 g
Resorcin	4 g
Distilled water	200 ml
30% aqueous anhydrous ferric chloride	25 ml
95% alcohol	200 ml
Conc. hydrochloric acid	4 ml

Dissolve the basic fuchsin and resorcin in the distilled water, bringing to the boil in an evaporating dish. While boiling, slowly add the aqueous anhydrous ferric chloride solution, stirring continuously. Continue for approximately 5 min. Cool and filter into a conical flask taking care that all the precipitate is collected. Discard the filtrate, dry the flask, and add the dried filter paper containing the precipitate to the flask. Add the alcohol and heat gently on a hot plate until the precipitate is dissolved. Remove the filter paper, add the conc. hydrochloric acid, cool and filter. Make up the final volume to 200 ml by pouring fresh 95% alcohol through the used filter paper. The purified basic fuchsin commonly used for Schiff's reagent gives inferior results.

Hart's modification

Weigert's solution diluted with 1% acid-alcohol. The proportions vary according to the avidity of the particular batch of stain prepared and should be calculated using a trial run. The usual proportions are Weigert's solution 5–20 ml, acid-alcohol 30–40 ml.

French's modification

Weigert's solution except for basic fuchsin 2 g; use 1 g each of basic fuchsin and crystal violet.

Sheridan's modification

Weigert's solution except for basic fuchsin; use 2 g each of crystal violet and dextrin.

Technique

1. Sections to water.
2. Treat with acidified potassium permanganate solution (see p. 149) for 5 min. Wash in water and bleach with 5% oxalic acid for approximately 1 min.
3. Having washed well in water, rinse in alcohol.
4. Stain in the elastin solution. The time will vary according to the batch and type of solution, e.g. Weigert's elastin solution will usually stain sufficiently well in 1–3 h at room temperature. Other elastin solutions may require overnight staining at room temperature.
5. Wash in water and differentiate in acid-alcohol until the background is clear of stain. Wash well in water. Note that with Sheridan's solution the green colouration of the elastin is enhanced by increased acid-alcohol differentiation.
6. Counterstain as required, e.g. neutral red, eosin or van Gieson.
7. Dehydrate, clear and mount as desired.

Results

Elastic fibres	dark blue-black (Weigert and Hart), dark blue-green (French), green (Sheridan)
Background	according to counterstain used

MODIFIED WEIGERT ELASTIN TECHNIQUE (Miller 1971)

Notes

The following stain for elastic fibres is a fairly rapid one and is used progressively.

Solutions

0.5% aqueous potassium permanganate
1% aqueous oxalic acid
Stain solution:

Victoria blue 4 R	1 g
New fuchsin	1 g
Crystal violet	1 g

Dissolve in 200 ml of hot distilled water and add in the following order:

Resorcin	4 g
Dextrin	1 g
Freshly prepared 30% aqueous ferric chloride	50 ml

Boil for 5 min and filter while still hot. Transfer the precipitate plus filter paper to the original flask and re-dissolve in 200 ml of 95% alcohol. Boil for 15–20 min. Cool, filter, and make up to a 200 ml volume with 95% alcohol. Finally add 2 ml of conc. hydrochloric acid.

Technique

1. Take sections to water.
2. Treat with potassium permanganate for 5 min.
3. Wash in water and bleach with oxalic acid for 2–3 min.
4. Wash well in water, then in 95% alcohol.
5. Place in either (a) undiluted stain for 1–3 h or (b) diluted stain (equal parts with 95% alcohol) overnight.
6. Wash in 95% alcohol then in water.
7. Counterstain as desired, e.g. van Gieson's stain in the usual manner (see p. 36).
8. Dehydrate, clear and mount as desired.

Results

Elastic fibres	black
Background	according to counterstain used

ORCEIN TECHNIQUE (Unna 1891)

Notes

This method shares with the Weigert-type techniques a remarkable selectivity for elastic tissue. Occasionally it fails to give good results and this can often be traced to a faulty batch of dye. The fact that it stains elastin a brown colour makes it less suitable than the Weigert methods for use with a van Gieson counterstain. The precise mechanism of orcein binding by elastin is not clear, although van der Waals forces are considered to be involved. As will be discussed in the Shikata technique for viral hepatitis antigen (see p. 258), following suitable pre-oxidation of tissue, orcein has a firm affinity for sulphur-containing compounds.

Staining solution

Dissolve synthetic orcein 1 g in 100 ml of 70% alcohol with the aid of gentle heat. Cool, filter and add 1 ml of conc. hydrochloric acid.

Technique

1. Sections to 70% alcohol.
2. Stain with the orcein solution for 1–2 h at 37°C.
3. Rinse in 70% alcohol, differentiate in 1% acid-alcohol if necessary, then wash in water.
4. Counterstain as required. Suitable counterstains are haematoxylin, 0.1% aqueous azure A or 1% aqueous methylene blue for 1–2 min. Alternatively, a yellow counterstain such as tartrazine gives effective contrast.
5. Dehydrate, clear and mount as desired.

Result

Elastin	dark brown
Background	according to counterstain used

ALDEHYDE FUCHSIN TECHNIQUE (Gomori, 1950b)

Notes

This is a popular method for elastin, staining both coarse and fine fibres strongly. It is less selective than other methods, demonstrating most tissue entities a similar colour. The underlying principle is obscure, although it has been stated that the combination of aldehyde and basic fuchsin demonstrates organically bound sulphur, e.g. sulphated mucins and insulin in β cells of the pancreas. Whether elastin contains such a sulphur moiety has yet to be firmly established.

No pre-oxidation is necessary to stain elastin or sulphated mucins. The staining is speeded up by pre-oxidation that also increases the number of tissue entities demonstrated, such as β cells of the pancreas. If periodic or peracetic acid is used as the oxidant, glycogen and neutral mucin are stained by Schiff's base formation. The solution can be capricious and there are various factors to be observed in its preparation. The basic fuchsin should have fine granule size (as for PAS); if in doubt use pararosanilin. Paraldehyde is prone to decompostion and only freshly opened samples should be used (Moment 1969). Following preparation the solution is allowed to 'blue' for at least 2 days at room temperature, preferably longer. This blueing has been attributed to the formation of acetaldehyde from acidic paraldehyde, which condenses with the amino groups of basic fuchsin moving the absorption spectrum to the longer wavelengths (Summer 1965). Older aldehyde fuchsin solutions will need filtering prior to use and staining times should be extended by 100%.

Various counterstains have been proposed for use with aldehyde fuchsin. Providing that a suitably contrasting one is used the final choice is not important. Van Gieson's solution is not suitable owing to the close colour similarity of the stained collagen fibres and elastin.

Solutions

Acidified potassium permanganate solution (see p. 49)

5% aqueous oxalic acid
Aldehyde fuchsin

Dissolve basic fuchsin 1 g in 100 ml of 60% alcohol. Add conc. hydrochloric acid 1 ml, and paraldehyde 2 ml. Allow to blue at room temperature for at least 2 days before using. Store at 4°C. The solution should keep for up to 1–2 months. Increased background staining is evidence of deterioration of the aldehyde fuchsin solution.

Technique

1. Sections to water.
2. Treat with the acid potassium permanganate solution for 1 min. Wash, bleach with the oxalic acid solution then wash well in water.
3. Rinse in 70% alcohol.
4. Stain with the aldehyde fuchsin solution for 4 min.
5. Rinse well in 70% alcohol, then in water.
6. Counterstain in either 0.1% aqueous methylene blue, 0.2% light green in 0.2% acetic acid or saturated tartrazine in Cellosolve (rinse subsequently in Cellosolve, not water) for 1 min.
7. Dehydrate, clear and mount in a DPX type mountant.

Results

Elastin, sulphated mucins (includes mast cells), β cells of pancreas and basophil cells of pituitary, some lipofuscins, gastric chief cells, hypothalamic neurosecretory cells, hepatitis B surface antigen	purple
Background	according to counterstain used

VERHOEFF'S TECHNIQUE (Verhoeff 1908)

Notes

This is a rapid method for staining elastic fibres a strong black colour. A disadvantage is that some expertise is necessary to stain the finer elastic fibres and obtain a well-differentiated background. The elastin staining is extracted by the van Gieson counterstain, therefore to obtain good results slightly underdifferentiate the Verhoeff stain in the ferric chloride solution. The principle of the technique is rather obscure. Both iodine and ferric chloride, with which the haematoxylin is combined, are oxidizing agents and it is this property that probably accounts for the production of a black dye with cationic properties (nuclei are also stained), rather than a simple dye–mordant–tissue mechanism.

Solutions

Lugol's iodine

2 g potassium iodide are dissolved in a few ml of distilled water; dissolve in this 1 g of iodine and finally make up to 100 ml volume with distilled water.

Verhoeff's stain:

5% alcoholic haematoxylin (freshly prepared solutions give stronger staining results)	20 ml
10% aqueous ferric chloride	8 ml
Lugol's iodine	8 ml

2% aqueous ferric chloride

Technique

1. Sections to alcohol.
2. Stain with Verhoeff's solution for 15 min (make up prior to use).
3. Wash in water and differentiate in 2% ferric chloride solution until the nuclei and elastic fibres are black and the background is still weakly stained.
4. Wash in water then in alcohol for approximately 5 min to remove iodine colouration of the background.
5. Wash in water and counterstain as desired with solutions such as van Gieson or neutral red for standard times.
6. Dehydrate, clear and mount as desired.

Results

Nuclei and elastic fibres	black
Background	according to counterstain used

ELASTASE DIGESTION (Fullmer 1958)

Notes

It may be desirable on occasion to confirm that the material reacting with elastin methods is elastin, and the use of elastase will be of assistance. Elastase is derived commercially from pig pancreas and is an expensive enzyme. We have found that the following technique works well although the time of digestion may need to be increased up to 18 h with certain material. Unlike collagenase, formalin fixation does not seem to inhibit the enzyme action in which elastin fibres are made soluble by fission of peptide linkages.

Solution

Dissolve 15 mg elastase (15–20 units/mg elastase) in 100 ml pH 8.8 buffer (see Buffer Tables).

Technique

1. Take two test sections plus suitable positive control sections to distilled water.
2. Treat one of the test and one of the positive control sections with the pre-heated enzyme for 6 h at 37°C. Duplicate sections are treated with pH 8.8 buffer only for the same time and temperature.
3. Wash all sections in water for several minutes.
4. Finally stain all sections with one of the preceding methods for elastic fibres.

5. Dehydrate, clear and mount as desired (if the aldehyde fuchsin technique is used, mount in one of the DPX-type mountants).

Results

Sections treated with the enzyme should show loss of elastic fibre staining when compared with the section treated with buffer only.

OXYTALAN FIBRES

First recognized by Fullmer & Lillie (1958), oxytalan fibres are composed of the microfibrillar component of elastic fibres with a morphology and (modified) histochemistry similar to that of elastic fibres. They are found in close association with tendons and ligaments and are particularly well seen in periodontal ligaments, where they insert into the cementum layers of teeth. They can be seen in the blood vessels of pregnant uteri (Manning 1974), and in the pathological cornea.

Table 3.1 Staining reactions of oxytalan and elastic fibres

Peracetic oxidized	Oxytalan fibres	Elastic fibres
Orcein	Brown (some)	Brown
Aldehyde fuchsin	Purple	Purple
Resorcin fuchsin	Purple-black (some)	Purple-black
Verhoeff's stain	Negative	Black
PAS	Negative	Magenta (weak)
Elastase digestion	Digested	Digested

OXYTALAN FIBRE DEMONSTRATION (from Alexander et al 1981)

Notes

An important feature of oxytalan histochemistry is that fibres react with some, but not all, elastic fibre techniques and then only after pre-oxidation techniques. Similarly, elastase will not digest oxytalan fibres unless this pre-oxidation step is applied. The most satisfactory dye for demonstration purposes is aldehyde fuchsin using peracetic acid or peroxymonosulphate as a pre-oxidant (Alexander et al 1981). Potassium permanganate can also be used but is less effective. The need for pre-oxidation in oxytalan fibre demonstration presumably denotes the presence of masking ethylene groups. When oxidized they either make available reactive sulphate radicals capable of ionic linkage or hydrogen bonding with appropriate dyes. It has also been suggested that there is a mucopolysaccharide present in the fibres that requires oxidation to open reactive bonds (Fullmer 1964). Table 3.1 was derived from Fullmer (1964), and Fullmer & Lillie (1958). It illustrates the reactions to various stains by oxytalan and elastic fibres using peracetic pre-oxidation.

Solutions

Peracetic acid:

    Glacial acetic acid   95.6 ml

30% (100 volumes) hydrogen peroxide	259 ml
Conc. sulphuric acid	2.2 ml

Add disodium hydrogen orthophosphate 0.04 g as a stabilizer, and allow to stand 1–3 days before use. The solution will keep for several months at 4°C.

10% aqueous potassium peroxymonosulphate*

Technique

1. Take duplicate paraffin sections of test material to distilled water.
2. Treat one section only with either peracetic acid for 30 min or potassium peroxymonosulphate for 60 min.
3. Wash well in water.
4. Carry out the aldehyde fuchsin stain for elastic fibres (see p. 58) on both sections according to the standard technique.
5. Dehydrate, clear and mount as desired.

Results

An increase in fibre staining in oxidized section, when compared to the un-oxidized section, will denote the presence of oxytalan fibres.

BASEMENT MEMBRANES (BASAL LAMINA)

Basement membranes (basal lamina) consist of muco-proteins associated with specialized reticulin fibres (collagen type IV). They normally underlie epithelial and blood capillary endothelial surfaces and may be particularly pronounced around hair follicles and epididymal tubules. The basal lamina must be breached, by definition, for an in-situ carcinoma to become infiltrating but this apparently simple event is confused by the fact that inflammation can also cause breaks in basement membranes and metastatic tumour may synthesize new basement membranes around groups of cells. Basement membranes can be demonstrated by trichrome methods, in which they take up the fibre stain. The periodic acid-Schiff (PAS) technique and its variant, the Allochrome method, or a modification of Gomori's hexamine-silver technique can all be used. Undoubtedly, the latter method gives the most precise demonstration of basement membranes. 3 μm paraffin sections are preferred. The PAS method used for basement membranes is essentially the same in principle as that described on page 135. It is necessary to extend the times of oxidation and Schiff reagent treatment by double and by up to half as much again respectively.

The proportion of fibres to mucoprotein varies in different tissues, with a consequent variation in staining reactions. For example, the basement membrane (basal lamina) of renal tubules is well shown by PAS (for the mucoprotein content). In the intestine, the basement membrane is poorly outlined by PAS, but well-shown by techniques for reticulin fibres. It has been shown (Laurie et al 1981) that at least two types of glycoprotein, fibronectin and laminin, may also be found in basement membranes.

---

* Obtainable as Caroat from Bayley Degusse Ltd., Stanley Green Trading Est., Cheadle Hulme, Cheadle, Cheshire.

MODIFIED HEXAMINE-SILVER TECHNIQUE (Gomori 1946, Jones 1957)

Notes

Periodate-formed aldehydes from carbohydrate-containing basement membranes will selectively reduce an alkaline hexamine-silver salt mixture. This technique is laborious but demonstrates the finer basement membranes such as those of the renal glomerulus better than other methods. Connective tissue fibres are also demonstrated to a variable degree. When demonstrating basement membranes of renal glomeruli, it is important to slightly over-impregnate with hexamine-silver. Take through a control section to test the efficacy of the solution. When dealing with renal tissue it is important to examine the glomeruli, not the tubules, to determine the end-point of the reaction. This is because the glomerular basement membrane (basal lamina) consists only of structural proteins and this is usually the primary site of interest in the study of glomerulonephritis, for instance. The tubular basement membrane also contains a reticulin element and will stain more readily.

Fixation is important; Bouin's fixative gives best results as impregnation times are shorter. Formalin is satisfactory but following long-standing fixation sections require prolonged impregnation in hexamine-silver. Formal sublimate fixation of tissue will result in relatively poor results, and it is better to avoid mercuric chloride-containing fixatives when using this technique.

Solutions

1% aqueous periodic acid.
Stock hexamine-silver solution
　　Mix 5 ml of 5% aqueous silver nitrate and 100 ml of 3% aqueous hexamine (synonyms: methanamine or hexamethylenetetramine). A white precipitate forms that dissolves on shaking. The solution will keep for a limited time (1–2 months) if stored in a dark container at 4°C.
Working solution
　　Dilute 2 ml of a 5% aqueous sodium borate solution with 25 ml of distilled water. Mix and add 25 ml of the stock hexamine-silver solution.
0.1% aqueous gold chloride
5% aqueous sodium thiosulphate (hypo)
0.2% light green in 0.2% acetic acid

Technique

1. Take sections to distilled water.
2. Treat with the periodic acid solution for 10 min.
3. Wash well in several changes of distilled water.
4. Place in pre-heated hexamine-silver solution in 56°C water bath. Examine after 20 min and subsequently at frequent intervals until the basement membranes are blackened; this will take from 25–40 min.
5. Wash well in several changes of distilled water.
6. Tone in 0.1% aqueous yellow gold chloride for 2–5 min.
7. Wash in water and treat with 5% hypo for 5 min.

8. Wash in water, counterstain in 0.2% light green in 0.2% acetic acid for 0.5–1 min.
9. Wash, dehydrate, clear and mount as desired.

Results

Basement membranes (basal lamina)	black
Background	green

An alternative is to counterstain with haematoxylin and eosin which provides a particularly useful stain for glomerular pathology.

ALLOCHROME TECHNIQUE (Lillie 1951)

Notes

This method is the PAS technique followed by a picro-methyl blue counterstain to give combined staining of basement membranes and connective tissue fibres in contrasting colours. We see little value in this method but it seems to enjoy some popularity.

Solutions

PAS solutions (see p. 135)
0.04% methyl blue in saturated aqueous picric acid

Technique

1. Sections to distilled water and treat with periodic acid and Schiff's reagent as for the PAS technique (see p. 135).
2. Stain the nuclei with an iron haematoxylin solution. Differentiate and blue.
3. Counterstain with the picro-methyl blue solution for 6 min.
4. Differentiate briefly in 95% alcohol. Dehydrate, clear and mount as desired.

Results

Nuclei	brown-black
Collagen and reticulin	blue
Cytoplasm and muscle	greenish-yellow
Basement membranes (basal lamina) and other periodate-reactive material	magenta

Table 3.2   Connective tissue staining results

Technique	Collagen	Reticulin	Elastin	Oxytalan	Basement Membranes	Muscle
Van Gieson	Red	—	—	—	—	Yellow
Trichromes	Blue	Blue	Red/Blue	—	Blue	Red
PTAH	Red	Red	Blue	—	—	Blue
Silver (untoned)	Brown	Black	—	—	—	—
Weigert's elastin	—	—	Blue-black	—	—	—

Table 3.2   *(continued)*

Technique	Collagen	Reticulin	Elastin	Oxytalan	Basement Membranes	Muscle
Weigert's with pre-oxidation	—	—	Blue-black	Blue-black	—	—
Sheridan's elastin	—	—	Green	—	—	—
Sheridan's with pre-oxidation	—	—	Green	Green	—	—
Orcein	—	—	Brown	—	—	—
Orcein with pre-oxidation	—	—	Brown	Brown	—	—
Aldehyde fuchsin	—	—	Purple	—	—	—
Aldehyde fuchsin with pre-oxidation	—	—	Purple	Purple	—	—
PAS	Weak	Magenta	Weak	—	Magenta	Voluntary and cardiac, magenta
Hexamine silver (Jones mod.)	—	—	—	—	Black	—

IMMUNOCYTOCHEMISTRY

In recent years there has been a greater reliance on the use of immunocytochemistry, at the expense of the tinctorial techniques, for the demonstration of muscle. For the general identification of both striated and smooth muscle fibres the antiserum to desmin is recommended, although false negativity can occur. Antisera to actin and myosin can be used in a similar manner but less reliably. Another marker, myoglobin, is only present in striated muscle (Elias 1990). Anti-vimentin (a general marker of mesenchymal tissues) will demonstrate neoplastic, as opposed to normal, muscle fibres.

With regard to the other connective tissues dealt with in this chapter, there are available a number of antisera for their demonstration. These include laminin and fibronectin for basement membranes, also elastin and some of the collagen subtypes, such as type IV. However, with the non-muscle elements it is debatable whether immunocytochemistry is worthwhile in the routine laboratory environment. Conventional techniques for collagen, reticulin and elastic fibres as well as basement membranes are still widely, and reliably, practised. There is, however, a need for a specific immunocytochemical marker for collagenous elements in soft tissue tumours to complement those currently in use for muscle.

REFERENCES

Alexander R A, Clayton D C, Howes R C, Garner A 1981 Effect of oxidation upon demonstration of corneal oxytalan fibres: a light and electron microscopical study. Medical Laboratory Sciences 38: 91–101

Baker J R 1966 Cytological technique, 5th edn. Methuen, London

Berry C L 1967 Myocardial ischaemia in infancy and childhood. Journal of Clinical Pathology 20: 38–41

Bohacek L G 1966 Acceleration of Mallory's phosphotungstic acid-haematoxylin staining for skeletal muscle fixed in formalin. Stain Technology 41: 101–103

Carle B N 1981 Autofluorescence in the identification of myocardial infarcts. Human Pathology 12: 643–646

Dubowitz V 1985 Muscle biopsy: a practical approach. Bailliere Tindall, London

Elias J M 1990 Immunohistopathology. A practical approach to diagnosis. ASCP Press, Chicago

Francis R 1982 Personal communication

French R W 1929 Elastic tissue staining. Stain Technology 4: 11

Fullmer H M 1958 Differential staining of connective tissue fibres in areas of stress. Science (New York) 127: 1240

Fullmer H M 1964 In: Provenza D V (ed) Oral histology inheritance and development. Pitman Medical, London

Fullmer H M, Lillie R D 1958 The oxytalan fibre: a previously undescribed connective tissue fibre. Journal of Histochemistry and Cytochemistry 6: 425–430

Gomori G 1937 Silver impregnation of reticulum in paraffin sections. American Journal of Pathology 13: 993

Gomori G 1946 A new histochemical test for glycogen and mucin. American Journal of Clinical Pathology 16: 177

Gomori G 1950a A rapid one-step trichrome stain. American Journal of Clinical Pathology 20: 661

Gomori G 1950b Aldehyde fuchsin a new stain for elastic tissues. American Journal of Clinical Pathology 20: 665

Gordon H, Sweets H H 1936 A simple method for the silver impregnation of reticulum. American Journal of Pathology 12: 545

Gray P, Pickle F M, Muser M D, Hayweiser J 1958 Oxazine dyes. I. Celestine blue with iron as a mordant. Stain Technology 31: 141

Green J 1960 Digestion of collagen and reticulin in paraffin sections by collagenase. Stain Technology 35: 273–276

Hart K 1908 Die Farbung der elastischen Fasern mit dem von Weigert angegebenen Farbstoff. Zentralblatt Für Allegemaine Pathologie und Pathologische Anatomie 19: 1

Heidenhain M 1915 Zeitschrift für wissenschaftliche Mikroskipie und für mikroskopische Technik 21: 1

Herovici C 1963 A polychrome stain for differentiating pre-collagen, from collagen. Stain Technology 38: 204–206

Ibeachum G I 1971 The storage of Weigert's iron haematoxylin. Medical Laboratory Technology 28: 117–120

James K R 1967 A simple silver method for the demonstration of reticulin fibres. Journal of Medical Laboratory Technology 24: 49–51

Jones D B 1957 Nephrotic glomerulonephritis. American Journal of Pathology 33: 313

Laidlaw G F 1929 Silver staining of skin and of its tumours. American Journal of Pathology 5: 239

Laurie G W, Lebold C P, Cournil I, Martin G R 1981 Immunohistochemical evidence for the intracellular formation of basement membranes collagen (type IV) in developing tissues. Journal of Histochemistry and Cytochemistry 28: 1267

Lendrum A C 1947 The phloxine-tartrazine method as a general histological stain and for the demonstration of inclusion bodies. Journal of Pathology and Bacteriology 59: 399

Lie J T 1968 Detection of early myocardial infarction by the acid fuchsin staining technic. American Journal of Clinical Pathology 50: 317–319

Lieb E 1948 Modified phosphotungstic acid-haematoxylin stain. Archives of Pathology 45: 559

Lillie R D 1951 The allochrome procedure: a differential method segregating the connective tissues, collagen, reticulin and basement membranes into two groups. American Journal of Clinical Pathology 21: 484

McFarlane D 1944 Picro-Mallory. An easily controlled regressive trichromic staining method. Stain Technology 19: 29

Mallory F B 1900 A contribution to staining methods. Journal of Experimental Medicine 5: 15

Mallory F B 1905 A contribution to the classification of tumours. Journal of Medical Research, Boston 13: 113–136

Manning P J 1974 The staining of elastic tissue and related fibres in uterine blood vessels. Medical Laboratory Technology 31: 115–125

Masson P 1929 Some histological methods. Trichrome stainings and their preliminary technique. Bulletin of the International Association of Medicine 12: 75

Miller P J 1971 An elastin stain. Medical Laboratory Technology 28: 148–149

Moment G B 1969 Deteriorated paraldehyde: an insidious cause of failure in aldehyde fuchsin staining. Stain Technology 44: 52–53

Montford P, Perez-Tanyayo R 1975 The distribution of collagenase in normal rat tissues. Journal of Histochemistry and Cytochemistry 22: 910–920

Poley R W, Fobes C D, Hall M J 1964 Fuchsinophilia in early myocardial infarction: a method for the demonstration of early myocardial infarction using acid fuchsin staining. Archives of Pathology 77: 325–329

Robb-Smith A H T 1937 Device to facilitate impregnation of reticulin fibrils in paraffin sections. Journal of Pathology and Bacteriology 45: 312–313

Scott D L, Salmon M, Walton K 1984 Reticulin and its related structural connective tissue proteins in the rheumatoid synovium. Histopathology 8: 469–479

Seki M 1932 Folia Anat Jap 10: 635

Selye H 1958 Chemical prevention of cardiac necroses. Ronald Press, New York

Sheridan W F 1929 Journal of Technical Methods Bulletin of International Association of Medical Museums 12: 123

Shum M W K, Hon J K Y 1969 A modified phosphotungstic acid-haematoxylin stain for formalin fixed tissues. Journal of Medical Laboratory Technology 26: 38–42

Slidders W 1968 A stable iron-haematoxylin solution for staining the chromatin of cell nuclei. Journal of Microscopy 90: Pt 1, 61–65

Summer B E H 1965 Experiments to determine the composition of aldehyde fuchsin solutions. Journal of the Royal Microscopical Society 84: 181–187

Terner J Y, Gurland J, Gaer S 1964 Phosphotungstic acid-haematoxylin: spectrophotometry of the lake in solution and in stained tissue. Stain Technology 39: 141–153

Unna P G 1891 Ueber 'Ichthyolfirnisse' Monatsh f. prakt. Dermat Hamb. XII: 49–56

van Gieson I 1889 Laboratory notes of technical methods for the nervous system. New York Medical Journal 50: 57

Verhoeff F H 1908 Some new staining methods of wide applicability, including a rapid differential stain for elastic tissue. Journal of American Medical Association 50: 876

Vice P 1968 Collagenase digestion for distinguishing neural from reticular fibres in silver stains. Stain Technology 43: 183–186

Weigert C 1898 Ueber eine Methode zur Farbung elastiche Fasern. Zentralblatt Für Allgemeine Pathologie und Patholgische Anatomie 9: 289

Weigert C 1904 Eine klein Verbesserung der Hamatoxylin-van Gieson Methods. Zeitschrift fur wissenschaftliche Mikroskipie und Fur mikroskipische Technik 21: 1

Wilder H C 1935 Improved technique for silver impregnation of reticulin fibres. American Journal of Pathology 11: 817–819

4. Intracellular granules

EOSINOPHIL CELLS

These cells were first described by Wharton-Jones in 1846 as 'coarse granule cells'. The term eosinophils was coined by Ehrlich in 1880. The granules are intensely acidophilic and stain well in an H & E preparation. They also stain with Congo red, the DMAB-nitrite reaction and amido black. In addition the two methods below give selective staining of the granules. Eosinophils may be present in any chronic inflammatory cell infiltrate but are particularly common in type I hypersensitivity reactions such as asthma and hay fever and may be recruited as part of the associated cellular reaction in neoplastic conditions such as Hodgkin's disease and histiocytosis X.

CARBOL CHROMOTROPE TECHNIQUE (Lendrum 1944)

Notes

This is an empirical, but remarkably selective, simple and reliable technique. The rationale is possibly that the presence of phenol lowers the pH of the solution and increases selectivity for the granules.

Staining solution

Melt 1 g phenol in a flask under hot water, add 0.5 g chromotrope 2R. Mix, dissolve the resultant sludge in 100 ml distilled water and filter. The solution keeps for up to 3 months.

Technique

1. Sections to water.
2. Stain the nuclei with one of the alum haematoxylin solutions (see p. 25). Differentiate and blue.
3. Stain with the carbol chromotrope solution for 30 min.
4. Wash, dehydrate, clear and mount as desired.

Results

Nuclei	blue
Eosinophil granules	red
Red blood cells	pale red

Paneth cell granules	rust-coloured
Enterochromaffin granules	weak brown

GIEMSA TECHNIQUE (Giemsa 1902)

Notes

This modified version of the original Giemsa technique gives good results on sections. Most acidophilic cells and eosinophils stain a similar colour. To achieve a good colour balance it is necessary to overstain initially with Giemsa, then slightly overdifferentiate in weak acetic acid until there is a general pink cast to the cells. This offsets the loss of eosinophilia and gain in basophilia which results upon alcohol dehydration. Decalcification of tissue with strong acids should be avoided as it results in a poor colour balance.

Solutions

Giemsa

This staining solution is readily available commercially but, to prepare a batch, the following formula may be used. Mix 7.36 g Giemsa dry stain in 500 ml glycerol heated to 50°C in a water bath. Leave for 30 min at 50°C with periodic mixing. Allow to cool and add 500 ml methanol (the acetone content is immaterial). Mix and filter.

Acetic acid differentiator

A convenient way of preparing the weak solution required is to take 1 ml of 1% acetic acid solution and dilute with 99 ml of distilled water.

Technique

1. Sections to distilled water.
2. Filter enough Giemsa stain into a Coplin jar filled with distilled water to render the solution a dark blue colour (0.5–1 ml). Stain with the solution for at least 20 min at 56°C until the section is an overall dark blue.
3. Rinse in distilled water and differentiate in weak acetic acid solution (approximately 1:10 000 v/v) until the section is predominantly pink in colour.
4. Rinse in distilled water, dehydrate, clear and mount as desired.

Results

Nuclei	purple
Azurophilic granules	blue
Eosinophil granules, red blood cells and other acidophil structures	pink

PANETH CELLS

It is a curious fact that while there is a legion of special stains for these cells, their demonstration is rarely called for in diagnostic histopathology. The cells were first described by Schwalbe in 1872 and later by Paneth, whose name they acquired. Paneth cells are in the bases of the crypts of Lieberkühn in the small bowel. Less often they can be seen in the appendix and proximal colon whilst in pathological conditions they can occur in the stomach (intestinal metaplasia) and large bowel (Paneth cell metaplasia in inflammatory bowel disease). The granules are similar to the zymogen granules of the pancreas in appearance, and their staining reactions are not dissimilar. The function of Paneth cells has not been resolved but it is well known that they contain zinc (Ham 1969). The granules contain lysozyme and it is postulated that these cells have an anti-bacterial role. For the best results prompt fixation is necessary to preserve the granules. Acid fixation will destroy the reactive elements, consequently neutral buffered formalin or formal calcium fixation is recommended although acidic fixatives can be used as secondary solutions if required. The cells are strongly acidophilic and can be readily seen in routine H&E sections. Two techniques are given below and their reactions to other staining methods are given in Table 4.1.

Table 4.1 Staining reactions of Paneth cells

Method	Colour
Phloxine-tartrazine	Red to orange
Fuchsin Miller	Red
DMAB-nitrite	Blue
MSB	Red
Giemsa	Red
Gram	Positive
PAS	Variable positive
PTAH	Blue
Amido black	Dark blue

PHLOXINE-TARTRAZINE TECHNIQUE (Lendrum 1947)

Notes

This technique for Paneth cells relies on over-staining with phloxine and progressive substitution by tartrazine. The method is not specific for the granules as most other acidophilic substances may also be demonstrated, e.g. fibrin and virus inclusion bodies. Muscle tends to retain the phloxine, although weakly.

Staining solutions

0.5% phloxine in 0.5% aqueous calcium chloride
Saturated tartrazine in Cellosolve (2-ethoxyethanol)
Mayer's haematoxylin (see p. 25)

Technique

1. Sections to water.
2. Stain nuclei with Mayer's haematoxylin solution. Differentiate and blue. Wash in water.
3. Stain with the phloxine solution for 10–15 min.
4. Wash in water, then in Cellosolve.
5. Treat with the tartrazine solution. At intervals, wash off in water and note remaining phloxine staining; repeat tartrazine staining until only red blood

cells and Paneth cell granules are strongly stained red. Finally, treat with the tartrazine solution for 3–4 s, sufficient to restain the background yellow.
6. Wash in Cellosolve, then xylene. Mount as desired.

Results

Nuclei	blue
Red blood cells and Paneth cell granules	red-orange
Muscle and keratin	pale red
Other tissues	yellow

AMIDO BLACK TECHNIQUE (Bower & Chadwin 1968)

Notes

This method is not specific but is highly selective and easy to carry out.

Solutions

0.5% amido black 10B (syn. naphthalene black) in equal parts of propylene glycol and distilled water
0.01% aqueous lithium carbonate
1% aqueous neutral red

Technique

1. Sections to water.
2. Stain with the amido black solution for 30 min.
3. Wash, differentiate in aqueous lithium carbonate solution until excess stain is removed.
4. Wash and counterstain with neutral red for 5 min. Wash.
5. Dehydrate, clear and mount as desired.

Results

Paneth cell granules, red blood cells, eosinophil granules	dark blue
Nuclei	red

GASTRIC GLAND CELLS

These cells are in the gastric fundus and body, and comprise epithelial lining cells, mucous neck cells, parietal (syn. oxyntic) cells and peptic (syn. chief, central or zymogen) cells. The demonstration of secretory cells of the stomach may be of use in highlighting gastric metaplasia in a Meckel's diverticulum (a congenital diverticulum of the ileum). Routinely these techniques are intended to show the normal histological structure of gastric mucosa and are useful for teaching purposes. The following two techniques are representative of the sparse literature. A more positive demonstration of the parietal cell content of the gastric mucosa is to utilize their significant content of NAD-diaphorase by enzyme histochemistry.

PAS-TOLUIDINE BLUE-AURANTIA TECHNIQUE (Cook 1962)

Notes

The rationale of the method depends on PAS reactivity of the epithelial lining and mucous neck cells. The RNA content of the peptic cells has a strong affinity for contrasting cationic dyes such as toluidine blue. The parietal cells take up the yellow counterstain aurantia. The dye aurantia is considered potentially explosive and the safety-conscious may prefer to use a more innocuous dye such as Milling yellow. When differentiating the toluidine blue in 70% alcohol, aim at underdifferentiation to avoid masking by the subsequent yellow dye. Dehydration in t-butanol avoids extraction of the toluidine blue.

Solutions

1% aqueous periodic acid
Schiff's reagent (see p. 135)
0.5% aqueous toluidine blue
0.25% aurantia in 50% alcohol or 2.5% Milling yellow 3G in Cellosolve

---

Technique

1. Sections to distilled water.
2. Apply the PAS technique: 5 min periodic acid and 15 min Schiff treatment. Wash well.
3. Stain the nuclei with iron haematoxylin (a celestine blue/Mayer's haematoxylin sequence also gives good results—(see p. 37). Differentiate and blue so the cell cytoplasm is left unstained. Wash.
4. Stain in the toluidine blue solution for 1 min.
5. Wash in water, then differentiate in 70% alcohol for up to 1 min until the peptic cells are blue and the background relatively clear.
6. Wash in water to stop the differentiation, and stain in the aurantia solution for 10 s, or wash in water then Cellosolve. Stain with the Milling yellow solution for 3–5 min (a gradual replacement of toluidine blue will occur with prolonged treatment).
7. Wash, blot dry, dehydrate in tertiary butanol or Cellosolve. Clear in xylene and mount as desired.

Results

Nuclei	blue-black
Epithelial and mucous neck cells	magenta
Peptic cells	blue
Parietal cells and red blood cells	yellow

METHASOL FAST BLUE-ALCIAN YELLOW-PYRONIN (Maxwell 1963)

Notes

This technique stains the gastric cells well. The mucin-containing cells are stained with alcian yellow, having first introduced acidic groups onto the component neutral mucin. This enables good colour contrast to be achieved using a blue dye and a red dye to stain the parietal and peptic cells respectively. The latter cell contains cytoplasmic RNA and binds the cationic pyronin.

Solutions

0.5% aqueous periodic acid
0.1% alcoholic methasol fast blue
10% aqueous sodium metabisulphite 100 ml (acidified with M hydrochloric acid 10 ml)
1% aqueous alcian yellow
0.01% aqueous lithium carbonate
2% aqueous pyronin (this may profitably be diluted to a 0.5% solution with distilled water, if overstaining occurs)

Technique

1. Sections to alcohol.
2. Stain with the methanol fast blue solution for 8–16 h at 60°C.
3. Wash in water, then differentiate in the lithium carbonate solution until the parietal cells are prominently shown against the background.
4. Wash well in distilled water, then treat with the periodic acid solution for 5 min.
5. Wash briefly in distilled water. Treat with acidified metabisulphite solution for 5 min.
6. Transfer direct to the alcian yellow solution for 10 min.
7. Wash in water and counterstain with pyronin solution for 30 s.
8. Wash, dehydrate, clear and mount as desired.

Results

Epithelial lining cells and mucous neck cells	yellow
Parietal cells	blue
Peptic cells	red

ANTERIOR PITUITARY CELLS

The adenohypophysis, the anterior lobe of the pituitary, is composed of a loose trabecular arrangement of glandular epithelial cells arranged around a blood sinusoidal system. The cells are divided into three groups by their staining reactions:

Chromophobe cells are the largest population, forming approximately 50% of the total. They have small nuclei and a scanty non-granular cytoplasm. At the electron microscope level a few secretory granules can be seen and it is thought that some of the cells secrete adrenocorticotrophic hormone (ACTH).

Acidophils account for 40% of the cell number; they are usually concentrated in the lateral wings of the anterior lobe. Acidophils have cytoplasmic granules; some of the cells secrete growth hormone and are termed somatotrophs whilst other cells, mammotrophs, secrete prolactin.

Basophils—these cells form 10% of the total. They are usually larger than acidophils, and are divided into two groups based on their staining reactions. Basophil-S cells are so-called because oxidation followed by alcian blue demonstrates sulphur-containing amino acids; basophil-R cells are named for their resistance to oxidation and subsequent alcian blue staining. The secretions of the two types of cell are different; S cells are thought to produce adrenocorticotrophic hormone (ACTH), while the R cell secretes thyrotrophic hormone (TSH), leuteinizing hormone (LH) and follicle-stimulating hormone (FSH).

The usual reason for investigating the cell population of the pituitary is to ascertain the presence or absence of a pituitary adenoma and to gain some insight into the cell constituents and the likely hormonal effects. A pituitary adenoma represents a neoplastic proliferation of one cell type, often at the expense of the remainder of the gland. The constituent cells may be secreting an excess of the relevant hormone or may be non-functional. The remainder of the gland may be compressed with a reduced output of hormones.

Most fixatives give acceptable staining results, although some people prefer mercuric chloride; we have noticed little difference. It is important to use thin sections—3–4 μm—especially for H&E. The staining reactions are shown in Table 4.2; besides the MSB technique, trichromes may be employed giving similar tinctorial results.

Table 4.2   Staining reactions of anterior pituitary cells

Cell type	MSB	Pontamine Sky blue eosin	PAS-OG	OFG	BR.AB-OFG
Chromophobes	—	Pale pink	Blue-grey	Pale blue-grey	Grey-green
Acidophils	Red	Red	Yellow	Yellow	Yellow
Basophil-R cell	Blue	Blue-purple	Magenta	Magenta	Magenta
Basophil-S cell	Blue	Blue-purple	Magenta	Magenta	Green-blue

KERENYI & TAYLOR'S (1961) PONTAMINE SKY BLUE METHOD

Notes

A simple method that demonstrates the component cells well.

Solutions

1% aqueous pontamine sky blue 5BX
Mayer's haematoxylin (see p. 25)
1% hydrochloric acid in 70% alcohol
0.5% ws eosin

Technique

1. Sections to water.
2. Stain in 1% aqueous pontamine sky blue for 2 min.
3. Wash in running water for 1 min.
4. Stain nuclei in Mayer's haematoxylin (see p. 25).

5. Rinse in tap water and differentiate nuclei in 1% acid-alcohol.
6. 'Blue' nuclei in running tap water for at least 5 min.
7. Stain in 0.5% aqueous eosin for 2 min.
8. Differentiate eosin in water, dehydrate, clear and mount in a synthetic resin medium.

Results

Nuclei	blue to blue-black
Basophils	bluish-purple
Acidophils	bright red
Chromophobes	pale pink

PAS ORANGE G FOR ANTERIOR PITUITARY CELLS (Pearse 1953)

Notes

This method is an extension of the PAS reaction, with basophils stained by Schiff's reagent, acidophils by orange G and the chromophobes by haematoxylin. Other PAS-positive structures also stain.

Technique

Steps 1–7 as in standard PAS method (see p. 135).

8. Stain in 2% orange G in 5% phosphotungstic acid for 20 s.
9. Differentiate in tap water until macroscopically the section is pale yellow. Check microscopically that only the red blood cells and acidophil cells are yellow.
10. Dehydrate, clear and mount as desired.

Results

Basophils	magenta
Acidophils	yellow
Red blood cells	yellow
Nuclei	blue-black
Chromophobes	pale blue-grey

ONE-STEP MSB FOR ANTERIOR PITUITARY CELLS (Lendrum et al 1962, Dawes & Hillier 1964)

Notes

This is a modification of the MSB method. It is an easy and reliable method requiring no differentiation and separating acidophils and basophils well.

Solutions

Yellow solution:

Martius yellow	100 mg

Absolute alcohol	95 ml
Distilled water	5 ml
Phosphotungstic acid	2 g

Red solution
1% brilliant crystal scarlet in 2.5% acetic acid.
Blue solution
0.5% aniline blue in 1% acetic acid.
Staining solution:

Yellow solution	45 ml
Red solution	30 ml
Blue solution	45 ml

The three solutions are filtered through separate filter papers into a single container in the order given above. The solution is allowed to stand for 3 days before use.

Technique

1. Sections to water.
2. Stain nuclei with celestine blue-haematoxylin (see p. 37).
3. Differentiate in acid-alcohol.
4. Blue in tap water.
5. Place in staining solution for 8 min.
6. Rinse rapidly in tap water and blot dry.
7. Dehydrate and mount as desired.

Results

Acidophils	red
Basophils	blue
Red blood cells	yellow
Nuclei	blue-black

ORANGE G-ACID FUCHSIN-GREEN (OFG) TECHNIQUE (Slidders 1961a)

Notes

A certain amount of expertise is needed to obtain good results, but colourful and clear-cut cell demonstration is possible. The staining of the basophils by acid fuchsin is progressive and should be continued until the cells, but not the background, are a well-defined red-purple.

Solutions

Saturated orange G in 2% phosphotungstic acid in 95% alcohol
0.5% acid fuchsin in 0.5% acetic acid
1.5% light green in 1.5% acetic acid

1% aqueous phosphotungstic acid
Iron haematoxylin solution (see p. 37)

Technique

1. Sections to water and stain the nuclei in an iron haematoxylin solution. Differentiate and blue. Wash in water, then in 95% alcohol.
2. Stain with the orange G solution for 2 min.
3. Rinse in distilled water and stain in the acid fuchsin solution for 2–5 min.
4. Rinse in distilled water, then treat with the phosphotungstic acid solution for 5 min.
5. Rinse in distilled water and stain in the light green solution for 1–2 min.
6. Wash in distilled water and blot dry.
7. Dehydrate, clear and mount as desired.

Results

Nuclei	blue-black
Basophils	red-purple
Red blood cells, acidophils	yellow
Chromophobes	pale blue-grey
Connective tissue	green

BR.AB-OFG METHOD FOR CELLS OF THE ANTERIOR PITUITARY
(Slidders 1961b)

Notes

This method is a development of the performic acid-alcian blue-PAS-orange G technique and separates the two types of basophil cell. Bromine is used instead of performic acid as in the PA-AB-OG method of Adams & Swettenham (1958). The rationale is that some sulphur-containing amino acids stain with alcian blue after bromine oxidation (hence 'S'), whilst other basophils do not so react to an oxidation-alcian blue sequence and are termed 'R' (resistant).

Solutions

Bromine water:

10% hydrobromic acid (aqueous)	45 ml
2.5% potassium permanganate (aqueous)	5 ml

Alcian blue:

Alcian blue	100 mg
Sulphuric acid (conc.)	1 ml
Glacial acetic acid	9 ml
Distilled water	90 ml

Carefully mix the dye and the sulphuric acid, stir with a glass rod. Slowly add the glacial acetic acid. Stir again. Make up to 100 ml with the distilled water and filter.

Technique

1. Sections to water.
2. Treat with bromine water for 5 min.
3. Wash in running tap water for 5 min.
4. Rinse in distilled water.
5. Stain in alcian blue solution for 1 h.
6. Wash well in tap water.
7. Proceed with the OFG method (see p. 77).

Results

Red blood cells, acidophils	orange-yellow
Basophils (S)	dark green-blue
Basophils (R)	magenta-red
Chromophobe cells	pale blue-grey
Nuclei	grey-blue

CARMOISINE-ORANGE G-WOOL GREEN TECHNIQUE FOR DIFFERENTIATING ACIDOPHIL CELLS (Brookes 1968)

Notes

The technique gives good results but requires a degree of expertise to obtain clear-cut colour differentiation of somatotrophic from lactotrophic pituitary acidophil cells.

Solutions

10% aqueous copper sulphate
1% carmoisine L in 1% acetic acid
Saturated orange G in 2% phosphotungstic acid in 95% ethanol
0.5% wool green S in 0.5% acetic acid

Technique

1. Sections to water and mordant in the copper sulphate solution for 2h at 44°C.
2. Wash well in tap water for 10–20 min, then in distilled water.
3. Stain with the carmoisine solution for 30 min.
4. Wash in distilled water, then in 95% alcohol.
5. Stain with the orange G solution for 5–30 min. Replacement of the carmoisine by the orange G in the somatotrophic cells will take place.
   This should be controlled by washing the slide at intervals in 2% phosphotungstic acid in 95% ethanol and examining microscopically.
6. Rinse well in distilled water.
7. Restain in the carmoisine solution for 5 min.
8. Rinse in distilled water and counterstain in the wool green solution for 10 min.
9. Rinse in distilled water, treat with 1% acetic acid for 2 min to remove excess wool green.
10. Dehydrate, clear and mount as desired.

Result

Somatotropes	yellow
Red blood cells, lactotropes	red
Basophils	green

METHYL BLUE-EOSIN TECHNIQUE (Mann 1894)

Notes

Colourful staining is obtained with this method, but unbalanced results can occur due to variation in dye batches. In such cases it is worthwhile experimenting with the proportions of methyl blue to eosin; for example 5% aqueous eosin instead of the 1% solution quoted may give better results.

Solutions

Methyl blue-eosin solution:

1% aqueous methyl blue (this solution should be freshly prepared)	35 ml
1% aqueous eosin ws yellowish	45 ml
Distilled water	100 ml

Differentiator
Add 5 drops of saturated potassium hydroxide in ethanol to 30 ml ethanol.

Technique

1. Sections to water.
2. Stain with the solution overnight at room temperature.
3. Rinse in distilled water.
4. Drain, slide, and differentiate sections in the alcoholic potassium hydroxide solution until a lighter, more precise result is obtained.
5. Rinse and dehydrate, clear and mount as desired.

Results

Nuclei and basophil cell granules	blue
Red blood cells and acidophil cell granules	red
Chromophobes	colourless

BASIC FUCHSIN-ALCIAN BLUE (Monroe & Frommer 1966)

Notes

The principle of this reaction is that tannic acid forms a mordant–dye complex with dyes having free amine radicals, in this case basic fuchsin, leading to strong staining of acidophil cells and weaker staining of delta basophil cells. Following phosphomolybdic acid treatment the beta basophils stain a blue-green colour. The technique produces good results provided the necessary expertise is acquired.

Solutions

10% aqueous tannic acid
1% basic fuchsin in 20% alcohol
1% aqueous alcian blue
1% aniline in 90% alcohol
1% aqueous phosphomolybdic acid

Technique

1. Sections to water.
2. Treat with the tannic acid solution for 15 min.
3. Wash well in water for 5 min.
4. Dilute the basic fuchsin solution with equal parts of distilled water and treat for several seconds, agitating the slide.
5. Wash in water.
6. Differentiate in the alcoholic aniline solution until the acidophil cells are red and the delta basophil cells pink.
7. Place in the phosphomolybdic acid solution for 30 s.
8. Wash in water, then stain in filtered alcian blue solution for 30 s.
9. Wash, dehydrate, clear and mount as desired.

Results

Acidophils	red
Beta basophils	blue-green
Delta basophils	purple
Chromophobes	colourless
Collagen	blue-green

THE PANCREAS

The organ is divided into two parts; the larger portion of the gland is exocrine. These cells are acidophilic and the cytoplasm contains zymogen granules that are involved in the production of digestive enzymes. Cells of the exocrine component are not difficult to demonstrate—they are easy to see in the conventional H&E, trichrome stains and phloxine-tartrazine methods. They are PAS-positive and react for the amino acids tyrosine and tryptophan (see p. 92 and p. 121 respectively). Zymogen granules are particularly well-shown with freeze-dried sections.

The smaller portion of the organ is endocrine—the islets of Langerhans are composed of groups of endocrine cells surrounded by exocrine glands. The islets of Langerhans are distributed throughout the organ but are found in greater number in the tail. The cells that make up the islets are of different types and each produces a specific hormone. At the present time four separate types of cell have been identified. The *A* (α_2) *cells* produce glucagon, the *B* (β) *cells* secrete insulin, the *D cells* (α_1) are thought to produce different hormones, mainly a somatostatin-like one, and the *C cells* are considered to be precursors of the alpha and beta cells. The conventional general staining methods cannot demonstrate the specific granules of the islet cells and can only be used as a guide when attempting to demonstrate these cells. The staining reactions of the general methods are given in Table 4.3.

Table 4.3   Staining reactions of the endocrine pancreas

Cell types	A-F mod.	Chrome haem.	Phlox. tart.	Grimelius	Hellerstrom Hellman	Lead haem.	Bodian
A cells (α_2)	Yellow	Red	Yellow	Positive	Negative	Positive	Positive
B cells (β)	Purple	Blue	Red	Negative	Negative	Negative	Negative
D cells (α_1)	Green	Red	Yellow	Negative	Positive	Positive	Positive

A variety of tumours of the pancreatic islets have been described and are best identified by the hormone they secrete. This may be by biochemical serum estimation or an immunocytochemical analysis on tissue sections when the lesion has been excised. Most such tumours are benign but malignant variants do occur and are best classified according to their hormonal product as insulinomas, glucagonomas, vipomas, somatostatinomas, pancreatic polypeptide-secreting tumours, carcinoid tumours and pancreatic gastrinomas.

Autolysis of the pancreas is rapid after death. The longer autolysis continues the less reliable are the staining techniques, so that often post-mortem material will not be satisfactory. For staining the islet cells, formalin and mercury fixation are best, except for the silver methods of Grimelius and Hellerstrom and Hellman and the Gomori haematoxylin technique, when Bouin is considered superior.

GOMORI'S CHROME ALUM-HAEMATOXYLIN (Gomori 1941)

Notes

This traditional method for islet cells is capricious. In our hands the alpha cells stain well, the beta cells inconsistently. The rationale is obscure.

Solutions

Haematoxylin
  Mix equal parts of 1% aqueous haematoxylin and 3% aqueous chrome alum. To a 100 ml volume add 5% aqueous potassium dichromate 2 ml and 0.5 M sulphuric acid 2 ml. Allow to stand for 48 h prior to use. The solution keeps for 4–8 weeks.
0.5% aqueous phloxine
3% aqueous sodium bisulphite
5% aqueous phosphotungstic acid

Technique

1. Sections to water, and if fixed in formalin, mordant in Bouin's solution overnight.
2. Wash well and treat with equal parts of 0.3% aqueous potassium permanganate and 0.3% sulphuric acid for 1 min.

3. Decolourize in sodium bisulphite solution (5% aqueous oxalic acid will do equally well).
4. Wash well in water, then stain with the haematoxylin solution for 15 min.
5. Wash in water, differentiate in acid-alcohol. Wash again, then blue. The differentiation should be prolonged until only the beta cell granules are stained a clear blue.
6. Stain with the phloxine solution for 5 min.
7. Wash in water, then treat with the phosphotungstic acid solution for 1 min.
8. Wash in water for up to 5 min (the phloxine staining will reappear). If the phloxine staining appears too heavy, differentiate in 95% alcohol.
9. Dehydrate, clear and mount as desired.

Results

A and D cells	red
B cells	blue
Exocrine zymogen cells	unstained to pale red

MODIFIED ALDEHYDE FUCHSIN STAIN (Halami 1952)

Notes

This is an extension of the original Gomori technique. It demonstrates D cells and gives a better staining of B cells. The sections are oxidized with Lugol's iodine before staining with aldehyde fuchsin. The observations to this stain on page 58 should be noted.

Solutions

Aldehyde fuchsin (see p. 58)
Lugol's iodine (see p. 59)
2.5% aqueous sodium thiosulphate (hypo)
Counterstain:

Light green	200 mg
Orange G	1 g
Phosphotungstic acid	500 mg
Glacial acetic acid	1 ml
Distilled water	100 ml

The solution keeps well.

Technique

1. Sections to water.
2. Oxidize with Lugol's iodine for 10 min.
3. Rinse in tap water and bleach with the sodium thiosulphate solution.
4. Wash in tap water followed by 70% alcohol.
5. Stain in aldehyde fuchsin stain for 15–30 min.
6. Wash in 95% alcohol followed by water.

7. Stain nuclei with celestine blue and haemalum sequence (see p. 37).
8. Wash in water, differentiate briefly in acid-alcohol and wash well in tap water.
9. Rinse with distilled water and counterstain with orange G-light green solution for 45 s.
10. Rinse briefly with 0.2% acetic acid followed by 95% alcohol.
11. Dehydrate, clear and mount as desired.

Results

B cells	purple-violet
A cells	yellow
D cells	green
Nuclei	blue-black

COMBINED PROTARGOL-ALDEHYDE FUCHSIN TECHNIQUE (Cook 1974, taken from Bodian 1936 and Gomori 1950)

Notes

This method makes use of the argyrophilia of both types of alpha cell to obtain contrast with subsequent staining of beta granules by aldehyde fuchsin. For the latter a pre-oxidation step is necessary. The protargol method gives strong argyrophilic demonstration of most tissue entities, notably nerve fibres and melanin. Sections are treated with protargol (a compound formed of gelatine and silver nitrate) in the presence of metallic copper. Cox (personal communication) suggested that the role of the copper is to produce nitric acid, causing the pH to fall and as a result slowing down the reaction with consequent lessened risk of over-impregnation. Following copper-protargol treatment, the sections are progressively reduced in a hydroquinone-gold chloride-oxalic acid sequence. Background precipitation is common in this technique, and thorough washing between the various stages will reduce this. Most sources of protargol have been unsatisfactory for this technique; we recommend Messrs. Roques of Paris, obtainable from Merck (UK).

Solutions

Aldehyde fuchsin solution (see p. 58)
Acidified potassium permanganate solution (see p. 49)
Copper-protargol solution
   Prepare fresh 50 ml of 1% aqueous protargol to which are added (in a Coplin jar) 2 g of clean copper foil cut into small (5 mm) pieces.
Primary reducer
   Hydroquinone 1 g; sodium sulphite 5 g; in 100 ml distilled water. Prepare fresh (the sodium sulphite acts as a stabilizer, allowing the solution to be kept for up to 2 days at 4°C).
1% aqueous gold chloride
0.1% light green in 0.2% acetic acid
5% and 2% aqueous oxalic acid
5% sodium thiosulphate (hypo)

Technique

1. Sections to distilled water.
2. Treat with the copper-protargol solution overnight at 37°C (exact time is not critical but do not leave for more than 48 h).
3. Wash in several changes of distilled water and reduce in hydroquinone for 10 min.
4. Wash well in distilled water. Thorough washing at this stage is most important and we suggest first in distilled water, then in tap water for several minutes and finally in distilled water again.
5. Treat with the yellow gold chloride for 5 min.
6. Wash well in several changes of distilled water.
7. Treat with the oxalic acid for 5 min (only at this stage should silver blackening be evident).
8. Fix in 5% hypo. Wash.
9. Treat with the acidified potassium permanganate solution for 1 min. Wash, then bleach with 5% aqueous oxalic acid. Wash well in water.
10. Rinse in 70% alcohol, and stain with the aldehyde fuchsin solution for 4–6 min.
11. Rinse well in 70% alcohol, then in water.
12. Counterstain if required in the light green solution for 1/2 min.
13. Wash, dehydrate, clear and mount in a synthetic resin.

Results

A and D cells (and nuclei to some degree)	black
B cells	purple
Background	green

MITOCHONDRIA

Mitochondria are cytoplasmic organelles consisting of 40% lipid, so that they are best preserved by fixatives such as osmium tetroxide and potassium dichromate. A solution we find particularly effective is that of Regaud (3% aqueous potassium dichromate 80 parts: formalin 20 parts). Extended fixation is recommended (4 days or so) and for best results tissue should be fresh at time of fixing. Cardiac muscle, kidney and liver show mitochondria to advantage. Thin paraffin sections should be used (3–4 μm).

The demonstration of mitochondria at light microscope level is not particularly rewarding. It is of little diagnostic significance except perhaps for the identification of 'ragged red fibres' in skeletal muscle fibres using a Gomori trichrome technique to identify abnormally large aggregates of mitochondria in mitochondrial myopathy. Giant mitochondria may be seen in liver biopsies from patients with alcoholic liver disease. Providing that the above points regarding fixation are observed, the following techniques can be used to demonstrate mitochondria: acid haematein (see p. 184), Sudan black (see p. 176), Luxol fast blue (see p. 352), PTAH (if preceded by treating the section with 5% aqueous ferric chloride for 24 h at room temperature—see p. 44). The Heidenhain and Altmann classic methods are described.

IRON HAEMATOXYLIN TECHNIQUE (Heidenhain 1896)

Notes

This technique demonstrates most structures simultaneously, employing differentiation until the desired constituent is shown to greatest advantage. Good results require practice and the novice may well find it advantageous to dilute the differentiator with equal parts of distilled water. This slows down differentiation making it easier to control. Gentle agitation of the slide during differentiation leads to more even results.

The basis of the method is that, following iron alum treatment, the section is stained with haematoxylin allowing a tissue–mordant–dye bonding to occur. On subsequent iron alum treatment competition with the bound haematoxylin for the tissue-binding sites occurs; the iron alum, being now in excess, is successful in progressively replacing the dye.

Solutions

5% aqueous ferric ammonium sulphate (iron alum)
0.5% haematoxylin in 10 ml ethanol and 90 ml distilled water (allow to ripen at least 6 weeks before use)

Technique

1. Sections to water.
2. Treat with the iron alum solution for 1 h at 56°C.
3. Wash in water, then treat with the haematoxylin solution for 1 h at 56°C.
4. Wash in water and differentiate in the iron alum solution at room temperature. This is best carried out in a Coplin jar and with microscopic control. Differentiate until the mitochondria are well-stained against a reasonably colourless background.
5. Wash well in water for several minutes.
6. Counterstaining is optional; suitable counterstains are eosin, tartrazine in Cellosolve, or light green in acetic acid using weak solutions for short periods of time.
7. Dehydrate, clear and mount as desired.

Results

Red blood cells, mitochondria and nuclei	blue-black
Background	clear, or according to the counterstain used

ALTMANN'S TECHNIQUE (Altmann 1894)

Notes

Champy's solution (potassium dichromate, osmium tetroxide, acetic acid) is often recommended for this method; other fixatives work equally well, e.g. Helly's and Regaud's solutions. After fixation, postchroming in 3% aqueous potassium dichromate for 3–7 days is usually specified. Following over-staining in aniline-acid fuchsin there is replacement differentiation with picric acid. A strong solution of acid fuchsin is necessary for a good result. Some variation in differentiation will occur in different parts of the section.

Solutions

Aniline-acid fuchsin
Add 5 ml aniline to 100 ml of heated distilled water. Mix well and add acid fuchsin to saturation (approximately 14% w/v). Allow to cool. Mix at intervals over 24 h. Filter.
Differentiator I:

Saturated alcoholic picric acid	20 ml
30% alcohol	80 ml

Differentiator II:

Saturated alcohol picric acid	10 ml
30% alcohol	80 ml

Technique

1. Sections to water.
2. Drain and flood with aniline-acid fuchsin. Heat until the steam rises three times over a period of 5 min (i.e. as for the Ziehl–Neelsen technique).
3. Rinse in water and differentiate in the picric-alcohol until the excess acid fuchsin staining is removed, then complete differentiation by treating with the weaker differentiator (picric-alcohol II). Control microscopically.
4. Rinse in water, dehydrate rapidly to avoid losing the picric acid background staining. Clear and mount as desired.

Results

Red blood cells, mitochondria and nuclei	red
Background (if Champy's fixative is used, lipids will be black)	yellow

RUSSELL BODIES

These occur in the cytoplasm of plasma cells and are seen frequently in cases of myeloma and rheumatoid arthritis. They vary in size and on occasion distend the cytoplasm of the cell. Staining bright pink with eosin in the same tone as red blood cells, they are distinguished by their smooth round shape. Mainly protein in content they are PAS-positive. Located in plasma cell cytoplasm they contain RNA. The staining reactions of Russell bodies are given in Table 4.4.

Table 4.4 Staining methods for Russell bodies

PAS reaction	Strongly positive
Millon reaction	Positive
Phloxine tartrazine	Bright red
Gram	Positive (with xylene-aniline diff.)
Methyl green-pyronin	Red

LYSOSOMES

These cytoplasmic inclusions are found in many cells, particularly in phagocytic cells such as macrophages and neutrophils. They are involved in enzymic break-down of phagocytosed material, and are membrane-bound cytoplasmic organelles containing many hydrolytic enzymes; the demonstration of one of these enzymes, acid phosphatase, is used as a lysosomal marker. The large lysosomes within neutrophils can be seen in Giemsa-stained preparations. Lysosomes increase in number in cells that are surviving under adverse conditions and therefore may be present in a wide range of degenerative processes and neoplasms. In the same manner as mitochondria, lysosomes are best studied using electron microscopy.

REFERENCES

Adams C W M, Swettenham K V 1958 The histochemical identification of two types of basophil cell in the normal human adenohypophysis. Journal of Pathology and Bacteriology 75: 95

Altmann R 1894 Die Elementarogranismen, 2nd edn. Veit, Leipzig

Bodian D 1936 A new method for staining nerve fibres and nerve endings in mounted paraffin sections. Anatomical Record 65: 89

Bower D, Chadwin C G 1968 Demonstration of Paneth cell granules using Naphthalene black. Journal of Clinical Pathology 21: 107

Brookes L D 1968 A stain for differentiating two types of acidophil cells in the rat pituitary. Stain Technology 43: 41

Cook H C 1962 Periodic acid-Schiff-Toluidine blue-Aurantia: a stain for the gland cells of the stomach. Stain Technology 37: 317

Cook H C 1974 Manual of histological demonstration techniques. Butterworths, London

Dawes R E, Hillier M H 1964 A one stage technique for differentiating the a and b cells of the anterior pituitary. Journal of Medical Laboratory Technology 21: 62

Giemsa G 1902 The azure dyes their purification and physiochemical properties. Znetbl Bakt Parasitkde (Abt 1) 31: 429. Cited from Bare (1970)

Gomori G 1941 Observations with differential stains on human islets of Langerhans. American Journal of Pathology 17: 395

Gomori G 1950 Aldehyde-fuchsin: a new stain for elastic tissue. American Journal of Clinical Pathology 20: 665

Halami N S 1952 Differentiation of the two types of basophils in an adenohypophysis of the rat and the mouse. Stain Technology 27: 61

Ham A W 1969 Histology, 6th edn. Lippincott, Philadelphia

Heidenhain M 1896 Noch einmal über die Darstellung der Centralkörper durch Eisenhamatoxylin nebst einigen allgemeinen Bemerkungen über die Hamatoxylinfarben. Z Wiss Mikrosk 13: 186

Kerenyi N, Taylor W A 1961 Niagara blue 4B as a fast simple stain for the adenohypophysis. Stain Technology 36: 169

Lendrum A C 1944 The staining of eosinophil polymorphs and enterochromaffin cells in histological sections. Journal of Pathology and Bacteriology 56: 441

Lendrum A C 1947 The phloxine-tartrazine method as a general histological stain and for the demonstration of inclusion bodies. Journal of Pathology and Bacteriology 59: 399

Lendrum A C, Foster D S, Slidders W, Henderson R 1962 Studies on the character and staining of fibrin. Journal of Clinical Pathology 15: 401

Mann G 1894 Ueber die Behandlung der Nerrenzellen fur experimental histolgische Untersuchnungen. Z.g. Wissensch Mikr. Brnschwg, xi: 479

Maxwell A 1963 The Alcian dyes applied to the gastric mucosa. Stain Technology 38: 286

Monroe C W, Frommer J 1966 A basic fuchsin-Alcian blue stain for the human hypophysis. Stain Technology 41: 248

Pearse A G E 1953 Histochemistry, theoretical and applied. Churchill, London

Slidders W 1961a The Fuchsin-Miller method. Journal of Medical Laboratory Technology 18: 36

Slidders W 1961b The OFG and Br AB-OFG methods for staining the adenohypophysis. Journal of Pathology and Bacteriology 82: 532

5. Proteins (amino acids) and nucleic acids

PROTEINS

Proteins are organic nitrogenous compounds forming one of the three basic constituents of tissues, with carbohydrates and lipids. The demonstration of proteins, unlike that of lipids and carbohydrates, does not hold a prominent place in practical histochemistry (nucleic acids being an exception to this rule). Proteins are part of every cell and tissue. On occasion it is necessary to determine if a protein is present and its precise nature. Proteins occur in tissues as either simple proteins (uncombined) or in combination with other constituents (e.g. lipids) as conjugated proteins. In histochemical terms the most important proteins are shown in Table 5.1.

Table 5.1 Proteins

Simple	Conjugated
Albumins	Nucleoproteins
Globulins	Mucoproteins
Fibrous, e.g. collagen, fibrin, elastin and keratin	Glycoproteins
	Chromoproteins
	Lipoproteins

Simple proteins are naturally occurring proteins yielding α-amino acids and derivatives on hydrolysis.

Conjugated proteins are compounds consisting of simple proteins in combination with non-protein constituents such as carbohydrates in glycoproteins, or lipids in lipoproteins.

Nucleoproteins are compounds of simple proteins, usually basic protein, in combination with nucleic acids.

DEMONSTRATION OF PROTEINS

The staining reaction of proteins and protein-containing substances depends upon their amino acid composition. The *fibrous proteins* are demonstrated by histological methods based on the physical configuration of their molecules, rather than their chemical composition, i.e. trichrome stains. *Amino acid* methods demonstrate the presence of part of the constituent amino acids and not the whole protein. A positive reaction is taken to indicate the presence of the protein. It is unlikely that free amino acids will remain in the tissue sections. Few dye methods are used routinely; those given below are the most useful. Table 5.2 lists the amino acid methods; a selection is given in detail. The DMAB-nitrite method for tryptophan is given on page 121.

Table 5.2   Amino acid staining methods. (This list is not complete; it gives only the more common methods.)

Millon reaction	Tyrosine (phenyl groups)	Pink
Sakaguchi	Arginine (guanidyl groups)	Orange-red
Mercury orange	Sulphydryl groups	Pale orange
DDD reaction	Sulphydryl groups. Disulphide linkages	Reddish-purple
Diazotization with acid	Tyrosine (phenyl groups)	Purple-red
DMAB-nitrite method	Trytophan (indole groups)	Deep blue
Performic acid-alcian blue	Disulphide groups	Dark blue
Ninhydrin-Schiff	Amino groups	Pink

Enzymes are proteins that catalyse specific reactions and are demonstrated using their specific activity (see Ch. 13). The future for the demonstration of specific proteins undoubtedly lies in the application of immunocytochemical techniques (see p. 281). The fundamental aspects of these techniques are described in Chapter 12.

TISSUE PREPARATION

The influence of fixatives on protein methods should be considered; formaldehyde for instance reacts with α-amino groups. Oxidizing agents used in fixatives will react with proteins—osmium for instance forms cross-links. In practical terms formaldehyde fixation should be used at a neutral pH and the time kept to a minimum; osmium tetroxide should be avoided (see Hopwood 1990). The best localization of proteins is obtained by using freeze-dried sections.

DEMONSTRATION METHODS

The staining methods that follow sometimes give a pale reaction product, also some of the techniques are destructive to tissue sections so care should always be taken. Where possible, positive controls should be employed, as well as an untreated duplicate section to serve as a negative control.

NINHYDRIN-SCHIFF FOR AMINO GROUPS (Yasuma & Itchikwa 1953)

Notes

Ninhydrin at neutral pH reacts with α-amino groups to form aldehydes that will re-colour Schiff's reagent.

Solutions

0.5% ninhydrin in absolute alcohol
Schiff's reagent (see p. 135)

Technique

1. Sections to 70% alcohol.
2. Treat with ninhydrin solution at 37°C overnight.
3. Wash in running tap water.

4. Treat in Schiff's reagent for 45 min.
5. Wash in running tap water.
6. Counterstain with an alum haematoxylin (see p. 25).
7. Wash in tap water; dehydrate, clear and mount as desired.

Results

Amino groups	magenta
Nuclei	blue

BLOCKING METHOD FOR AMINO GROUPS (Stoward 1963)

Notes

This is a deamination technique, for which the absence of a ninhydrin-Schiff reaction is positive confirmation of the presence of amino groups.

Solution

Sodium nitrite	1 g
3% sulphuric acid	30 ml

Technique

1. Sections to distilled water.
2. Immerse in a freshly prepared solution that has been pre-cooled for 48h at 4°C.
3. Wash in distilled water.
4. Leave sections in distilled water for 4 h at 60°C.
5. Employ the ninhydrin-Schiff method above in conjunction with an untreated section.

Result

Amino groups are positive after the ninhydrin-Schiff method above and negative after the blocking method/ninhydrin-Schiff method.

MILLON REACTION FOR TYROSINE (Baker 1956)

Notes

This is a histochemical modification of Millon's biochemical test and demonstrates the presence of hydroxyphenyl groups. The phenyl is first converted into nitrosophenol that combines with mercury to produce a coloured reaction product. Tyrosine is the only amino acid that contains hydroxyphenyl groups. The colour reaction is pale pink. Great care, and possibly luck, is required to keep the sections on the slides; be sure to take more than one section through the method and use a section adhesive. Pancreas is a good positive control tissue.

Solutions

Solution A

10 g of mercuric sulphate is added to a mixture of 90 ml distilled water and 10 ml of conc. sulphuric acid, and dissolved by heating. After cooling to room temperature 100 ml of distilled water is added.

Solution B

0.25 g of sodium nitrite is dissolved in 10 ml of distilled water.

Working solution

5 ml of solution B is added to 4 ml of solution A.

Technique

1. Sections to distilled water.
2. Immerse sections in the reagent in a small beaker and bring to the boil; gently simmer for 2 min.
3. Allow to cool to room temperature.
4. Wash in three changes of distilled water, 2 min each.
5. Dehydrate, clear, and mount as desired.

Result

Tyrosine-containing proteins   red or pink

DIAZOTIZATION-COUPLING FOR TYROSINE (Glenner & Lillie 1959)

Notes

This method employs 8-amino-1-naphthol-5-sulphonic acid ('S' acid) as a coupling amine for the diazonium nitrites produced by nitrosation of tyrosine. It is necessary to carry out both incubation stages in the dark and at a low temperature. In our hands this gives better and stronger results than the previous technique.

Solutions

Incubating solution A:

Sodium nitrite	3.5 g
Acetic acid (conc.)	4.4 ml
Distilled water	47 ml

Incubating solution B:

8-amino-1-naphthol-5-sulphonic acid	0.5 g
Potassium hydroxide	0.5 g
Ammonium sulphamate	0.5 g
70% alcohol	50 ml

Technique

1. Sections to distilled water.
2. Place sections in incubating solution A at 4°C for 24 h in the dark.

3. Rinse in four changes of distilled water at 4°C.
4. Transfer sections to incubating solution B at 4° for 1 h in the dark.
5. Wash in three changes of 0.1 M HCl, 5 min each.
6. Rinse in running tap water for 10 min.
7. Counterstain if required in alum haematoxylin (p. 25).
8. Dehydrate, clear and mount as desired.

Results

Tyrosine-containing proteins   purple-red

PERFORMIC ACID-ALCIAN BLUE FOR DISULPHIDE (SS) AND SULPHYDRYL (SH) GROUPS (Adams & Sloper 1955)

Notes

Some proteins contain sulphydryl/disulphide groups. These are produced by the amino acids cysteine, cystine and methionine. The disulphide linkage is between two sulphur atoms (-S-S-) and the sulphydryl grouping is between a sulphur and a hydrogen atom (-S-H-). Both these sulphur-containing groups can be demonstrated by several techniques, of which this is the best. The performic acid is freshly prepared and allowed to stand for 1 h before use. The washing stage following oxidation is critical; the washing needs to be thorough but the sections have a tendency to wash off. Basophils of the anterior pituitary and keratin make good control tissues. The conventional Schmorl reaction (see p. 203) will also demonstrate sulphur-containing amino acids, but less precisely.

Solutions

Performic acid:

98% formic acid	40 ml
100 vol. hydrogen peroxide	4 ml
Conc. sulphuric acid	0.5 ml

Alcian blue solution:

Alcian blue	1 g
98% sulphuric acid	2.7 ml
Distilled water	47.2 ml

Technique

1. Sections to water; blot to remove surplus water.
2. Stand sections in performic acid for 5 min.
3. Wash well in tap water for 10 min.
4. Dry in 60°C oven until just dry.
5. Rinse in tap water.
6. Stain in alcian blue solution at room temperature for 1 h.
7. Wash in running tap water.
8. Counterstain (e.g. neutral red) if required.

9. Wash in tap water.
10. Dehydrate, clear and mount as desired.

Results

Disulphide and sulphydryl groups   blue
(The intensity of the reaction depends on the amount of disulphide/sulphydryl
present.)
Nuclei (if counterstained)   red

BLOCKING OF SS AND SH GROUPS (Taken from Chèvremont & Fréderick 1943)

Notes

This is applied with the above technique to confirm (using duplicate sections) the nature of the positive groups. The underlying principle is that any SS groups present are first reduced to SH. The formed, and any pre-existing SH groups are next blocked with a mercury salt that condenses specifically with those groups.

Solutions

20% aqueous sodium dithionite (freshly prepared)
Mercuric chloride solution (saturated aqueous)

Technique

1. Treat duplicate sections with the freshly prepared sodium dithionite solution for 30 min at 37°C.
2. Wash well in water 10 min. Treat with the mercuric chloride solution for 24 h at room temperature.
3. Wash well in water and carry out the appropriate technique concurrently with untreated sections.

SAKAGUCHI REACTION FOR ARGININE (Baker 1947)

Notes

The guanidyl groups react with α-naphthol and a red colour is developed in the presence of a strong alkali. Sections for this method should be at least 10 μm thick; best results in our hands are obtained with sections 15 μm thick, showing the weak colour better. The method tends to be destructive to sections.

Solutions

Incubating solution:

1% sodium hydroxide	2 ml
1% α-naphthol in 70% alcohol	2 drops
1% sodium hyperchlorite in distilled water	4 drops

Pyridine-chloroform solution:

Pyridine	30 ml
Chloroform	10 ml

Technique

1. Sections to alcohol.
2. Rinse in 70% alcohol.
3. Flood slide with incubating solution for 15 min.
4. Drain and gently blot dry.
5. Immerse in pyridine-chloroform solution for 2 min.
6. Mount in fresh pyridine-chloroform solution and ring coverslip.

Result

Arginine   orange-red

NUCLEIC ACIDS

Interest in nucleic acids has developed due to their involvement in chromosomes and their role in protein synthesis. There are two types of nucleic acid, deoxyribonucleic acid (DNA) and ribonucleic acid (RNA). Basic dyes show an increased avidity for the nuclei of malignant cells. This can be shown to be due to an increase in DNA content and often to an increase in chromosomal number. The staining of DNA can be standardized using the Feulgen or Gallocyanin reactions described below; the degree of DNA increase can then be calculated. Non-malignant nuclei can show a simple doubling or quadrupling of chromosome number with time, liver being a good example of this. Malignant cell nuclei often show an irregular increase in chromosome number termed 'aneuploidy'. The degree of aneuploidy has been used both as evidence for the presence of a malignant clone of cells and as a parameter in the estimation of the prognosis of some types of malignant disease. Nucleic acids are polynucleotides. A nucleotide is a phosphoric ester of a nucleoside that is the condensation product of a purine or pyrimidine nitrogenous base with a pentose or deoxypentose sugar. Both DNA and RNA contain the purine bases adenine and guanine, but the pyrimidine bases differ in that cytosine and thymine are present in DNA, and cytosine and uracil in RNA. As will be seen, the sugar differs in the two types of nucleic acids: in DNA the sugar content is deoxyribose and in RNA ribose. On hydrolysis the nucleic acids yield phosphate groups, sugars and the nitrogenous bases. The demonstration of nucleic acids depends upon the reaction of dyes with phosphate groups, and the production of aldehydes from the deoxyribose sugar in DNA. Phosphate group reactivity is commonly shown as a basophilia with cationic dyes such as methylene blue. At a low (3–4) pH both DNA and RNA are selectively stained, but are undoubtedly better shown by the methyl green-pyronin technique.

DNA DEMONSTRATION

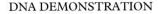

The most reliable histochemical technique for DNA is the Nucleal test, introduced

by Feulgen & Rossenbeck, that depends on the presence in DNA of a deoxyribose sugar.

FEULGEN REACTION (Feulgen & Rossenbeck 1924)

Notes

The method utilizes mild hydrolysis with M HCl in which aldehyde groups are liberated by the breaking of the purine-deoxyribose bonds. As in the PAS reaction, the aldehydes re-colour Schiff's reagent, producing the magenta colour in the nuclear chromatin. RNA is depolymerized by the hydrolysis and takes no part in the reaction. Fixation is important, e.g. Bouin's fixative will cause over-hydrolysis during fixation so is unsatisfactory as a fixative for this reaction. Other fixatives are acceptable and the hydrolysis time is adjusted accordingly. Thin rapidly fixed blocks give superior results. The hydrolysis stage is critical and is usually carried out at 60°C in M HCl. Although many alternative hydrolysing solutions are available, none produces better results. During hydrolysis a stronger reaction is obtained as the time is increased until the optimum is reached. If the hydrolysis is continued the reaction becomes weaker due to depolymerization of DNA. In cases of doubt some slides should be hydrolysed at different times. Active aldehydes occur naturally in the tissues in lipids and connective tissue fibres. These Schiff-positive structures may be present in the tissue section, and a control section should be left in distilled water while the test section is hydrolysed. The optimal times for hydrolysis are given in Table 5.3.

Table 5.3   Feulgen hydrolysis times in pre-warmed M HCl at 60°C

Fixative	Time (min)
Carnoy 6.3.1; Regaud-sublimate	8
Chrome-acetic, Regaud	14
Flemming	16
Formaldehyde vapour	30–60
Formalin, Formal-sublimate, Helly	8
Newcomer	20
Susa	18
Zenker, Zenker-formal	5

Solutions

M hydrochloric acid:

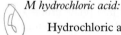

Hydrochloric acid (conc.)	8.5 ml
Distilled water	91.5 ml

Schiff's reagent (see p. 135)

Technique

1. Sections to distilled water.
2. Rinse sections in M HCl at room temperature for 1 min.
3. Place sections in M HCl at 60°C (see Table 5.3).

4. Rinse sections in M HCl at room temperature for 1 min.
5. Transfer sections to Schiff's reagent for 30 min.
6. Wash in tap water for at least 10 min.
7. Counterstain if required in 1% light green 2 min or sat. tartrazine in Cellosolve 1 min (we recommend the latter).
8. Wash in water if counterstained in light green, or in Cellosolve if tartrazine has been used.
9. Dehydrate, clear and mount as desired.

Results

DNA	magenta
Cytoplasm (depending on counterstain used)	green or yellow

NAPHTHOIC ACID HYDRAZIDE-FEULGEN FOR DNA (Pearse 1951)

Notes

This technique utilizes the aldehydes produced by hydrolysis by coupling them to a diazonium salt.

Solutions

M hydrochloric acid:

Hydrochloric acid (conc.)	8.5 ml
Distilled water	91.5 ml

NAH solution:

2-hydroxy-3-naphthoic acid hydrazide	50 mg
Absolute alcohol (ethanol)	47 ml
Acetic acid (conc.)	3 ml

Fast blue B solution:

Fast blue B	50 mg
Veronal acetate buffer, pH 7.4	50 ml

This solution must be freshly prepared.

Technique

1. Sections to distilled water.
2. Rinse briefly in M HCl.
3. Place sections in M HCl at 60°C (as for the Feulgen technique).
4. Rinse sections in M HCl at room temperature for 1 min.
5. Rinse sections in distilled water for 1 min.
6. Rinse sections in 50% alcohol for 1 min.
7. Place sections in NAH solution at room temperature for 3–6 h.
8. Rinse sections in 50% alcohol for 10 min.
9. Rinse sections in 50% alcohol for 10 min.
10. Rinse sections in 50% alcohol for 10 min.

11. Rinse sections in distilled water for 1 min.
12. Place sections in fresh fast blue B solution for 3 min.
13. Dehydrate, clear and mount as desired.

Result

DNA   blue to bluish-purple
Protein material   purplish-red

RNA/DNA DEMONSTRATION

Ribonucleic acid methods are not specific; they depend upon the non-specific property of their affinity for basic dyes. The basophilia is produced by the acidic, i.e. phosphate, groups in the nucleic acids. Methyl green is the most selective basic dye for nucleic acids. It is an impure dye and chloroform extraction is necessary to remove the crystal and methyl violet impurities. When treated in this way and used at an acid pH it appears to be specific for DNA. This is due to spatial alignment of phosphate radicals of the DNA to the NH_2 groups on the methyl green molecules. Pyronin binds to the RNA by the normal electrostatic mechanism, i.e. cationic dye to anionic nucleic acid, but there is no spatial alignment.

METHYL GREEN-PYRONIN METHOD (Pappenheim 1899, Unna 1902)

Notes

This method employs methyl green to demonstrate DNA and pyronin to stain RNA. The selectivity of pyronin for RNA is not high, but with carefully controlled conditions and careful differentiation the use of pyronin produces acceptable results for RNA and is particularly useful for the identification of plasma cells that have a high cytoplasmic concentration of RNA related to the synthesis of immunoglobulin molecules. We have found that rinsing in 93% alcohol, followed by absolute alcohol, gives better results than the usual acetone-xylene treatment (Warford 1982).

Staining solution

2% aqueous methyl green (chloroform washed)	9 ml
2% aqueous Pyronin Y	4 ml
Acetate buffer pH 4.8	23 ml
Glycerol	14 ml

Mix well before use.

Technique

1. Sections to water.
2. Rinse in acetate buffer pH 4.8.
3. Place in the staining solution for 25 min.
4. Rinse in buffer.

5. Blot dry or rinse in 93% alcohol.
6. Dehydrate, clear and mount as desired.

Results

DNA	green-blue
RNA and acid mucins	red

The following variation by Elias (1969) has worked well in our hands.

Solutions

Methyl green:

Methyl green	1 g
Acetate buffer pH 4.1	200 ml

Wash in chloroform until completely free of traces of methyl violet.

Staining solution:

Methyl green solution	100 ml
Pyronin Y	0.2 g

The solution is well stirred and stored at 4°C and filtered before use.

Technique

1. Sections to distilled water.
2. Place in the staining solution at 37°C for 1 h.
3. Rinse in distilled water at 1°C for 2 s.
4. Blot sections dry.
5. Rinse in tert-butanol.
6. Dehydrate in two changes of tert-butanol for 5 min.
7. Clear and mount as desired.

Results

DNA	green-blue
RNA and acid mucins	red

HITCHCOCK-EHRICH TECHNIQUE (Hitchcock & Ehrich 1930)

Notes

This method, based on the previous technique, has the advantage of being quick
and simple, but is more capricious than the methyl green-pyronin method. It uses
malachite green and acridine red. The authors recommend Zenker-acetic fixation,
but the method works after formalin fixation if the staining time is extended.

Solution

Malachite green 0.3 g in 15 ml distilled water. Acridine red 0.9 g in 45 ml distilled
water. Mix before use.

Technique

1. Sections to distilled water.
2. Stain in the solution for 1–5 min.
3. Wash in distilled water.
4. Dehydrate, clear and mount as desired.

Results

DNA   blue-green
RNA   red

GALLOCYANIN-CHROME ALUM METHOD (Einarson 1932, 1951)

Notes

Gallocyanin forms a red cation lake with chromium potassium sulphate. The dye lake combines with phosphate groups of nucleic acids to form a tissue–mordant–dye compound. The method demonstrates both nucleic acids, so the use of extraction techniques is necessary to isolate a specific nucleic acid. The staining is progressive and needs no differentiation. It is better not to counterstain and to avoid the use of celloidin. The method is of accepted specificity for the nucleic acids when used at a low pH (below 1.0).

Solution

Chrome alum   5 g
Distilled water   100 ml

Chrome alum is dissolved in distilled water, gallocyanin added and the solution slowly heated until it boils. Allow to boil for 5 min, cool to room temperature, adjust the volume to 100 ml and filter before use.

Technique

1. Sections to water.
2. Stain in gallocyanin-chrome alum solution (18–48 h).
3. Wash in tap water.
4. Dehydrate, clear and mount as desired.

Results

RNA, DNA   grey-blue

EXTRACTION METHODS FOR NUCLEIC ACIDS

Specific control of the staining methods discussed is possible by using extraction techniques (Table 5.4). These techniques remove or denature nucleic acids, leaving other tissue structures unaffected. Extraction is either enzymatic or chemical.

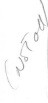

Enzymatic methods use deoxyribonuclease and ribonuclease and are specific with suitable controls.

Table 5.4 Extraction of nucleic acids

Solution	Conc.	Temp (°C)	Extracted	Type of method
Ribonuclease	0.1%	37	RNA	Enzyme
Deoxyribonuclease	0.08%	37	DNA	Enzyme
Perchloric acid	5%	60	RNA,DNA	Acidic
Perchloric acid	10%	4	RNA	Acidic
Trichloracetic acid	4%	90	RNA,DNA	Acidic
Hydrochloric acid	M HCl	37	RNA, DNA	Acidic

Ribonuclease

The enzyme splits RNA into its component nucleotides and is produced from fresh beef pancreas (Brachet 1940). A crude source of the enzyme is found in saliva (Bradbury 1956). Whilst removing RNA, the Feulgen reaction is unaffected. Mercuric chloride and potassium dichromate fixation of tissue inhibit ribonuclease digestion.

Deoxyribonuclease

There is less need for this enzyme as there are specific methods for DNA. One potential use is the selective demonstration of viral DNA as the capsids resist the penetration of deoxyribonuclease, unlike normal cell nuclear DNA (Lucia et al, 1984). It acts only on fixed tissues and is specific for nuclear DNA extraction. The Feulgen reaction is negative after treatment. Mercuric chloride and potassium dichromate fixation inhibit digestion.

Chemical extraction

Various acids can be used to extract nucleic acids from tissue sections. Depending upon the acids and the conditions used, either RNA or both RNA and DNA can be removed.

ENZYME EXTRACTION OF RNA (Brachet 1940)

Solution

Ribonuclease	8 mg
Distilled water	10 ml

Technique

1. Sections of test and controls to distilled water.
2. Place test slide and positive control slide in ribonuclease solution; place negative control slide in distilled water, both at 37°C for 1 h.

3. Wash in distilled water.
4. Apply methyl green-pyronin method (see p. 98).

Results

Test slide and positive control slide	RNA negative, DNA green
Negative control slide	RNA red, DNA green

ENZYME EXTRACTION OF DNA (Brachet 1940)

Solution

Deoxyribonuclease	10 mg
0.2 M Tris buffer, pH 7.6	10 ml
Distilled water	50 ml

Method

1. Test and control sections to distilled water.
2. Place test section and positive control slide in extraction solution, and negative control section in Tris buffer pH 7.6 only, both at 37°C for 4 h.
3. Wash in running tap water.
4. Stain both sections by the Feulgen method (see p. 96).

Results

Test section and positive control section	DNA negative
Negative control section	DNA magenta

NUCLEIC ACID EXTRACTION OF RNA WITH PERCHLORIC ACID

Note

Perchloric acid at a raised temperature extracts both RNA and DNA. RNA is removed more rapidly enabling its differential extraction, if low temperatures are used as follows.

Solution

Perchloric acid conc.	5 ml
Distilled water	45 ml
1% aqueous sodium carbonate	

Technique

1. Sections of test and control to distilled water.
2. Treat sections with the perchloric acid at 4°C for 18 h (duplicate negative control sections are placed in distilled water).
3. Rinse in distilled water.
4. Transfer to the sodium carbonate solution for 5 min.

5. Wash in tap water.
6. Apply methyl green-pyronin method (see p. 98).

Results

RNA is extracted in the treated sections.
DNA is not extracted but polymerized, which will cause it to become pyroninophilic.

NUCLEIC ACID EXTRACTION OF RNA AND DNA WITH PERCHLORIC ACID

Solution

Perchloric acid conc.	2.5 ml
Distilled water	47.5 ml
1% aqueous sodium carbonate	

Technique

1. Sections of test and control to distilled water.
2. Treat sections with the perchloric acid at 60°C for 20 min (duplicate negative control sections are placed in distilled water).
3. Rinse in distilled water.
4. Transfer to the sodium carbonate solution for 5 min.
5. Wash in tap water.
6. Apply methyl green-pyronin method (see p. 98).

Results

RNA and DNA are extracted in the treated sections.

NUCLEOLAR ORGANIZER REGION (NOR) DEMONSTRATION

'NORs' are composed of loops of DNA that transcribe for RNA and are related to cell nucleolus formation. There is a relationship between the amount present in cell nuclei, and the proliferative activity of the component cells. Not surprisingly this has led to much endeavour to relate this relationship to neoplastic lesions, using NOR quantitation. Areas of effort include lymphomas (Crocker & Nar 1987)and melanocytic lesions (Crocker & Skilbeck 1987). Normal glandular cell nuclei contain up to three NORs whereas carcinoma cell nuclei may contain up to eight. The value and efficacy of NOR demonstration in disease is questionable, and the attempt to assign quantitative parameters difficult. The technique that has evolved is the AgNOR technique.

AgNOR TECHNIQUE (Ploton et al 1986)

Notes

It is important to use thin (3 μm) sections and to observe scrupulous distilled water washing of the slides and any glassware used for preparing the solutions. When making the NOR count at the conclusion of staining, it is important to focus up and down carefully, to achieve full particle separation in any NOR aggregates. The rationale of the technique is that NORs are associated with sulphydryl group-containing proteins (nucleolin) that are argyrophilic (Rowlands 1988).

Solution

2% gelatin in 1% aqueous formic acid	1 part
50% aqueous silver nitrate	2 parts

Technique

1. Take thin paraffin sections to distilled water. Wash well.
2. Treat sections with gelatin-silver nitrate solution for 50 min in the dark.
3. Wash well in distilled water.
4. Dehydrate, clear and mount as desired.

Results

NORs	black intranuclear dots
Background	pale yellow-brown

REFERENCES

Adams C W M, Sloper J C 1955 Technique for demonstrating neurosecretory material in the human hypothalamus. Lancet 1: 651
Baker J R 1947 The histochemical recognition of certain guanidine derivatives. Quarterly Journal of Microscopical Science 88: 115
Baker J R 1956 The histochemical recognition of phenols especially tyrosine. Quarterly Journal of Microscopical Science 97: 161
Brachet J 1940 La detection histochemique des acides pentose-nucleiques. Comptes Rendus des Seances de la Societe de Biologie et de Sans Filiales 133: 88
Bradbury S 1956 Human saliva as a convenient source of ribonuclease. Quarterly Journal of Microscopical Science 97: 323
Chèvremont M, Fréderick J 1943 Une nouvelle méthode histochimique de mise en evidence des substances à fraction sulfhydrile. Archives of Biology 54: 589
Crocker P, Nar P 1987 Nucleolar organiser regions in lymphomas. Journal of Pathology 151: 111–118
Crocker P, Skilbeck N Q 1987 Nucleolar organiser regions associated proteins in cutaneous melanocytic lesions: a quantitative study. Journal of Clinical Pathology 40: 885–889
Einarson L 1932 A method for progressive selective staining of Nissl and nuclear substances in nerve cells. American Journal of Pathology 8: 295
Einarson L 1951 On the theory of gallocyanin-chromalum staining and its application for quantitative estimation basophilia. Acta Pathologica et Microbiologica Scandinavica 81: 256
Elias J M 1969 Effects of temperature, post-staining rinses and ethanol butanol dehydrating mixtures on methyl green pyronin staining. Stain Technology 44: 201
Feulgen R, Rossenbeck H 1924 Mikroskopisch-chemischer Nachweis einen Nucleinsarus von Typus der Thymonuclinsaure und die darauf berhende elektive Färbung. Von Zellkernen in Microscopischen Prepäraten Zeitshrift Physiology Chemistry 135: 203

Glenner G, Lillie R D 1959 Observations on the diazotization-coupling reaction for the histochemical demonstration tyrosine: metal chelation and formazan variants. Journal of Histochemistry and Cytochemistry 7: 416

Hitchcock C H, Ehrich W 1930 A new method for differential staining of plasma cells and of other basophilic cells. Archives of Pathology 9: 625

Hopwood D 1990 In: Bancroft J D, Stevens A (eds) Theory and practice of histological techniques, 3rd ed. Churchill Livingstone, Edinburgh

Lucia H L, Livolsi V A, Lowell D M 1984 A histochemical method for demonstrating papilloma virus infection in paraffin-embedded tissue. American Journal of Clinical Pathology 82: 589–593

Pappenheim A 1899 Vergleichende Untersuchungen über die elementare Zusammensetzung des rothen Knockenmarkes einiger Säugenthiere. Virchow's Archiv fur Pathologische Anatomie Physiologie 157: 19

Pearse A G E 1951 Review of modern methods in histochemistry. Quarterly Journal of Microscopical Science 92: 393

Ploton D, Menager M, Jeannesson P, Humber G, Pigeon F, Adnett J J 1986 Improvement in the staining and in the visualization of the argyrophilic proteins of the nucleolar organizing regions at the optical level. Histochemical Journal 18: 5–14

Rowlands D C 1988 Nucleolar organiser regions in cervical intraepithelial neoplasia. Journal of Clinical Pathology 4: 1200–1202

Stoward P J (1963) D Phil Thesis. University of Oxford

Unna P G 1902 Eine modifikation der Pappenheimschen Färbung auf Granoplasma. Monatschefte für Praktische Dermatologie 35: 76

Warford A 1982 Personal communication

Yasuma A, Itchikawa T 1953 Ninhydrin-Schiff and alloxan-Schiff staining. Journal of Laboratory and Clinical Medicine 41: 296

6. Abnormal protein deposits

AMYLOID

Amyloid was given its name by Virchow in the 1850s and indicates a starch-like material. Amyloidosis describes a condition in which a deposition of amorphous congophilic material occurs extracellularly in tissues. Organs such as the liver, spleen and kidneys may become enlarged, pale and have a 'waxy' appearance. Earliest deposits of amyloid are seen in the walls of blood vessels and, if infiltration continues, the structure is replaced and its function lost. It is usual today for amyloidosis to be diagnosed at a relatively early stage. Most surgical material we see contains small deposits in the walls of blood vessels. Amyloidosis is a disease process in which histochemistry is a useful aid in diagnosis. This gives the laboratory worker considerable responsibility because the staining methods have to be of the highest standard. In the last 35 years a considerable amount of information regarding the nature and origin of amyloid has been published and several aetiological factors identified, however the detailed pathogenesis is still incompletely understood.

Classification

Many classifications have appeared over the years to keep pace with biochemical, clinical and histopathological developments. The Reimann, Koucky and Eklund (1935) system has needed to be substantially modified by current information.

AL amyloid (primary amyloid) is almost always associated with a monoclonal band in the serum and the patient usually already has, or will develop, multiple myeloma or a related disorder. The amyloid is derived from the variable region of the Ig light chain. The tissues characteristically involved are of parenchymal origin such as blood vessel walls, muscle, skin, tongue and heart muscle, but deposits can be widely dispersed.

AA amyloid (secondary amyloid) occurs in association with a wide range of predisposing or co-existent diseases. These are usually long-standing chronic infections, such as tuberculosis, osteomyelitis and leprosy. The chronic inflammatory diseases rheumatoid arthritis and ulcerative colitis also produce deposits of amyloid. AA amyloid is most frequently found in the kidney, spleen, liver and adrenals, but it can also be seen in lymph nodes, intestine and pancreas. The AA amyloid is derived from an acute phase protein called 'serum amyloid A' protein.

Tumour-forming or tumour-associated amyloid is found in tumours of the diffuse endocrine system, particularly medullary carcinoma of the thyroid.

Familial amyloid can be seen in cases of cardiomyopathy and polyneuropathy.

Here the amyloid is derived from pre-albumin and occurs in myocardium of the heart.

Senile amyloid can be seen in the heart, brain (in senile plaques and walls of small blood vessels) and seminal vesicles. Alzheimer's disease is characterized by amyloid plaques within the cerebral structure.

Experimental amyloid is produced in animals by repeated casein injections.

Chemical composition and ultrastructure

The composition of amyloid has been a matter of speculation for many years. This has been caused by the reactivity of amyloid to carbohydrate techniques and the problems encountered in separating a true amyloid deposit from tissue structure. In recent years analyses of pure amyloid have shown that it consists of over 95% protein and between 1 and 5% carbohydrate. The carbohydrate content is mainly mucopolysaccharide, as heparan sulphate, chondroitin sulphate and dermatan sulphate (Bitter & Muir 1966, Muir & Cohen 1968). The variable chemical content of amyloid, caused by its origin, site and mode of production, affects its histological staining reactions but not its ultrastructure. The protein component has been shown to have high levels of tryptophan and tyrosine.

Amyloid has a unique ultrastructure. Under the electron microscope it appears as unbranched fibrils with no specific orientation. Each fibril consists of two electron-dense filaments 2.5–3.5 nm in diameter separated by a 2.5 nm inter-space, giving the whole fibril a diameter of 8–10 nm and a variable length that may be up to several microns (Francis 1990). These fibrils are usually found in extracellular spaces. Amyloid fibrils have been subjected to many investigations to locate an amino acid that could be used for demonstration, but to date the histochemist can only identify the proteins tryptophan and tyrosine. Eanes & Glenner (1968) showed that the amyloid fibril protein is arranged in an anti-parallel beta pleated sheet. If the pleated sheet structure is damaged by enzymatic action then the standard characteristics of amyloid—its fibrillar structure and Congo red binding with green birefringence—are lost. It has become clear that amyloid fibrils can be formed from at least six protein groups: these groups are shown below in Table 6.1, modified from Francis (1990). In addition there is also a separate non-fibrillar protein common to all the amyloid subtypes called amyloid P protein that is derived from a normal circulating protein called serum amyloid P protein.

Technique (general points)

It is well-recognized that amyloid deposits are best shown using cryostat or free-floating frozen sections, but in the routine surgical laboratory this is not usually practical. In our hands fixation does not appear critical, though in the past many of our colleagues preferred mercuric chloride-containing solutions. Long fixation over a period of years in formalin reduces the intensity of the staining reactions due to methylene bridge formation. Two of the techniques, the methyl green and DMAB-nitrite method, give their best results if applied to unfixed tissue. Cut sections containing amyloid appear to lose some of their reactivity on storage so test and control sections should be freshly cut. Not all deposits will react to staining methods in the same way. Large deposits of amyloid give a far less intense staining reaction than small deposits in vessel walls. AA amyloid produces brighter

Table 6.1   Protein groups in amyloid

Protein group	Origin	Classification
AA amyloid	Derived from serum amyloid A protein, an acute phase protein	Secondary to chronic inflammatory diseases, familial Mediterranean fever, experimentally induced in animals
AL amyloid (immunoglobulin-derived)	Immunoglobulin light chains from plasma cells & related cells	(Primary), multiple myeloma
Pre-albumin	Pre-albumin (serum)	Cardiac amyloid, senile amyloid, familial neuropathy
Diffuse endocrine system amyloid (polypeptide hormone-derived)	Calcitonin, insulin, glucagon, etc.	Insulinomas, medullary carcinoma, pituitary adenomas
A4 protein (chromosome 21)	Probably derived from an intra-membranous protein	Alzheimer's disease
β_2-microglobulin	HLA Class I antigens on cell surfaces of lymphoid and other cells	Patients on long-term renal haemodialysis

results and gives a more consistent appearance to histochemical methods than AL and other types of amyloid. On occasion AL and experimentally produced amyloid have failed to react with staining methods in our hands despite showing the characteristic ultrastructure. Therefore, positive control sections should always be used.

Microscopical appearance

In formalin sections amyloid appears as a homogeneous material staining pink-red with eosin (eosinophilic). It is weakly PAS-positive, staining green or blue with trichromes and khaki with van Gieson. It is weakly autofluorescent and birefringent. None of these methods is specific for amyloid. Using an H&E stain, small amounts of amyloid can easily be confused with other homogeneous pink-staining material such as hyaline, old collagen and fibrinoid or missed altogether. These small deposits of amyloid are difficult to see, and specialized methods are employed. At this stage it is worth considering the methods available to demonstrate amyloid (Table 6.2).

Table 6.2   Methods for amyloid

Type of method	Utilizes
Metachromasia and polychromasia	Crystal violet, methyl violet and methyl green
Selective staining	Congo red, Sirius red and related dyes
Fluorescence	Thioflavine T & S, Congo red and other fluorochromes
Polarization	Congo red, Sirius red, toluidine blue
Enzyme methods	Pepsin and other enzymes
Protein technique	DMAB-nitrite
Immunocytochemical	Use of specific antisera
Electron microscopy	Ultrastructure studies

STAINING METHODS

Iodine

Amyloid can be demonstrated in fresh tissue with iodine. The tissue is rinsed in 1% acetic acid before being treated with Gram's iodine. Amyloid deposits stain a deep brown colour. Further treatment with 10% sulphuric acid will change the colour to blue-violet. This method has traditionally been used in the post-mortem room to demonstrate macroscopically visible deposits. Fixation affects the reaction but fresh frozen sections can be treated in the same way, and if they are mounted in an iodine-glycerol mixture they will show amyloid as a purple colour.

Metachromatic or polychromatic methods

Methyl violet was first used to demonstrate amyloid as long ago as 1875 by Cornil and, with crystal violet and dahlia, has enjoyed considerable popularity. The use of these dyes is often called 'metachromasia' but this is not strictly accurate as the differential staining of amyloid is almost certainly due to the dye 'mixture' having more than one component (Cohen 1967). A correct term would be 'polychromatic' staining. Conventional metachromatic dyes such as thionin and toluidine blue do not give good results, although removal of the protein moiety by pepsin digestion will enhance toluidine blue staining (Windrum & Kramer 1957). Using a 0.1% toluidine blue at pH 5.7 with 0.1 M magnesium chloride and staining for 1 h, Mowry & Scott (1967) obtained a weak red birefringence effect with amyloid. Generally, none of these methods is satisfactory as they are non-specific (mucins also stain purple-red), and the results are often less satisfactory when mounted but we have experience of one case of idiopathic liver amyloidosis where the results with crystal violet were superior to those by the Congo red polarizing microscopy technique! Frozen sections give brighter and more easily differentiated staining than fixed sections regardless of whether or not crystal or methyl violet is used. Staining with these dyes is considered even less reliable with AL amyloid deposits. The following techniques are those that have given the best results in our hands.

CRYSTAL VIOLET TECHNIQUE (Hucker & Conn 1928)

Notes

Ammonium oxalate is added to the crystal violet solution to enhance the polychromatic effect. The slides should be examined wet before mounting as some loss of staining brightness subsequently occurs. Alcohol dehydration destroys the purple-red staining and is best avoided and an aqueous mountant used instead. The recommended one is a modified Apathy's solution, which helps to keep diffusion of dye into the mountant and subsequent fading to a minimum (avoid glycerol-jelly for these reasons).

Solutions

Staining solution

　　2 g crystal violet is dissolved in 20 ml 95% alcohol. Add 80 ml of 1% aqueous ammonium oxalate. Dissolve with the aid of gentle heat. Cool and filter.

Modified Apathy mountant (Highman 1946)

Dissolve 20 g gum arabic and 20 g cane sugar in 40 ml of distilled water using gentle heat (56°C). Add 20 g potassium acetate and 0.1 g thymol. Mix and allow to stand at room temperature to dissolve. Place in a 56°C oven and filter through a coarse (Green's) filter paper into another container also in the oven. The solution will have a tendency to set due to evaporation of solvent; this is avoided by adding pre-warmed distilled water.

Technique

1. Sections to water.
2. Stain with the crystal violet solution for 2–3 min.
3. Wash and differentiate in 0.2% acetic acid. Control differentiation using the microscope followed by washing in water for 10–30 s. Aim at removing the excess dye only.
4. Wash in water and mount in the modified Apathy's solution.

Results

Amyloid, certain mucins, colloid, renal hyaline material	red-purple
Background	blue

FORMIC ACID-CRYSTAL VIOLET TECHNIQUE (Fernando 1961)

Notes

Formic acid is used both as the diluent and differentiator for the dye and serves to accentuate the polychromatic effect. The author recommended that Helly and Bouin's fixatives should be avoided. His mountant is similar in its action to the Highman modification of Apathy's solution, but is non-setting and requires sealing with varnish. When checking differentiation it is better to rinse in distilled, as opposed to tap, water otherwise the amyloid takes on a bluish tinge.

Solutions

1% crystal violet in 3% formic acid
Mountant:

Dextrin	16.7 g
Sucrose	16.7 g
Sodium chloride	10 g
Thymol	0.01 g
Distilled water	100 ml

Mix constituents and heat in a porcelain dish with constant stirring until dissolved. Cool and filter through a coarse (Green's) filter paper.

Technique

1. Sections to alcohol.

2. Blot dry. Stain in filtered crystal violet solution for 10 min.
3. Drain and blot dry.
4. Differentiate in 1% aq. formic acid 1–3 min (nearer 1 min). Rinse in distilled water.
5. Mount either in the specified mountant or in modified Apathy's solution.

Results

Amyloid, some mucins, hyaline material	purple-red
Background tissue	blue

METHYL GREEN TECHNIQUE (Bancroft 1963)

Notes

Primary staining in methyl violet is followed by partial replacement staining with methyl green (extracted). Methyl green acts as a combined differentiator and counterstain; the time is shortened if partial differentiation in acetic acid is applied prior to the methyl green treatment. Only frozen sections give acceptable results.

Solutions

1% aqueous methyl violet
2% aqueous methyl green
   Extract with chloroform as for the methyl green-pyronin technique (see p. 112).

Technique

1. Sections to water.
2. Stain with the methyl violet solution for 2 min.
3. Wash in water and briefly (20 s) differentiate in 1% acetic acid. Wash in water.
4. Treat with the methyl green solution for 5–10 min until sufficient differentiation of methyl violet staining of the background has occurred.
5. Wash in water and mount in modified Apathy's solution.

Results

Amyloid, some mucins, hyaline material	purple-red
Nuclei	green
Background	clear

STANDARD TOLUIDINE BLUE (STB) METHOD (Wolman 1971, from Francis 1990)

Notes

This method stains many tissue components—including amyloid—an orthochromatic blue colour. Amyloid is distinguished by its striking dark red birefringence. Cooper (1974) found the mechanism of binding to be that of Congo red. Some tissue components, for example cartilage matrix, mast cell granules and other connective tissue mucopolysaccharides, stain metachromatically purple with toluidine blue that gives anomalous yellow-green polarization colours. This latter effect is probably an electrochemical bonding and can be minimized if the staining solution is saturated with sodium chloride (Cooper 1974). Occasional amyloid deposits, especially those of endocrine origin, are negative with this method and minimal deposits are sometimes difficult to visualize.

Staining solution

1% toluidine blue in 50% isopropanol

Technique

1. Well-deparaffinized sections to water, removing fixation pigment where necessary.
2. Stain in the toluidine blue solution 30 min at 37°C.
3. Blot section carefully then place in absolute isopropanol for 1 min.
4. Clear and mount as desired.

Results

Amyloid and many other tissue components stain an orthochromatic blue colour, but when examined under polarized light amyloid gives a dark red birefringence.

CONGO RED METHODS

It is well recognized that amyloid has an affinity for Congo red. Initially Congo red was used as a clinical test for amyloid. Bennhold described the first satisfactory Congo red stain. Many modifications have appeared over the years and the most useful and reliable are given below. The dye is highly selective for amyloid but not specific as collagen, elastic fibres, hyaline and corpora amylacea of brain and prostate will also stain. Congo red dye forms non-polar hydrogen bonds with amyloid. It is also a fluorochrome and will impart a red fluorescence to amyloid.

An important feature of Congo red staining is the red to green birefringence seen when using polarized light. This is due to the parallel alignment of the dye molecules on the linearly arranged amyloid fibrils (Wolman & Bubis 1965). This apple green birefringence effect was first noted by Divry & Florkin (1927) and is widely regarded as the most effective technique for the demonstration of amyloid (Missmahl & Hartwig 1953, Cohen 1967). It is not truly specific, as cellulose (Puchtler et al 1962) and young Haversian bone (Reissenweber 1969) will also exhibit Congo red-green birefringence. It has also been shown when using fixatives such as Carnoy, alcohol or Bouin that connective tissue fibres can give this effect (Klatskin 1969). In practice, Congo red-green birefringence is a reliable index for the presence of amyloid. Heptinstall (1974) reported that the green birefringence may be lacking in thin sections and recommended 6 μm thickness. A weak birefringence with Congo red staining of amyloid may occur and this requires other confirmatory techniques.

There have been many important developments in the Congo red technique, and these will be dealt with in chronological order. Other similar dyes have been tried, and of these, Sirius red has been the most successful. Whatever variant is used, frozen sections give brighter staining than paraffin sections.

HIGHMAN'S CONGO RED TECHNIQUE (Highman 1946)

Notes

An alcoholic solution of Congo red is used. Differentiation is easier to control than in the original Bennhold method and we suggest that Highman's is the method of choice out of the several allied ones in use. It is preferable to slightly underdifferentiate the Congo red as weakly reacting deposits of amyloid may be lost by over-zealous differentiation. When using this approach any non-specific background staining can be readily identified by the absence of green birefringence when examined by polarizing microscopy.

Solutions

0.5% Congo red in 50% alcohol
0.2% potassium hydroxide in 80% alcohol

Technique

1. Section to water (or alcohol).
2. Stain with the Congo red solution for 5 min. Drain.
3. Differentiate with the potassium hydroxide solution for 15–20 s until the background is clear (see Notes).
4. Wash in water, stain nuclei with an alum haematoxylin. Differentiate and blue.
5. Dehydrate, clear and mount as desired.

Results

Eosinophils, amyloid, elastin, keratin	orange-red
Nuclei	blue
Background	relatively clear

ALKALINE CONGO RED TECHNIQUE (Puchtler et al 1962)

Notes

This is a progressive method, requiring no differentiation step. Salts act as ionic competitors for the dye, and background (polar) staining is eliminated; only the non-polar binding of Congo red occurs. The main disadvantages of the method lie in its complexity and the short bench-life of the solutions used.

Solutions

Stock alcoholic sodium chloride solution
   Saturated sodium chloride in 80% alcohol (keeps well).

Working solution:

Stock solution	50 ml
1% aqueous sodium hydroxide	0.5 ml

Mix and filter, use within 15 min.

Stock Congo red stock solution

Saturated Congo red in 80% alcohol saturated with sodium chloride (keeps fairly well).

Working staining solution:

Stock solution (Congo red)	50 ml
1% aqueous sodium hydroxide	0.5 ml

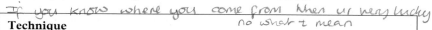

Technique

1. Sections to water.
2. Stain the nuclei with an alum haematoxylin. Differentiate and blue.
3. Treat with the alcoholic sodium chloride-hydroxide solution for 20 min. Drain.
4. Stain with the Congo red solution for 20 min. Rinse with alcohol.
5. Dehydrate, clear and mount as desired.

Results

Eosinophils, amyloid, elastin, keratin	orange-red
Nuclei	blue
Background	clear

HIGH pH CONGO RED TECHNIQUE (Eastwood & Cole 1971)

Notes

This is an ingenious and simple technique using Congo red at pH of 10.0, at which level binding of the dye by ionic forces, i.e. background staining, will not occur. Therefore differentiation is minimal. In practice, it seems that the post-staining rinsing in alcohol is critical; too long a rinse gives false negative or weak results, whilst too short a rinse causes background staining.

Staining solution

Dissolve 0.5 g Congo red in 100 ml of 50% buffered ethanol. A suitable buffer (pH 10.0) is as follows:

0.1 M glycine (mol. wt. 72.07)	30 ml
0.1 M sodium chloride (mol. wt. 58.5)	30 ml
0.1 M sodium hydroxide (mol. wt. 40)	40 ml

Technique

1. Sections to water.
2. Stain nuclei with an alum haematoxylin solution. Differentiate and blue.
3. Stain with the Congo red solution for 10–20 min.

4. Wash in 70% alcohol until the background is clear.
5. Dehydrate, clear and mount as desired.

Results

Eosinophils, amyloid, elastin, keratin	orange-red
Nuclei	blue

POTASSIUM PERMANGANATE-CONGO RED METHOD FOR AMYLOID
(Wright et al 1977)

Notes

This is a simple technique for distinguishing between the AL and AA forms of amyloid. The method is based on the altered affinity of some amyloid for Congo red after exposure to potassium permanganate and dilute sulphuric acid. Romhanyi (1972) demonstrated that amyloid fibrils were either resistant or sensitive to trypsin digestion. The resistant type was AL or immunoglobulin-derived and the sensitive type was described earlier as AA amyloid. Wright et al (1977) modified the technique by using a potassium permanganate-oxalic acid sequence instead of trypsin. In our experience this concept is of doubtful validity as we have obtained inconsistent results.

Solutions

Acidified potassium permanganate:

0.5% potassium permanganate	25 ml
0.3% sulphuric acid	25 ml

0.5% oxalic acid

Technique

1. Sections to water.
2. Treat sections with acidified potassium permanganate for $2\frac{1}{2}$ min.
3. Bleach with 0.5% oxalic acid until the section is colourless.
4. Rinse thoroughly in tap water.
5. Stain section by a Congo red method (see p. 114).

Results

AL, senile and familial polyneuropathy-associated amyloids	show positive Congo red staining
AA amyloid and β_2-microglobulin-associated amyloid	no Congo red staining

SIRIUS RED TECHNIQUE (Llewellyn 1970)

Notes

This technique is a variation on the Congo red technique of Puchtler et al (1962) (see above) using Sirius red. The dye is similar to Congo red in that it is a 'direct cotton dye' and was introduced, amongst others, as a suitable alternative to Congo red (Sweat & Puchtler 1965). The method is similar in principle to the alkaline Congo red technique incorporating various salts to enable progressive staining; it claims the added advantage that the solutions are simplified and more stable. Unfortunately, the solutions are not stable and their preparation requires expertise. Some workers have also experienced subsequent fading of the stained amyloid.

Solution

Dissolve 0.5 g Sirius red F3B in 45 ml distilled water. Add absolute alcohol 50 ml and 1% aqueous sodium hydroxide 1 ml. With vigorous mixing, slowly add sufficient 20% aqueous sodium chloride to produce a fine precipitate (using a strong backlight) and keeping the amount of added salt solution to the bare minimum (up to 4 ml). Allow to stand overnight and filter.

Technique

1. Sections to water.
2. Stain the nuclei with an alum haematoxylin. Differentiate and blue.
3. Wash in water, then 70% alcohol.
4. Stain with the Sirius red solution for 1 h.
5. Wash well in tap water. Dehydrate, clear and mount as desired.

Results

Eosinophils, amyloid, elastin, keratin	deep red
Nuclei	blue
Background	colourless

SECONDARY FLUORESCENT STAINING

The first use of fluorescent techniques for the demonstration of amyloid was by Chiari (1947), who used dyes such as thiazine red, euchrysin 26NV and thioflavine S. This type of method did not become popular until Vassar & Culling (1959) introduced thioflavine T. These two workers claimed specificity of staining for amyloid but it has become increasingly evident that many other substances also exhibit secondary fluorescent staining (Rogers 1965, Porteous et al 1966).

Several workers have attempted to increase the selectivity of thioflavine T for amyloid; for example, Mowry & Scott (1967) used a 0.1% solution of thioflavine T at pH 5.7 containing 0.4 M magnesium chloride. Burns et al (1967) lowered the pH of the dye solution from 3.6 to 1.2. This latter group of workers found that at this low pH only a few substances, other than amyloid, exhibited a yellow fluorescence with short wavelength blue ultraviolet light. In our experience thioflavine T fluorescence can only be safely used as a confirmatory method, in that a substance yielding a negative thioflavine fluorescence is most unlikely to be amyloid. The converse is not necessarily true. Thioflavine T is frequently used as a screening method.

In a correctly adjusted fluorescence microscope amyloid deposits fluoresce strongly and can easily be seen at low magnification. Other fluorochromes are used with success, notably Congo red and thioflavine S. Congo red has the advantage over both thioflavine dyes that with careful differentiation little non-specific staining will be seen. The Congo red method and two versions of the thioflavine T method are given below.

THIOFLAVINE TECHNIQUE (Vassar & Culling 1959)

Notes

Thioflavine T has an affinity for amyloid, the rationale of which has not been definitely established but is probably an electrostatic one. The solution deteriorates over a period of months and keeps better in a dark container. The fluorescence of the stained amyloid will gradually fade on storage of the sections; for best results examine a recently stained section. Whilst sections may be mounted in glycerol, satisfactory results can be obtained by using a DPX-mountant (avoid Canada balsam as this exhibits autofluorescence). The fluorescent colour of thioflavine-stained amyloid depends on the type of barrier filter used. Both iodine quartz and mercury vapour systems give good results.

Solution

Mayer's haematoxylin (see p. 25)
1% aqueous thioflavine T

Technique

1. Sections to water.
2. Stain with Mayer's haematoxylin for 2 min (to mask nuclear fluorescence). Wash in water.
3. Stain with the thioflavine solution for 3 min. Wash in water.
4. Differentiate out excess fluorochrome in 1% acetic acid for 20 min.
5. Wash well in water, blot dry. Dehydrate, clear and mount in a DPX-type mountant.

Results

a. Using a mercury vapour lamp with a red suppression filter (BG38), exciter filter (UG1) and barrier filter (K430):

    Amyloid, elastin, etc.   silver-blue

b. Using an iodine quartz or mercury vapour lamp with exciter filter (BG12) and barrier filter (K530):

    Amyloid, elastin, etc.   yellow

pH 1.4 THIOFLAVINE T (Burns et al 1967)

Notes

Low pH staining increases the selectivity by favouring the fluorochromic fraction binding to amyloid while depressing non-amyloid fluorochrome staining.

Technique

As given in the previous method but using a freshly prepared 0.5% thioflavine T in 0.1 M hydrochloric acid.

Results

Amyloid, Paneth cells	silver-blue or yellow according to filters used

CONGO RED AS A FLUORESCENCE METHOD FOR AMYLOID (Cohen et al 1959, Puchtler & Sweat 1965)

Notes

Congo red used as a fluorochrome demonstrates amyloid. Other tissue components stain, but by using a more dilute Congo red stain and differentiating well, other congophilic material is barely discernible. It is possible to overdifferentiate, but this rarely happens in practice.

Solutions

Congo red:

Congo red	0.1 g
Absolute alcohol	50 ml
Distilled water	50 ml

Differentiator:

Potassium hydroxide	0.2 g
Absolute alcohol	80 ml
Distilled water	20 ml

Technique

1. Sections to water.
2. Stain with the Congo red solution for 1 min.
3. Wash in tap water.
4. Differentiate in differentiator solution until all the section appears colourless.
5. Wash in water.
6. Dehydrate through clean alcohol and clear in fresh xylene.
7. Mount in DPX or fluoro-free mountant.

Results

Amyloid deposits	orange to red fluorescence

Table 6.3 Amyloid demonstration methods

Method	Evaluation of method	Comments
Crystal violet	Not sensitive or highly selective	Easy and quick in experienced hands. Never use alone.
Toluidine blue	Sensitive with polarization	Positive with polarization. Not to be used alone.
Congo red	Sensitive and highly selective with polarizing microscopy	The best technique if used in conjunction with polarizing microscopy.
Thioflavine T or Congo red as fluorescent dye	Sensitive but not specific	Screening method, confirmation of result required with polarization/ Congo red.
Alcian blue	Sensitive, but not specific	Time-consuming. Looks good, selective.
DMAB-nitrite	Moderately sensitive and selective	Confirms a high tryptophan content.
Electron microscopy	Distinctive fibrils	The final arbiter.
Immunocyto-chemistry	Specific	May replace Congo red in due course when a more comprehensive panel of antisera becomes available.

OTHER STAINING METHODS

Many dyes have been tried in an attempt to find a specific method for amyloid. Most of these attempts have concentrated on staining the mucopolysaccharide content rather than the proteins present in deposits.

ALCIAN BLUE TECHNIQUE (Lendrum et al 1972)

Notes

Pennock et al (1968) used alcian blue at pH 1.0 and 5.7 with added magnesium ions. The drawback to their method is that mucin is also stained by the alcian blue. This staining varies depending upon the pH of the alcian blue and the molarity of the magnesium salt. The method below, which uses 0.5% alcian blue and sodium sulphate to suppress background staining, has proved reliable in our hands. Alcian blue at pH 1.0 stains recent amyloids bright green. The colour is rendered fast by alkalization in borax.

Solutions

Acetic-alcohol (prepare fresh):

95% ethanol	45 ml
Distilled water	45 ml
Acetic acid (conc.)	10 ml

Alcian blue solution (prepare fresh):

1% alcian blue in 95% ethanol	45 ml
1% aqueous hydrated sodium sulphate	45 ml
Acetic acid	10 ml

Allow to stand for 30 min before use.

Saturated borax in 80% alcohol

Technique (slightly modified)

1. Sections to water.
2. Rinse in the acetic-alcohol solution.
3. Stain with the alcian blue solution for 2 h. Rinse in the acetic-alcohol, then in water.
4. Alkalinize in the borax solution for at least 30 min. Wash in water.
5. Apply van Gieson's technique (see p. 36).
6. Rinse in distilled water or alcohol. Dehydrate, clear and mount in a DPX-type mountant.

Results

Recent amyloid, some colloids	bright green
Old amyloid	paler green or non-reactive
Collagen	red
Muscle	yellow

DMAB-NITRITE TECHNIQUE (Adams 1957)

Notes

Tryptophan, when treated with p-dimethylaminobenzaldehyde (DMAB), produces b-carboline and this, when oxidized by sodium nitrite, forms an insoluble blue pigment. This is of value when a suspected amyloid deposit, showing Congo red staining, gives only weak birefringence. Only tryptophan-rich substances such as amyloid and fibrin react, other Congo red-positive materials like elastin do not. Deposits giving positive Congo red staining and a positive DMAB-nitrite reaction are most likely to be amyloid (Cooper 1969). The diffuse endocrine system amyloid is low in tryptophan content however, and thus DMAB-negative. Lengthy formalin fixation will cause a negative reaction. The technique employs a strong acid, and it will be found useful to mount sections on slides using an adhesive, and to prepare the reagents in a well-ventilated atmosphere.

Solutions

5% DMAB in conc. hydrochloric acid
1% sodium nitrite in conc. hydrochloric acid
1% aqueous neutral red

Technique

1. Take a known positive control and the test sections to alcohol. Celloidinize.
2. Harden the celloidin film in water, then rinse in distilled water and drain.
3. Treat with the DMAB-HCl solution for 1 min. Drain.
4. Transfer sections to the sodium nitrite-HCl for 1 min with continuous agitation.

5. Wash in water for 30s, then in 1% acid-alcohol for 15 s. Wash well. Counterstain in the neutral red solution for 5 min.
6. Wash, dehydrate, clear and mount as desired.

Results

Tryptophan-rich tissues, i.e. amyloid, fibrin, fibrinoid, Reinke crystals, Paneth cell granules, eosinophil cell granules   dark blue
Nuclei   red

ENZYME METHODS

Amyloid deposits in paraffin sections seem little affected by enzymes. Cooper (1974) tried eleven enzymes and found that the routine staining methods were little changed in their reactivity to amyloid following treatment. Work using unfixed cryostat sections, however, shows that some types of amyloid are affected by enzyme activity and others are not. AL amyloid, for instance, shows resistance to all types of enzymes whereas AA amyloid in unfixed sections can be sensitive to digestion. This difference accords with their behaviour in staining methods.

PEPSIN DIGESTION

This is a useful adjunct to the standard techniques. Amyloid is not digested by low pH pepsin treatment, whereas other tissue components are. Absence or presence of digestion can be subsequently confirmed by counterstaining the sections with light green; failure of the background tissues to stain is taken as evidence of digestion.

Notes

Sections are mounted on slides with an adhesive. The pepsin powder should be fresh (several weeks shelf-life) as we have experienced technique failure due to deteriorated samples.

Solutions

Digestion solution
0.2 g pepsin is dissolved in 40 ml of 0.02 M HCl, giving a solution of pH 1.6
Highman's Congo red solution and differentiator (see p. 114)
Counterstain
0.2% light green in 0.2% acetic acid.

Technique

1. Two sections of known control material and two test sections to distilled water.
2. Treat one section of each pair with the pre-heated pepsin solution and the remaining two sections with 0.02 M hydrochloric acid only for 4 h at 37°C.

3. Wash sections well in water for several minutes.
4. Carry out the Congo red technique on all sections, differentiating as appropriate and staining the nuclei with alum haematoxylin. Wash well.
5. Counterstain all sections with the light green solution for 30 s.
6. Wash, dehydrate, clear and mount as desired.

Results

Amyloid in both treated and untreated sections	pale red
Non-amyloid in the treated section	colourless
Non-amyloid in the untreated section	green
Nuclei	blue

IMMUNOCYTOCHEMISTRY

Being largely protein in nature, amyloid should be ideal material for demonstration by immunocytochemical means. Unfortunately, because of its inherently diverse nature, the epitopes present will vary so that no one antiserum can act as a universal marker for amyloid. This is particularly the case with the AL type of amyloid which is less consistently demonstrable than, say, the AA form (Francis 1990).

The antigenic variability of amyloid is undoubtedly the main reason immunocytochemistry is not a commonplace method for its detection, and a pan-amyloid marker remains a desirable future development. There is still a role for immunocytochemistry, either when the Congo red-green birefringence effect is equivocal or to identify the precise type of amyloid present, which the tinctorial methods are unable to do with any certainty.

The following is a brief account of the range of appropriate antisera now available for use with conventionally prepared paraffin sections:

AA protein—can be successfully employed for the demonstration of the secondary type of amyloid.

Immunoglobulin light chains (kappa-lambda) are used for the demonstration of AL amyloid, but are unreliable. A negative result does not rule out AL amyloid as this is derived from the variable region of homogeneous light chains that also varies from patient to patient (van de Kaa et al 1986). A more profitable course might be to use a combined approach of Congo red and light chain positivity, with anti-AA protein negativity.

Amyloid P component—a glycoprotein present in all types of amyloid except that which occurs in the CNS plaques of Alzheimer's disease. Unfortunately it is not a particularly sensitive marker and is, moreover, not specific for amyloid. It is found, for example, in elastic tissue (Elias 1990).

β_2-microglobulin—a polypeptide occurring normally in cell membranes. It is particularly linked to renal dialysis-associated amyloidosis where it presents in various tissues including synovium (Fitzmaurice et al 1991). Generally it is not considered a reliable amyloid marker (Elias 1990).

Pre-albumin—not very reliable as a general amyloid marker (Francis 1990), but will demonstrate the type found in the familial polyneuropathies. As with the anti-amyloid P component, Alzheimer disease-associated deposits are negative.

ELECTRON MICROSCOPY

Amyloid has an ultrastructure that appears unchanged despite the tissue origin, the type of amyloid or the age of the deposit. The amyloid fibril structure is unique, enabling the electron microscopist to confirm that a suspect deposit is amyloid.

SUMMARY

In the surgical laboratory today it is rare to receive a case with massive deposits of amyloid and, as Francis (1990) states, 'the cases today involve material with minimal deposits often only in the walls of blood vessels'. The needle biopsy and other small biopsy techniques are responsible for early diagnosis along with the clinical awareness of the disease. In both our laboratories the rectal biopsy appears to be the clinicians' method of choice. The small biopsy has both advantages and drawbacks; recently deposited amyloid reacts more intensely with staining solutions than long-standing deposits, so that the demonstration is easier. On the other hand the amount of tissue is small and orientation important, so that considerable care is required. In the staining of rectal biopsies it must be remembered that mucin is also present and will be reactive with polychromatic, metachromatic and possibly other methods.

The laboratory has at its disposal an ever increasing number of staining methods for the demonstration of amyloid, but in reality at the current time only the Congo or Sirius red techniques with polarization should be used for diagnosis (Table 6.3). The other methods are useful confirmatory techniques, unless of course one is fortunate enough to have access to an electron microscope, which would take priority.

FIBRIN AND FIBRINOID

Fibrin is an insoluble fibrillar protein formed from plasma fibrinogen; it contains basic amino acids which give it a strong acidophilia. In its early stages of development it is seen as fine threads, later becoming a homogeneous mass. Fibrin occurs in tissues where damage is due to an acute inflammatory reaction, particularly of serous membranes, which produces a transfer of fluid and plasma proteins from damaged blood vessels; the plasma fibrinogen polymerizes forming insoluble fibrin.

Fibrinoid is similar in appearance, being an amorphous, eosinophilic material. Its staining reactions are as for fibrin with occasional variations. It appears in tissues in different locations from fibrin, being often seen within blood vessel walls where the vessel has undergone necrosis, in glomerulonephritis and connective tissue disease. There is doubt about the true nature of fibrinoid—the consensus is that it is a mixture of fibrin with additional proteins from blood plasma; alternatively fibrinoid may be fibrin that has undergone an ageing process (Lendrum et al 1962).

Demonstration of fibrin

Fibrin is seen stained bright red in an H&E preparation, and is PAS-positive. It is orthochromatic, monorefringent and weakly autofluorescent. Due to its tryptophan content it is DMAB-nitrite-positive (see p. 121). In practice many staining methods demonstrate it; some are listed in Table 6.4. Fibrin itself does not always react to dyes in the same way: long-standing deposits tend to stain in a similar manner to collagen. The method of choice is the MSB of Lendrum et al (1962) that is given below. Formalin fixation is usually adequate although better results are obtained with trichrome-type methods if Helly's solution is used.

Table 6.4 Staining reactions of fibrin

Stain	Fibrin
MSB (and other trichromes)	Red
PAS	Magenta
PTAH	Blue
Gram–Weigert	Blue-black
Phloxine-tartrazine	Red
DMAB-nitrite	Blue
Schmorl	Blue
Fuchsin-Milling yellow	Red
Acid picro-Mallory	Red
Eosin	Red
van Gieson	Yellow

MARTIUS YELLOW-BRILLIANT CRYSTAL SCARLET-SOLUBLE BLUE (MSB) (Lendrum et al 1962)

Notes

This method initially uses a small molecule yellow dye, which, when combined with phosphotungstic acid in alcoholic solution, will selectively stain red cells. It is possible that early deposits of fibrin will also take up the dye, the phosphotungstic acid blocking subsequent staining of other tissue structures. A medium-sized molecule red dye is then used to stain muscle and mature fibrin. The staining of collagen is prevented by the phosphotungstic acid used earlier. Additional treatment with aqueous phosphotungstic acid removes any red staining from collagen fibres. A large molecule blue dye is then applied to stain collagen and old fibrin. Lendrum et al (1962) strongly recommend the use of mercuric chloride fixation; in its absence post-fixation in Helly is advisable. Thin sections are necessary to achieve satisfactory results with the method.

Solutions

0.5% martius yellow (syn. naphthol yellow) in 2% phosphotungstic acid in 95% alcohol
1% brilliant crystal scarlet 6R (syn. crystal ponceau) in 2.6% acetic acid
1% aqueous phosphotungstic acid
0.5% soluble blue (syn. aniline blue ws) in 1% acetic acid

Technique

1. Sections to water and stain the nuclei with a suitable iron haematoxylin solution (see p. 86). Rinse in 95% alcohol.
2. Stain with the martius yellow solution for 2 min. Wash briefly in water.
3. Stain with the brilliant crystal scarlet solution for 10 min. Wash in water.
4. Treat with the phosphotungstic acid solution for 5–10 min. Wash in water.

5. Stain with the soluble blue solution for 10 min. Wash in water and blot dry.
6. Dehydrate, clear and mount as desired.

Results

Fibrin	red
Muscle	paler red
Nuclei	blue-black
Collagen	blue
Red blood cells	yellow

FUCHSIN-MILLING YELLOW TECHNIQUE (Slidders 1961)

Notes

This is similar in principle to the previous technique. Acid fuchsin staining is followed by phosphotungstic acid and progressive replacement and counterstaining with the dye Milling yellow. Fibrin is clearly shown against the yellow background; it is possible to displace much of the red dye in the muscle with the counterstain.

Solutions

1% acid fuchsin in 2.5% acetic acid
1% aqueous phosphotungstic acid
2.5% Milling yellow 3G in Cellosolve

Technique

1. Sections to water and stain the nuclei with a suitable iron haematoxylin solution (see p. 37).
2. Treat with the acid fuchsin solution for 3–5 min.
3. Rinse in water. Treat with the phosphotungstic acid solution for 5 min. Wash in water.
4. Rinse well in Cellosolve.
5. Differentiate and counterstain in the Milling yellow solution until only the fibrin is deeply stained red. This usually takes from 30 min to 1 h.
6. Rinse in Cellosolve. Clear and mount as desired.

Results

Fibrin	bright red
Muscle	very weak red
Nuclei	blue-black
Background (e.g. collagen, red blood cells)	yellow

ACID PICRO-MALLORY TECHNIQUE (Lendrum 1949)

Notes

This is similar in principle to the trichrome techniques; it stains fibrin strongly and muscle weakly.

Solutions

0.2% orange G in saturated alcoholic picric acid
1% acid fuchsin in 3% trichloracetic acid
1% aqueous phosphomolybdic acid
2% aniline blue ws in 2% acetic acid

Technique

1. Sections to water and stain the nuclei with a suitable iron haematoxylin solution (see p. 37). Differentiate so that the background is reasonably clear.
2. Rinse in 95% alcohol and stain with the picro-orange solution for 2 min.
3. Wash in water for 5–10 s until only the red blood cells are yellow.
4. Treat with the acid fuchsin solution for 5 min.
5. Wash briefly in water, then treat with equal parts of the picro-orange solution and 80% alcohol for a few seconds.
6. Differentiate in the phosphomolybdic acid solution for 5–10 min.
7. Wash in water. Stain with the aniline blue solution for 5–10 min.
8. Wash, dehydrate, clear and mount as desired.

Results

Fibrin	bright red
Muscle	paler red
Nuclei	blue-black
Collagen	blue
Red blood cells	yellow-orange

TRYPSIN DIGESTION (Glynn & Loewi 1952)

Notes

Using trypsin at an alkaline pH the authors claim that although fibrin is digested, fibrinoid and collagen are not. In our limited experience with the technique, reasonably good results are obtained although it is often necessary to extend times of treatment. Formalin fixation is satisfactory.

The usual source of enzyme is beef pancreas. In human tissue the spermatozoon acrosome is rich in trypsin, where it is largely responsible with hyaluronidase for the breakdown of the zona pellucida of the ovum during fertilization.

Digestion solution

Dissolve 0.1% trypsin in pH 8.0 phosphate buffer and add 1% w/v calcium chloride.

Technique

1. Two sections of positive control material and the test material to water.
2. Rinse well in distilled water.
3. Treat one test and one positive control section with the pre-heated trypsin

solution for 3 h at 37°C. The remaining duplicate sections are treated with pH 8.0 buffer only, for the same time and temperature.
4. Wash all sections well in water for 5–10 min.
5. Carry out a suitable technique for fibrin (the MSB technique gives good results).
6. Dehydrate, clear and mount as desired.

Results

If the MSB technique is used subsequent to digestion:

Fibrin in undigested sections	red
Fibrin in digested sections	not stained

IMMUNOCYTOCHEMISTRY

Antisera for the immunocytochemical demonstration of fibrin (anti-fibrinogen) are widely available—either with FITC for immunofluorescence, or with peroxidase for immunoperoxidase techniques. Their principal use is in renal pathology and both types of label have their adherents.

Davison et al (1973) contrasted the use of tinctorial techniques, electron microscopy and immunocytochemistry for the demonstration of fibrin in tissue sections. Their conclusions were that only immunocytochemistry afforded results that were truly specific. As might be imagined, the dye methods were more subjective and even electron microscopy could show false positivity if immunoglobulin deposits were present.

REFERENCES

Adams C W M 1957 A p-dimethylaminobenzaldehyde nitrite method for the histochemical demonstration of tryptophan and related compounds. Journal of Clinical Pathology 10: 56
Bancroft J D 1963 Methyl green as a differentiator and counterstain in the methyl violet technique for the demonstration of amyloid. Stain Technology 38: 336
Bitter T, Muir H 1966 Mucopolysaccharides of whole human spleens in generalised amyloidosis. Journal of Clinical Investigation 45: 963
Burns J, Pennock C A, Stoward P J 1967 The specificity of the staining of amyloid deposits with thioflavine T. Journal of Pathology and Bacteriology 94: 337
Chiari H 1947 Ein Beitrag zur sekundaren Fluoreszensdesogen localen Amyloids. Mikroscopie 2: 79
Cohen A S 1967 Amyloidosis. New England Journal of Medicine 277: 522
Cohen A S, Calk E, Levine C I 1959 Analysis of histology and staining reactions of casein induced amyloidosis in the rabbit. American Journal of Pathology 35: 971
Cooper J H 1969 An evaluation of current methods for the diagnostic histochemistry of amyloid. Journal of Clinical Pathology 22: 410
Cooper J H 1974 Selective amyloid staining as a function of amyloid composition and structure. Laboratory Investigation 31: 232
Davison A M, Thomson D, MacDonald M K, Rae J K, Utterly W S, Clarkson A R 1973 Identification of intrarenal fibrin deposition. Journal of Clinical Pathology 26: 102–112
Divry P, Florkin M 1927 Sur les propriétés optiques de l'amyloide. Comptes Rendus de Séances de la Société de Biologie et Ses Filiales 97: 1808
Eanes E D, Glenner G G 1968 X-ray diffraction studies on amyloid filaments. Journal of Histochemistry and Cytochemistry 16: 673

Eastwood H, Cole K R 1971 Staining of amyloid by buffered Congo red in 50% ethanol. Stain Technology 46: 208

Elias J M 1990 Immunohistopathology: a practical approach to diagnosis. ASCP Press, Chicago

Fernando J C 1961 A durable method of demonstrating amyloid in paraffin sections. Journal of the Institute of Science Technology 7: 40

Fitzmaurice R J, Bartley C, McClure J, Ackrill P 1991 Immunohistological characterisation of amyloid deposits in renal biopsy specimens. Journal of Clinical Pathology 44: 200

Francis R J 1990 Amyloid. In: Bancroft J D, Stevens A (eds) Theory and practice of histological techniques. Churchill Livingstone, Edinburgh

Glynn L E, Loewi G 1952 Fibrinoid necrosis in rheumatic fever. Journal of Pathology and Bacteriology 64: 329

Heptinstall R H 1974 Pathology of the kidney, 2nd edn. Vol 2. Little & Brown, Boston

Highman B 1946 Improved methods for demonstrating amyloid in paraffin sections. Archives of Pathology 41: 559

Hucker G J, Conn H J 1928 A quick stain for staining Gram-positive organisms in the tissues. Archives of Pathology 5: 828

Klatskin G 1969 Non-specific green birefringence in Congo-red stained tissues. American Journal of Pathology 56: 1

Lendrum A C 1949 Staining of erythrocytes in tissue sections; a new method and observations on some of the modified connective tissue stains. Journal of Pathology and Bacteriology 61: 442

Lendrum A C, Fraser D S, Slidders W, Henderson R 1962 Studies on the character and staining of fibrin. Journal of Clinical Pathology 15: 401

Lendrum A C, Slidders W, Fraser D S 1972 Renal hyalin: a study of amyloidosis and diabetic fibrinous vasculosis with new staining methods. Journal of Clinical Pathology 25: 373

Llewellyn B D 1970 An improved Sirius red method for amyloid. Journal of Medical Laboratory Technology 27: 308

Missmahl H P, Hartwig N 1953 Polarisation-optische Untersuchungen an der Amyloidsubstanz. Archive für Pathologische Anatomie 324: 489

Mowry R W, Scott J E 1967 Observations on the basophilia of amyloids. Histochemie 10: 8

Muir H, Cohen A S 1968 In: Mandema E, Ruinen L, Scholten J G, Cohen A S (eds) Symposium on amyloidosis. Excerpta Medica, Amsterdam

Pennock C A, Burns J, Masserella G 1968 Histochemical investigation of acid mucosubstances in secondary amyloidosis. Journal of Clinical Pathology 21: 578

Porteous I B, Beck J S, Curie A R 1966 The pituitary acidophil: a comparison of its staining reactions with anti-human growth hormone and thioflavine T. Journal of Pathology and Bacteriology 91: 539

Puchtler H, Sweat F 1965 Congo red as a fluorescence stain for microscopy of amyloid. Journal of Histochemistry and Cytochemistry 13: 693

Puchtler H, Sweat F, Levine M 1962 On the binding of Congo red by amyloid. Journal of Histochemistry and Cytochemistry 10: 355

Reimann H A, Koucky R F, Eklund C M 1935 Primary amyloidosis limited to tissue of mesodermal origin. American Journal of Pathology 11: 977

Reissenweber N J 1969 Dichroism with Congo red. A specific test for amyloid? Virchow's Archives (Pathol Anat) 347: 254

Rogers D R 1965 Screening for amyloid with the thioflavin T fluorescent method. American Journal of Clinical Pathology 44: 59

Romhanyi G 1972 Differences in ultrastructation organisation of amyloid as revealed by sensitivity or resistance to induced proteolysis. Virchow's Archives (Pathol Anat) 357: 29

Slidders W 1961 The Fuchsin-Miller method. Journal of Medical Laboratory Technology 18: 36

Sweat F, Puchtler H 1965 Demonstration of amyloid with direct dyes. Archives of Pathology 80: 613

van de Kaa C A, Hol P R, Huber J, Linke R P, Kooiker C J, Gruys E 1986 Diagnosis of the type of amyloid in paraffin wax embedded tissue sections using antisera against human and animal amyloid proteins. Virchow's Archives (Pathol Anat) 408: 649

Vassar P S, Culling F A 1959 Fluorescent stains with special reference to amyloid and connective tissue. Archives of Pathology 68: 487

Windrum G K, Kramer H 1957 Fluorescent microscopy of amyloid. Archives of Pathology 63: 373

Wolman M 1971 Amyloid its nature and molecular structure: comparison of a new toluidine blue polarised light method with traditional procedures. Laboratory Investigation 25: 104

Wolman M, Bubis J J 1965 The cause of the green polarisation colour of amyloid stained with Congo red. Histochemie 4: 351

Wright J R, Calkins E, Humphrey R L 1977 Potassium permanganate reaction in amyloidosis. Laboratory Investigation 36: 274

7. Carbohydrates

A simple carbohydrate molecule is a monosaccharide such as glucose that plays a central role in nutrition but is highly soluble and difficult to demonstrate within tissues. Glycogen, a polysaccharide, represents a store of food in liver and muscle and consists of a long chain of sugar molecules. Shorter and more complex chains of sugar molecules may be covalently linked to protein and lipid molecules forming glycoproteins and glycolipids respectively. The carbohydrate component modifies the function of the main protein or lipid molecule.

MUCINS

CONNECTIVE TISSUE MUCINS

The gel-like consistency of much of the extracellular connective tissue is due to the presence of glycosaminoglycans. These are long unbranched chains of disaccharides where one of two sugars in the repeating disaccharide unit is an amino sugar (such as N-acetyl glucosamine or N-acetyl galactosamine). Usually the amino sugar is sulphated and the second sugar is a uronic acid. Hence these molecules usually carry a high negative charge. Most glycosaminoglycans are linked to protein molecules to form proteoglycans. Hyaluronic acid is the exception in that it is not linked to a protein molecule and lacks sulphated sugars. It is probably the most primitive form of glycosaminoglycan in evolutionary terms, being found particularly in the early embryo and in a variety of adult tissues and fluids.

EPITHELIAL MUCINS

Epithelial mucins consist of a variety of glycoproteins. These consist of a protein molecule attached to an oligosaccharide by an amino sugar linkage. The oligosaccharide may consist largely of mannose groups or have a more complex structure with branched chains containing amino sugars and sialic acid terminal groups.

NEUTRAL MUCINS

These are epithelial mucins with no reactive acid radical but with free hexose groups present, i.e. glycoprotein with high mannose oligosaccharide. They are found in gastric mucosa, prostate gland and, to a variable extent, in goblet cells elsewhere. They are PAS-positive but do not stain with alcian blue.

ACID MUCINS: SULPHATED

Strongly acidic (connective tissue)

These proteoglycans, with one exception (keratan sulphate), contain sulphated glucuronic acid moieties. They react at low pH levels (0.5) with cationic dyes, are PAS-negative and occur in tissues such as skin, cartilage, bone, blood vessel walls and umbilical cord. In this group are chondroitin-4-sulphate, chondroitin-6-sulphate (chondroitin sulphates A and C), dermatan sulphate, heparin/heparan sulphate and keratan sulphate.

Strongly acidic (epithelial)

These mucins react similarly to the above group in their reactions with cationic dyes but are PAS-positive and epithelial in origin. An example of this type of mucin has been reported in bronchial serous glands (Lamb & Reid 1970).

Weakly acidic

These mucins are mainly epithelial in origin and stain with cationic dyes at pH 1.0. They are found, for example, in goblet cells of the colonic mucosa.

ACID MUCINS: CARBOXYLATED

N-acetyl sialomucin (sialidase-labile sialomucin)

These mucins are epithelial in origin and contain a sialic acid molecule that reacts at pH levels of 2.0 and above with cationic dyes, the bonding taking place with carboxyl groups. They are identified by their ready extraction with the enzyme sialidase, are PAS-positive and are present in salivary and bronchial glands.

N-acetyl-O-acetyl sialomucin (sialidase-resistant sialomucin)

This group is composed almost entirely of sialomucins that are resistant to sialidase extraction. These mucins are also epithelial in origin and react, in terms of alcian blue staining, similarly to the enzyme-labile sialomucins. They are found in colonic goblet cells and are PAS-negative.

Hyaluronic acid

This glycosaminoglycan, i.e. connective tissue mucin, is found in umbilical cord. The reactive site is a carboxyl group that stains with pH 2.5 alcian blue, but is PAS-negative.

ACID MUCINS: SULPHATED SIALOMUCINS

This is a controversial group, the existence of which has yet to be fully established. Histochemically they give reactions for sulphated mucins and yet are extracted by sialidase. They have been reported in prostatic tumours (Hukill & Vidone 1967), sheep colon (Kent & Marsden 1963) and malignant synovioma (Cook 1973).

MUCINS AND PATHOLOGY

The different staining characteristics of mucins can be useful in diagnostic histopathology. Thus the presence of epithelial type-mucin in the tissues may support the diagnosis of an invasive adenocarcinoma whereas connective tissue mucin production may be increased in a non-specific tissue reaction. It is clearly important to be able to distinguish between these two categories.

Intestinal metaplasia in the stomach can be readily identified using alcian blue staining at an acid pH for acid non-sulphated mucin and the high iron diamine reaction to demonstrate sulphated mucins. Normal gastric mucin consists largely of neutral non-sulphated mucins.

Filipe (1972) proposed the idea that the reduction in sulphated glycoproteins (and an increase in sialomucin) in intestinal mucosa was an indicator of premalignant change in carcinoma of the large bowel. It has subsequently been argued that this change may be a consequence rather than a precursor of neoplasia. It may still be of some value as a marker of a premalignant change although it is somewhat variable.

FIXATION AND PROCESSING

Most routine fixatives are suitable; neutral buffered formalin is recommended, but Bouin's is not recommended (Cook 1959, Goldstein 1962, Allison 1973). This, however, does not apply to the component mucins of the mucopolysaccharidoses where alcohol or acetone fixation is employed. Decalcification procedures affect the histochemical reactions and must be chosen with care. Charman & Reid (1972), in a survey, considered that the best histochemical results with mucins could be obtained following either formic acid, sodium formate or EDTA treatment. Freeze-dried tissues are the best basis for the demonstration of mucins, but paraffin processing is satisfactory and is normally used. Floating out sections on 70% alcohol as opposed to water may on occasion be advisable when studying connective tissue mucins, as diffusion from the section may occur into the water. Details of staining techniques for mucins are given below and their staining reactions in Table 7.1.

Table 7.1   Significant techniques for mucins and glycogen

	SAB	LAB	PAS	BPAS	HID	D	Si	Hy
Polysaccharide								
Glycogen	−	−	+	±	−	dig	−	−
Hyaluronic acid	+	−	−	−	−	−	−	dig
Mast cells	±	+	−	−	+	−	−	−
Neutral mucin	−	−	+	−	−	−	−	−
Sialomucin								
a. enzyme labile	+	−	+	−	−	−	dig	−
b. enzyme resistant	+	−	−	+	−	−	−	−
Strongly sulphated								
a. connective tissue	V	+	−	−	+	−	−	Vdig
b. epithelial	V	+	+	−	+	−	−	−
Weakly sulphated	+	+	V	−	+	−	−	−

Key: SAB = standard (pH 2.5) alcian blue; LAB = low (0.2) pH alcian blue; PAS = periodic acid-Schiff; BPAS = borohydride-saponification-PAS; HID = high iron diamine; D = diastase digestion; Si = sialidase digestion; Hy = hyaluronidase digestion; dig = digested; V = variable reaction; + = stained; − = unstained; ± = weakly stained.

GENERAL TECHNIQUES

See Figure 7.1 for mucin identification scheme.

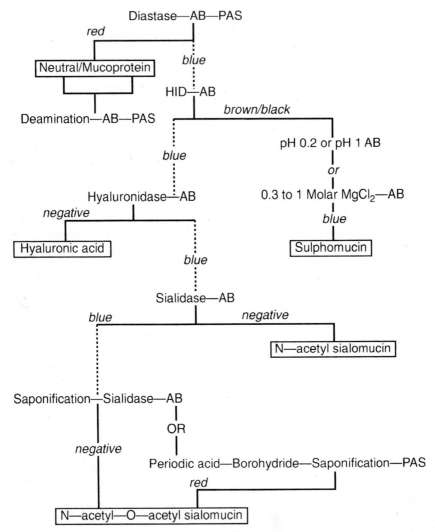

Fig. 7.1   Mucin identification scheme.

PAS TECHNIQUE

Neutral mucins react positively with the PAS technique, as do sialidase-labile sialo-mucins (Quintarelli et al 1960). Weakly sulphated mucins vary in reactivity whilst the connective tissue's strongly sulphated mucins and hyaluronic acid are negative. Scott & Dorling (1969) showed that 1:4 linked uronic acid-containing mucins, such as chondroitin sulphate, may give a positive Schiff reaction by employing a long pre-oxidation step. For normal demonstration purposes it is unimportant whether the McManus (below) or the Hotchkiss variant is used. Glycogen will react positively, and in frozen sections lipidopolysaccharides, i.e. sphingomyelin, may also react.

PERIODIC ACID-SCHIFF TECHNIQUE (PAS) (Schiff 1866 McManus 1946)

Notes

Substances containing vicinal glycol groups or their amino or alkylamino derivatives are oxidized by periodic acid to form dialdehydes, which combine with Schiff's reagent to form an insoluble magenta compound. Such substances are of the carbohydrate group and this method is used in their indentification.

In Schiff's reagent the chromophoric groups of basic fuchsin are broken by sulphuration to form a colourless solution. In the presence of free aldehyde groups an insoluble coloured compound similar, but not identical, to the original dye is formed. Periodic acid is the oxidant used to avoid over-oxidation of the formed aldehydes to carboxyl groups and thereby producing a weak or negative reaction. For basement membranes (basal lamina), longer times than for the conventional PAS technique should be used to give the best results, i.e. periodic acid 10 min, and 20–25 min in Schiff reagent. The use of post-Schiff sulphite rinses to reduce background colouration is not necessary, provided washing in running water is thorough and that the alkalinity of the tap water is not too high.

Table 7.2 lists substances that might be expected to react with the PAS technique.

Table 7.2   PAS-positive substances in tissue

α–antitrypsin	Amoebae and *Balantidium coli*	Amyloid (weakly)
Basement membranes	Cellulose	Cerebrosides
Chitin	Collagen (weakly)	Corpora amylacea
Elastin (weakly)	Fibrin	Fibrinoid
Fungi	Gastric mucous neck cells	Glycogen
Granular cell myoblastoma	Lipofuscins (some)	Lymphoblasts
Melanosis coli pigment	Megakaryocytes	Muscle type Z fibres
Mycobacterium avium intracellulare	*M. leprae* (weakly)	Myelocytes
Neutral mucin	Neutrophils	Organisms, various
Paneth cell granules	Pancreatic zymogen granules	Pituitary basophils
Plasma and serum	Platelets	Reticulin
Russell bodies	Sialomucins (N-acetyl)	Starch
Thyroid and pituitary colloid		

Solutions

1% aqueous periodic acid
Schiff's reagent:

Basic fuchsin (for Feulgen and Gomori)	1 g
Distilled water	200 ml
Potassium or sodium metabisulphite	2 g
Analar conc. hydrochloric acid	2 ml
Decolourizing charcoal	2 g

Bring the distilled water to the boil, remove flame (to avoid excessive effervescence), and add the basic fuchsin. Mix, cool to 50°C and add the meta-bisulphite. Mix and cool to room temperature before adding the hydro-chloric acid and charcoal. Leave overnight in the dark at room temperature. Filter and store at 4°C in a dark container. In use it will change from colourless to pale yellow to pink due to loss of sulphur dioxide, causing restoration of the basic fuchsin colour. When this happens the solution should be discarded.

Technique

1. Sections to distilled water.
2. Treat with the periodic acid solution for 5 min (see Notes).
3. Rinse well in distilled water.
4. Treat with Schiff's reagent for 15 min (see Notes).
5. Wash in running tap water for 5–10 min (this intensifies the colour reaction).
6. Stain nuclei with Harris's haematoxylin solution (see p. 125). Differentiate and blue.
7. Dehydrate, clear and mount as desired.

Results

PAS-positive material (see below)	magenta
Nuclei	blue or blue-black

THE MILD PAS TECHNIQUE

The mild PAS technique uses a weak periodic oxidation step to demonstrate the N-acetyl sialomucins selectively (Roberts 1977). This concept is based on the biochemical observation (Clancy & Whelan 1967) that sialic acid side chains are more rapidly oxidized by periodate than other sugars. The weak oxidation can be achieved by treating sections with 0.01% aqueous periodic acid instead of the usual 1% solution.

LECTINS

Another means of demonstrating sugars, free and in their nitrogenated form, in tissue is to take advantage of their specific lectin affinities. Lectins are proteins of non-immune origin, mainly from plants but also from certain animal tissues such as eels and snails, which are capable of binding to sugars in tissue preparations. Each iso-lectin binds to a particular sugar, but different lectins bind to tissue moieties to varying degrees, even though they may have the same sugar specificity.

There are many different types of lectin in histochemical use: examples of commonly used ones are concanavilin A (from jack bean), wheatgerm, Helix pomatia (from snail), and gorse. These have an affinity for mannose, glucosamine, galactosamine and fucose sugars respectively. Ulex europeus I, which is extracted from gorse, is of some practical importance. It can be used as a marker for endothe-lial cells and tumours of vascular origin although it is not specific (Leathem 1990, personal communication). Peanut agglutinin identifies both macrophages and histiocytes as well as the Reed–Sternberg cells of Hodgkin's disease. More specifically, lectins (leuko-agglutinin) have been used to identify the β 1-6 complex type oligosaccharide grouping on tumour cells and identify that its presence correlates with an increased metastatic potential (Dennis et al 1987). The technique employs a variety of labels, immunoperoxidase being probably the most popular in direct or indirect form. This is either a direct application to the slide of a conjugated lectin, or an indirect approach where there is an initial lectin treatment with a subsequent conjugated anti-lectin treatment.

LECTINS TECHNIQUE USING ULEX EUROPEUS I

Notes

The various solutions should be prepared fresh for consistent results. A range of lectins is supplied by Sigma Chemical Ltd. Antisera to the lectins are available from Dako Ltd. These are not the only suppliers but their reagents have worked well in our hands. Controls are important; positive and negative should be stained with the test material.

Solutions

3% hydrogen peroxide in methanol
Trypsin
  Dissolve 0.1 g trypsin and 0.1 g calcium chloride in 100 ml distilled water that has been pre-heated to 37°C. Adjust PH to 7.8 using 0.1 M sodium hydroxide solution.
UEA I lectin
  Dissolve 10 mg/1 ml buffer and add 1 mM each of calcium chloride, magnesium chloride and manganese chloride (activators for the reaction).
Anti-lectin antiserum
  Dilute 1:100 with buffer.
Biotinylated swine anti-rabbit antiserum
  Dilute 1:1500 with buffer.
ABC reagent
  Prepared as per kit instructions (AB Complex—HJRP kit, Dako Ltd.).
Diaminobenzidine-hydrogen peroxide
  Dissolve 5 mg DAB in 10 ml buffer and add 0.1 ml of 1% hydrogen peroxide.
Buffer—0.05 M Tris-HCl-saline pH 7.6

Technique

1. Sections to water.
2. Treat with hydrogen peroxide-methanol for 10 min.
3. Wash in water, then treat with trypsin for 12 min at 37°C.
4. Wash in water. Rinse with buffer for 5 min.
5. Treat with lectin solution for 30 min. A negative control is used, treating a duplicate section with lectin solution to which has been added a 0.1 M concentration of fucose.

6. Wash in buffer. Treat with anti-UEA for 30 min.
7. Wash in buffer. Treat with biotinylated secondary antiserum for 30 min.
8. Wash in buffer. Treat with ABC reagent for 30 min.
9. Wash in buffer. Treat with DAB reagent for 5 min.
10. Wash in buffer, then in water.
11. Stain the nuclei in an alum haematoxylin, differentiate and blue.
12. Dehydrate, clear and mount as desired.

Results

Lectin-positive material (UEA I for endothelial cells)	brown
Nuclei	blue

METACHROMASIA

The ability to react metachromatically is a property of both carboxylated and sulphated mucins, while neutral mucins are *orthochromatic*. *Metachromasia* is a property exhibited by negatively charged entities (polyanions) with certain cationic dyes. They react to form dye polymers that have a different absorption characteristic from the normal dye (monomer) and a different colour emission. For example, azure A exhibits a purple-red metachromasia and a blue orthochromasia, i.e. non-metachromasia colour. This is known as a *hypsochromic* shift in light absorption. It is a shift in absorption toward the shorter wavelengths of light with a consequent shift in colour emission towards the longer wavelengths of light (the opposite reaction is termed bathochromic). Metachromatic dyes such as azure A and toluidine blue may be used at a varying pH in a similar manner to alcian blue. *Metachromasia* below pH 4.0 indicates the presence of sulphated mucins, above 4.0 hyaluronic acid also reacts (Spicer 1960). Precise mucin identification by metachromatic dyes is difficult and unreliable and is little used in critical work. One important use for metachromatic staining is the demonstration of the labile mucins found in the mucopolysaccharidoses. Here the usual techniques for mucins give unsatisfactory results, with the exception of the low pH alcian blue method.

AZURE A TECHNIQUE (Hughesdon 1949)

Notes

This reliable technique produces a reasonably alcohol-fast metachromasia to a wide range of acidic mucins. The alcohol-fast metachromasia is attributed to a pre-oxidation step using potassium permanganate, and the bright staining effect to uranyl nitrate as a differentiator (the sialomucins giving a particularly bright metachromasia). Poor results can usually be traced to unsatisfactory batches of dye.

Solutions

1% aqueous potassium permanganate
5% aqueous oxalic acid

0.2% aqueous azure A
0.2% aqueous uranyl nitrate

Technique

1. Sections to water.
2. Treat with the potassium permanganate solution for 5 min.
3. Wash in water. Bleach with the oxalic acid solution.
4. Wash well in water for several minutes.
5. Stain with the azure A solution for 5 min.
6. Wash briefly in water. Differentiate in the uranyl nitrate solution for 10–30 s with agitation until a lighter general staining effect is achieved.
7. Wash in water and blot dry. Dehydrate, clear and mount in a DPX-type mountant.

Results

Mucins	purple-red
Background	blue

RELEASING PROTEIN-BOUND CARBOHYDRATE

DEAMINATION TECHNIQUE (From Lillie 1954)

Notes

On occasions a particular carbohydrate moiety is prevented from reacting histochemically by the protein fraction to which it is chemically bound. This is often the case when dealing with mucoproteins where removal of the protein amino groups allows the 'unmasked' carbohydrate, such as sialic acid, to react with suitable dyes.

The technique described is useful and employs van Slyke's reagent to destroy protein groups. The rationale of the technique is that nitrous acid formed by the action of acetic acid on sodium nitrite releases nitrogen which converts the primary amino groups to hydroxyl groups. The combined alcian blue-PAS, if carried out post-deamination, shows a change from a PAS to an alcian blue reactivity in suitable material. Deamination can be used in histological practice for blocking acidophilic reactions (which are invariably amino group based).

One incidental effect of deamination is that cell nuclei become alcianophilic. This is presumably because in the absence of the nuclear proteins the large alcian blue molecules are able to enter the intermicellar spaces of the nucleic acids and link with negatively charged phosphate radicals. Celloidinization of slides may be necessary to avoid section loss during treatment, but remove the celloidin film prior to alcian blue staining.

Solutions

van Slyke's reagent:

Sodium nitrite 6 g in 35 ml distilled water
Add 5 ml acetic acid and mix. Prepare fresh.

1% alcian blue in 3% acetic acid.
1% aqueous periodic acid
Schiff's reagent (see p. 135)

Technique

1. Two test and two positive control sections to distilled water.
2. Treat one section of each with the van Slyke reagent for 15 h at room temperature. The remaining duplicate sections should be treated with 5% acetic acid for the same period.
3. Wash all sections in water for 5–10 min.
4. Carry out the combined alcian blue-PAS technique (see p. 149).
5. Dehydrate, clear and mount as desired.

Results

Deaminated material containing previously masked polyanions will show a loss of PAS positivity and a gain in alcian blue reactivity.

SOUTHGATE'S MUCICARMINE (Mayer 1896 Southgate 1927)

Notes

This is an earlier empirical technique and has enjoyed considerable vogue for mucin staining. It is useful for staining fungi such as *Cryptococcus neoformans* but for mucin demonstration it has little to commend its use. It uses a complex solution, has a lengthy staining time and is imprecise in staining. It has been shown (Cook 1968) that neutral mucins stain weakly or not at all. The strongly sulphated mucins are variable in their reaction, whilst the other acidic mucins (particularly hyaluronic acid) stain strongly. In its favour is the fact that, like alcian blue, it seems specific for mucins.

The solution incorporates aluminium salts and the rationale of staining is one of a positively charged carmine–mordant complex bonding with the negatively charged acid mucins. The nuclei are well-stained to avoid subsequent masking by the mucicarmine. Ehrlich's haematoxylin is not used as it stains some mucins.

Staining solution

Grind 1 g carmine and place in a large (500 ml) conical flask. Add 100 ml of 50% alcohol and mix. Add 1 g aluminium hydroxide, mix and add 0.5 g anhydrous aluminium chloride. Mix and boil gently for $2\frac{1}{2}$ min. Cool and filter. Store at 4°C where it will keep for 6 months or so.

Technique

1. Sections to water
2. Stain the nuclei with an alum haematoxylin solution (see Notes). Differentiate well in acid-alcohol and blue.

3. Stain with the mucicarmine solution for 20 min.
4. Wash in water, dehydrate, clear and mount as desired.

Results

Mucins	red
Nuclei	blue

METHODS FOR CARTILAGE

Demonstrating cartilage is principally done by staining the component mucins of the dense matrix. These mucins are connective tissue in type, mainly of the strongly acidic sulphated group. Some hyaluronic acid is also present.

Techniques such as aldehyde fuchsin (see p. 58), high iron diamine (see p. 152), low pH alcian blue (see p. 147) and high molarity magnesium chloride alcian blue (see p. 147) give good results. Cartilage matrix is also PAS-positive, due to the presence of glycoprotein. Glycogen, which is present in the chondrocyte lacunae, is also PAS-positive. *Metachromasia* is usually strong with dyes such as thionin, toluidine blue and azure A (see p. 138). Safranin exhibits a bathochromic metachromasia staining cartilage yellow, against the red non-cartilaginous elements. H&E staining of cartilage is variable, the basophilia (haematoxyphilia) is more pronounced when Ehrlich's solution is used. There are no important aspects of fixation and preservation to note. The floating out of paraffin sections may need to be carried out on warm 70% alcohol rather than water, to avoid the diffusion of mucoid material.

METHODS FOR MAST CELLS

Mast cells were described by von Recklinghausen in the early 1870s and subsequently demonstrated by Ehrlich in 1877. They are found in loose connective tissue such as the external muscle layers of the gastrointestinal tract and in fibroadenosis of the breast. They are also found as mucosal mast cells in the lamina propria of the intestines. Contrary to belief, they are not seen to any great extent in normal human skin, where they can be located around dermal blood vessels, nerves and skin appendages.

The characteristic granules are not easily distinguished in an H&E preparation of human tissue; they are more readily distinguished in animal tissue. The granules are rich in heparin, a strongly sulphated acid mucin; hence their metachromasia and reactions with low pH alcian blue and aldehyde fuchsin techniques. Mucosal mast cells are smaller than the connective tissue mast cells, with less pronounced granules and containing less heparin and histamine. In certain species, e.g rat, there is also a high content of 5-hydroxytryptamine (5HT) so that the appropriate histochemistry will be obtained (see p. 226). In human tissue this is not significant. Most fixatives are suitable, with mercuric chloride and alcoholic solutions, particularly Carnoy, giving the best results. Besides the two techniques to be described in detail, the following methods may be used: alcian blue—either low pH such as 0.2 or 0.5, or with added electrolyte such as 0.4 M magnesium chloride (see p. 147); Giemsa (see p. 70); aldehyde fuchsin; azure A (see p. 138); methyl green-pyronin (see p. 98); chloroacetate esterase (see p. 313).

THIONIN TECHNIQUE (Cook 1961)

Notes

The method makes use of the alcohol-resistant metachromasia exhibited by mast cell granules to give highly selective staining. The alkaline pH of tap water is used as a diluent for the stain and aids the metachromatic effect. Slightly overdifferentiate in the acetic acid for the best results.

Staining solution

Prepare a stock 0.6% aqueous thionin solution, and into a Coplin jar filled with tap water filter approximately 0.5 ml of dye solution.

Technique

1. Sections to water.
2. Stain with the solution for 20–30 min.
3. Wash, differentiate in 0.2% acetic acid until only the cell nuclei and mast cell granules are stained purple, controlling microscopically.
4. Wash in water, dehydrate clear and mount in a DPX-type mountant. Alternatively rinse in alcohol and counterstain in saturated tartrazine in Cellosolve for 30s. Wash in alcohol, clear and mount as desired.

Results

Mast cell granules	purple
Cell nuclei	blue
Background	clear if not counterstained, yellow if counterstained

PINACYANOL TECHNIQUE (Bensley 1952)

Notes

This method gives clear-cut results allied to a simple staining technique. Unfortunately, the staining solution is complex and the dye expensive. Staining is by the interaction of pinacyanol with erythrosin; the resultant precipitate ('erythrosinate') is highly selective when dissolved in alcohol for mast cell granules. The reaction is probably a polychromatic one.

Solutions

Stock solution

Allow 0.1. g pinacyanol to dissolve in 100 ml distilled water (with initial mixing) overnight in the dark. Dissolve 0.1 g erythrosin in 100 ml distilled water and add 75 ml of this to the pinacyanol solution with agitation. A precipitate will appear that will increase as more erythrosin solution is added (a drop at a time with constant mixing). If too much erythrosin is added poor results will be obtained. To determine when the optimal precipitate has been produced, test by adding one drop of solution to a Whatman number 1 filter paper. When the resultant diffusion ring is just faintly pink then precipitation is complete. If not pink, continue adding a few more drops of erythrosin solution with constant mixing. Do not overshoot. Finally, filter the solution discarding the filtrate and drying the deposit on the filter paper at 37°C. When dry, dissolve the precipitate in 150 ml of ethanol and store at 4°C in a dark bottle. The stock solution should keep for up to 1 year.

Working solution:

Stock solution	5 ml
30% ethanol	45 ml

Mix and discard after use.

Technique

1. Sections to water.
2. Stain with the solution for 20–30 min.
3. Blot dry, differentiate if necessary in 95% alcohol, clear and mount as desired.

Results

Mast cell granules	purple-red
Cell nuclei	blue

ALCIAN BLUE-SAFRANIN METHOD FOR MAST CELLS (Csaba 1969)

Notes

This method is said to differentiate between the mast cells containing heparin and those with histamine (Csaba 1969).

Staining solution

Alcian blue	0.9 g
Safranin	0.045 g
Ferric ammonium sulphate	1.2 g
Acetate buffer pH 1.42 (see Appendix 3)	250 ml

Technique

1. Sections to tap water.
2. Stain in the alcian blue-safranin solution for 15 min.
3. Rinse in tap water.
4. Dehydrate in tertiary butyl alcohol, clear and mount in DPX.

Results

Mast cells containing biogenic amines (histamine)	blue
Mast cells containing heparin	red

METHODS FOR MESOTHELIOMA

This tumour arises most frequently in the pleura but also in peritoneum and pericardium. It is not common but is of interest histochemically as it often presents diagnostic problems that can often be solved by using the appropriate supportive techniques. In exfoliative cytology, it is virtually impossible to differentiate mesothelioma cells from primary lung adenocarcinoma cells in serous fluid smears.

It has been shown that hyaluronic acid is present in a small but significant number of cases of mesothelioma (Wagner et al 1962), as is glycogen (Wagner et al 1962, Cook 1973). These tumours show a cellular picture varying from fibroblast-type cells to epithelial-type cells with well-marked glandular spaces; there is often a mixture of the two elements. Fibroblast-type tumour cells rarely show either hyaluronic acid or glycogen. Any hyaluronic acid present is likely to be in small amounts. In our experience it is sometimes necessary to conserve the mucin present by floating out paraffin sections on alcohol rather than water to prevent diffusion of the mucin. It is also worth applying the dialyzed iron-Perls technique besides alcian blue, as it is a more sensitive marker for scanty deposits of acid mucin.

The following is a scheme for demonstrating the presence of hyaluronic acid or glycogen in a suspected mesothelioma. It is important that only mucin contained in or produced by the tumour cells be considered, and not that present as a non-specific stromal inflammatory reaction. Immunocytochemistry also has an important role to play in the diagnosis of this tumour (see Ch. 12).

Technique

1. Tissue blocks are paraffin processed in the conventional manner. Twelve serial sections are floated out on warm water in the usual way and picked up on serially numbered acid-alcohol washed slides (see p. 32). A duplicate set of sections is floated out on warm 70% alcohol. All slides are then heat-dried.
2. Sections from both sets of slides (alcohol and water floated-out) are stained by the standard alcian blue method (see p. 146), dialysed iron-Perls (see p. 148) and by alcian blue-PAS and diastase alcian blue-PAS (see p. 149). The two sets of alcian blue and dialyzed iron-Perls treated sections are examined microscopically and sections selected for subsequent hyaluronidase digestion, based on which method evidenced the greatest amount of mucin. Where possible, floating out sections on water is preferable to alcohol as the latter incurs a greater degree of section loss from the slide during staining.
3. Selected test sections, with positive control sections, are subjected to hyaluronidase digestion (see p. 160) followed by either the alcian blue or dialyzed iron-Perls technique (whichever had proved better). Any material digested by the enzyme is stained to differentiate sulphated from carboxylated acid mucin. Sometimes it is necessary to confirm hyaluronic acid (carboxylated) is present rather than sulphated mucins.

Interpretation of histochemical results with alcian blue and dialyzed iron-Perls techniques

Positive staining by tumor cells that is abolished by prior hyaluronidase digestion is most likely to be due to the presence of hyaluronic acid. This finding supports a diagnosis of mesothelioma. Acid mucin present in tumour cells and not digested by the enzyme would indicate an epithelial neoplasm.

Alcian blue-PAS technique

The PAS result is significant in this instance; a positive reaction that was abolished by prior diastase digestion indicates glycogen in the tumour cells. This finding supports a diagnosis of mesothelioma, although not as significant a parameter as the presence of hyaluronic acid. Alternatively, should the PAS-positive material be undigested by diastase treatment, then it would denote the presence of neutral mucin. This finding would not support a diagnosis of mesothelioma and would indicate an adenocarcinoma. Such a conclusion would be further supported if, besides neutral mucin, the tumour cells contained acid mucin that was unaffected by hyaluronidase digestion (as previously mentioned).

METHODS FOR THE MUCOPOLYSACCHARIDOSES

Notes

In the various types of mucopolysaccharidosis glycosaminoglycans (GAG) are deposited in abnormal amounts in the various connective tissues, also in such cells as histiocytes and hepatocytes. It will be remembered that for their demonstration it is necessary to avoid aqueous solutions during fixation, processing and section preparation. Consequently it is important to liaise, beforehand, with the clinician taking the specimen so that cryostat sections can be cut.

Besides the techniques to be described the abnormal GAG may be satisfactorily demonstrated using low, i.e. pH 0.2, alcian blue. Suggested positive control materials are normal heart valve and aorta, if positive mucopolysaccharidosis material is not available.

TECHNIQUE FOR FRESH FROZEN SECTIONS (Dorling 1980, Crow et al 1983)

Solutions

Saturated azure A in absolute alcohol
Saturated azure A in 70% alcohol

Technique

1. Prepare 15 μm thick fresh cryostat sections (preferably using snap-frozen tissue, although this is not essential).
2. Place in the azure A in absolute alcohol solution for 10 min.
3. Transfer to the azure A in 70% alcohol solution for 5–10 min.
4. Dehydrate rapidly through absolute alcohol, clear and mount in a synthetic mountant.

Results

    Glycosaminoglycans   red-purple
    Tissue background   blue

TECHNIQUE FOR PARAFFIN SECTIONS (Gardner 1968)

Solution

0.25% toluidine blue in pH 4.5 buffer (see Buffer tables)

Technique

1. Paraffin sections from tissue fixed 3 hours in Carnoy's fluid (and floated out on alcohol) are taken to alcohol and blotted dry.
2. Stain with the toluidine blue solution for 10 s only.
3. Blot dry, dehydrate, clear and mount in a synthetic mountant.

Results

    Glycosaminoglycans   red-purple
    Tissue background   blue

METHODS FOR ACID MUCINS

ALCIAN BLUE TECHNIQUE

Notes

This dye—first used in the dyeing of cotton—was introduced by Haddock (1948). It was subsequently presented as a histochemical technique by Steedman (1950). Alcian blue, alcian yellow, and the mixtures of the two known as alcian green 2 GX and alcian green 3 BX, are copper phthalocyanin dyes containing positively charged groups capable of salt linkage with certain polyanions.

These polyanions consist of sulphate and carboxyl radicals of acid mucins; the phosphate radicals of nucleic acid do not react. Consequently acid mucins are stained intensely and permanently. Although certain insoluble calcium deposits in tissue will stain through their non-protein-bound phosphate radicals, the staining of mucins by the alcian dyes can be safely regarded as specific. The standard solution for staining acid mucins is 1% alcian blue in 3% acetic acid.

Varying the pH of the solution produces more information concerning the types of acid mucin present. At a pH of 0.2 strongly sulphated mucins are ionized and react, at pH 1 weakly and strongly sulphated mucins react, whilst at pH 2.5 most acid mucins will stain. A word of caution: using pH staining variation it is not always possible to obtain clear-cut demarcation of different mucins. Better results may sometimes be obtained using varying electrolyte molarities of alcian blue solutions, the critical electrolyte concentration (CEC) effect. The CEC-type techniques rely, according to the originators, on electrolytes such as magnesium chloride when incorporated into the staining solution, competing with alcian blue molecules for points of attachment with acid mucins. The point at which staining ceases, due to electrolyte competition, is the CEC point and varies according to the substrate used. For example, below a molarity of 0.06 magnesium chloride both carboxyl and sulphate groups stain with alcian blue. Above a molarity of 0.2–0.3 only sulphate radicals should stain (Scott & Dorling, 1965, Scott et al 1968, Dorling 1969).

Alcian blue solutions should be filtered before use; they slowly deteriorate with age and should be discarded after 6 months. Low pH and CEC stain solutions deteriorate more rapidly and are prepared prior to use. Celloidin is strongly stained by the alcian dyes and should be avoided. Staining times are not critical and the ones specified are ample. Counterstaining should be minimal to avoid masking any weak alcian blue reactions.

VARYING pH TECHNIQUE

Solutions

pH 3.1: dissolve 1 g alcian blue in 100 ml of 0.5% acetic acid
pH 2.5: dissolve 1 g alcian blue in 100 ml of 3% acetic acid
pH 1.0: dissolve 1 g alcian blue in 100 ml of 0.1 M hydrochloric acid
pH 0.2: dissolve 1 g alcian blue in 100 ml of 10% sulphuric acid
0.5% aqueous neutral red

Technique

1. Sections to distilled water.
2. Filter on the appropriate dye solution and leave for 5 min.
3. If the lower pH solutions are being used, drain and blot dry to prevent any alteration in staining due to water washing. Otherwise wash in water briefly.
4. Counterstain in 0.5% aqueous neutral red for 2–3 min.
5. Wash in water. Dehydrate, clear and mount as desired.

Results

At pH 3.1 and 2.5 most acid mucins (excepting some of the strongly sulphated group)	blue
At pH 1.0 only weakly and strongly sulphated acid mucins	blue
At pH 0.2 only the strongly sulphated group	blue
Nuclei	red
Background	pale red to colourless

CRITICAL ELECTROLYTE CONCENTRATION TECHNIQUE (CEC)
(Scott & Dorling 1965)

Solutions (these should be prepared fresh for use)

0.05% alcian blue in 0.2 M acetate buffer pH 5.8 (see Appendix 3)
Prepare a range of different molarity electrolyte solutions with the above, using magnesium chloride ($MgCl_2$ $6H_2O$ M.W. = 203:30). Having calculated the amount of salt required, add to the 0.05% alcian blue solution, mix well and

filter. Note that the magnesium chloride is a deliquescent salt and is stored under airtight conditions. The following range of varying molarity magnesium chloride-alcian blue solutions is suggested as a useful workable scheme:

0.06 Molar	(1.22 g in 100 ml of buffered alcian blue solution)
0.2–0.3 Molar	(6.09 g in 100 ml of buffered alcian blue solution)
0.5–0.6 Molar	(10.15 g in 100 ml of buffered alcian blue solution)
0.7–0.8 Molar	(14.21 g in 100 ml of buffered alcian blue solution)
0.9–1.0 Molar	(18.27 g in 100 ml of buffered alcian blue solution)

Technique

1. Take five identical sections to water.
2. Stain one section in each of the different alcian blue solutions overnight, i.e. 16–18 h.
3. Wash in water and counterstain in 0.5% aqueous neutral red, 2–3 min.
4. Wash in water, dehydrate, clear and mount as desired.

Results

0.06 M MgCl$_2$-alcian blue	all acid mucins stain blue and there is a weak background reaction
0.2/0.3 M MgCl$_2$-alcian blue	weakly and strongly sulphated mucins stain blue only
0.5/0.6 M MgCl$_2$-alcian blue	strongly sulphated acid mucins stain blue only
0.7/0.8 M MgCl$_2$-alcian blue	heparin/heparan sulphate and keratan sulphate stain blue only
0.9/1.0 M MgCl$_2$-alcian blue	keratan sulphate stains blue only

DIALYZED IRON-PERLS TECHNIQUE (Hale 1946)

Notes

The use of dialyzed iron-Prussian blue reaction to visualize acid mucins is a more sensitive technique than alcian blue, but produces non-specific staining (Casselman 1962, Korhonen & Makela 1968). Whilst strong colouration of acid mucins is certainly afforded, we prefer the simpler alcian blue technique for routine use, although the dialyzed iron-Perls technique is useful for scanty deposits of acid mucins. As with the alcian blue technique, it is possible to combine with the PAS method to afford a similar tinctorial distinction between acid and neutral mucins. The rationale of the method is that at a low pH (1.9) colloidal iron is selectively adsorbed on to acidic groups of mucin. The adsorbed iron is subsequently visualized by forming Prussian blue with potassium ferrocyanide. As any haemosiderin present in the tissue will also react, it is important to take through a duplicate control section that is treated with the ferrocyanide-hydrochloric acid mixture only. Consequent colouration should be borne in mind when assessing the results of the test section. It will be found that a shorter-than-usual application of ferrocyanide-hydrochloric acid is necessary to avoid an undesirable heavy reaction with the colloidal iron and consequently heavier background. The dialyzed iron solution deteriorates with time and should not be used when more than 3 months old.

Solutions

Stock dialyzed (colloidal) iron solution (Bancroft 1975)
  Add 2.2 ml of 29% aqueous ferric chloride to 125 ml of boiling distilled water and stir well. When the colour darkens, allow to cool. Store at 4°C.
Working dialyzed iron solution:

Dialyzed iron solution	20 ml
Conc. acetic acid	5 ml
Distilled water	15 ml

2% aqueous potassium ferrocyanide
2% hydrochloric acid
1% aqueous neutral red

Technique

1. Test and a duplicate control section to distilled water.
2. Treat the test section only with the dialyzed iron-acetic acid solution for 10 min.
3. Wash well in several changes of distilled water.
4. Treat both test and control sections with a filtered solution of equal parts of potassium ferrocyanide and hydrochloric acid for 10 min.
5. Wash well in distilled water.
6. Counterstain with neutral red for 5 min.
7. Dehydrate, clear and mount in a synthetic resin.

Results

Acid mucins, haemosiderin	dark blue
Collagen	pale blue
Nuclei	red

In the duplicate control section (not treated with dialyzed iron) only haemosiderin will be blue.

SEPARATING ACID FROM NEUTRAL MUCINS

COMBINED ALCIAN BLUE-PAS TECHNIQUE (Mowry 1956)

Notes

This is a useful technique for distinguishing between acid and neutral mucins, demonstrating most mucins in a single preparation. In practice a negative result, i.e. alcian blue and PAS-negative, means a given substance is unlikely to be a mucin. The rationale of the method is that acid mucins stain first with alcian blue and are unable to react with the subsequent PAS. Following on with the PAS, only neutral mucins and carbohydrates such as glycogen will stain red.

When a haematoxylin nuclear stain is used it is important to stain lightly to prevent cytoplasmic staining action as a potential source of confusion with the alcian blue. Mayer's haematoxylin is suitable. Alcian green and yellow are not suitable for this combined technique as they are easily masked by the PAS.

Solutions

1% alcian blue in 3% acetic acid
1% aqueous periodic acid
Schiff's reagent (see p. 135)
Mayer's haematoxylin (see p. 25)

Technique

1. Sections to distilled water.
2. Treat with the alcian blue solution for 5 min.
3. Wash well in distilled water.
4. Treat with the periodic acid solution for 5 min.
5. Wash well in distilled water. Then treat with Schiff's reagent for 15 min.
6. Wash in running water for 10 min.
7. Stain the nuclei with Mayer's haematoxylin solution. Differentiate and blue (see Notes).
8. Dehydrate, clear and mount as desired.

Results

Acid mucins	blue
Neutral mucins (and glycogen)	red
Mixtures	purple
Nuclei	pale blue

METHODS FOR NEUTRAL MUCINS

These are widely occuring carbohydrates of epithelial origin not possessing histo-chemically demonstrable anionic radicals, for example they do not stain with alcian blue. The reactive side chain hexose groups permit their demonstration with PAS-based techniques. One such has already been described (the combined alcian blue-PAS technique, see p. 149) and a blockade-PAS reaction is given below, together with a technique employing carmine staining. Although neutral mucins and mucoprotein react in a similar manner histochemically, there are fundamental differences. The latter, in contrast to neutral mucin, may be derived from epithelium or connective tissue and has a dominant protein moiety that may mask a reactive polyanion such as sialic acid (see p. 139).

PHENYLHYDRAZINE-PAS FOR NEUTRAL MUCIN (Spicer 1961)

Notes

Aldehydes produced from neutral mucins can be blocked by phenylhydrazine so that they are subsequently Schiff-negative; acid mucins are not blocked. The rationale of this differential blockade devolves on the negatively charged phenylhy-drazine molecules being repelled by negatively charged polyanions such as those of N-acetylated sialomucin and so not blocked. Neutral mucins being electrostatically neutral, do not repel the phenylhydrazine, with which they condense and become Schiff-negative. Other normally PAS-positive substances such as glycogen and mucoproteins are also blocked. The phenylhydrazine solution is prepared fresh; the dry reagent itself has a reasonably long shelf-life at room temperature. As is usual with this type of method one set of slides is treated with phenylhydrazine and another set with solvent only so that final comparisons can be made.

Solutions

1% aqueous periodic acid
5% aqueous phenylhydrazine hydrochloride
Schiff's reagent (see p. 135)

Technique

1. Positive control and test sections to distilled water.
2. Treat all sections with periodic acid for 5 min.
3. Wash well in distilled water and treat the positive control and test sections with phenylhydrazine for 1 h. Duplicate sections are allowed to remain in distilled water for that period.
4. Wash the treated sections in running water for 5 min, then rinse well in distilled water.
5. Treat all sections with Schiff's reagent for 15 min.
6. Wash in running tap water for 5–10 min.
7. Stain the nuclei with a suitable haematoxylin such as Harris's solution (see p. •••). Differentiate and blue as per usual.
8. Dehydrate, clear and mount as desired.

Results

Neutral mucins	negative
Periodate-reactive acid mucins	magenta
Nuclei	blue

CARMINE FOR NEUTRAL MUCINS (Berger & Pizzolato 1975)

Notes

A simplified Best's carmine solution is employed in this technique for neutral mucin, which is stained a bright red colour along with glycogen. To a lesser degree cell nuclei, elastin and keratin will also stain. The authors' suggested rationale is that of hydrogen bonding of the carmine by hydroxyl groups on the neutral mucin complexes. As with Best's carmine technique (see p. 162) the high (12.0) pH of the solution prevents dye-to-tissue binding based on ionic interactions alone. The carmine solution may be used for staining or preceded by alcian blue staining to give a combined demonstration of acid and neutral mucins in a similar manner to the combined alcian blue-PAS technique (see p. 149). The technique is easy to perform and seems, in our limited experience, to give reproducible results.

Solutions

1% alcian blue in 3% acetic acid

Carmine solution
Dissolve 1 g potassium carbonate in 100 ml of 70% alcohol, then add 1 g carmine and mix thoroughly. Filter. The solution remains stable for up to 3 days at 4°C.

Technique

1. Sections to water.
2. Stain with alcian blue for 5 min.
3. Wash in water, then in 70% alcohol.
4. Stain with the carmine solution for 30–45 min.
5. Wash in 95% alcohol (washing in water will extract the stain), then in absolute alcohol. Clear and mount as desired.

Results

Neutral mucin and glycogen	red
Cell nuclei, keratin and elastin	pale red
Acid mucins	blue

METHODS FOR SULPHATED MUCINS

HIGH IRON DIAMINE FOR SULPHOMUCINS (Spicer 1965)

Notes

Sulphated mucins are clearly and specifically demonstrated by this method, the standard technique for the demonstration of this large and complex group of substances. The rationale is that, by treating sections with a mixture of certain diamine salts and ferric chloride, a black-brown cationic complex is formed that bonds to sulphate-containing moieties. The specificity of the technique is due to the low (1.4) pH of the reactant solution, at which pH level carboxylated moieties are non-ionized. It is important that the times of treatment are not exceeded, otherwise non-sulphated mucins progressively react. Following the staining of sulphomucins with high iron diamine, counterstaining with a pH 2.5 alcian blue solution stains carboxylated mucins a contrasting blue colour. It is convenient to use the ferric chloride as a 60% solution, but discard when more than a few weeks old. A heavy background staining is evidence of a deteriorated ferric chloride solution or diamine salt (dry). The shelf-life of the latter is approximately one year.

Solutions

High iron diamine:

N, N-dimethyl-meta-phenylenediamine dihydrochloride*	120 mg
N, N-dimethyl-para-phenylenediamine dihydrochloride*	20 mg
Distilled water	50 ml
Ferric chloride (60% BDH solution)	1.4 ml

---

* Obtainable from Phase Separations Ltd., Deeside, Clwyd.

Dissolve the two diamine salts simultaneously in the distilled water, then add to the ferric chloride solution and mix. (The mixing is conveniently done in a Coplin jar.)

1% alcian blue in 3% acetic acid

0.5% aqueous neutral red

Technique

1. Positive control and the test sections to distilled water.
2. Treat all sections with the high iron diamine solution for 18–24 h.
3. Wash well in running water.
4. Stain with the alcian blue solution for 5 min.
5. Wash in water, stain nuclei with the neutral red solution for 2–3 min.
6. Wash in water, dehydrate, clear and mount as desired.

Results

Sulphated mucins	black/brown
Carboxylated mucins	blue
Nuclei	red

COMBINED ORCEIN-ALCIAN BLUE (Singh & Gorton 1989)

Notes

This is an alternative to the high iron diamine-alcian blue technique for separating sulphomucins from sialomucins and has the advantage of a shorter treatment time. The rationale is that sulphur groups in the protein core of glycoproteins are oxidized by potassium permanganate, and the sulphonate residues that are formed will bind the orcein dye. Sialomucins are stained blue by subsequent alcian blue treatment (see p. 146). The technique used is a Shikata orcein variant (see p. 258) but with an orcein staining of 4 h at room temperature (instead of the usual 1.5 h at 37°C); the tartrazine staining is omitted.

Results

Sulphomucins are brown and sialomucins are blue.

COMBINED ALDEHYDE FUCHSIN-ALCIAN BLUE (Spicer & Meyer 1960)

Notes

This method depends on the greater affinity of sulphated mucins for aldehyde fuchsin as opposed to that of carboxylated mucins (neutral mucins do not stain unless pre-oxidants such as periodic acid are used). If alcian blue staining follows, sulphated mucins will not stain as they will have taken up the aldehyde fuchsin comparatively strongly; only the carboxylated mucins stain blue. Pre-oxidants, such as iodine or potassium permanganate, are unnecessary for the reaction. (For a discussion of the rationale of aldehyde fuchsin and the general points appertaining to the preparation of aldehyde fuchsin, see p. 58.) Despite aldehyde fuchsin staining not being specific for sulphated mucins (elastin will also stain), it is a successful and reliable technique, but does have the disadvantage of utilizing a complex solution having a limited shelf-life.

Solutions

Aldehyde fuchsin solution (see p. 58)
1% alcian blue in 3% acetic acid

Technique

1. Sections to 70% alcohol.
2. Treat with the aldehyde fuchsin solution for 20 min.
3. Rinse well in 70% alcohol, then in water.
4. Stain with the alcian blue solution for 5 min.
5. Wash in water. Dehydrate, clear and mount in a synthetic mountant.

Results

Strongly sulphated mucins	deep purple
Elastin, weakly sulphated mucins	purple
Carboxylated mucins	blue

ALUMINIUM SULPHATE-ALCIAN BLUE TECHNIQUE (Heath 1961)

Notes

Certain dyes—such as thionin, toluidine blue, methylene blue, nuclear fast red and alcian blue—when dissolved in an aluminium sulphate solution will stain sulphated mucins. Heath (1961) attributed this to the formation of mordant-type chelate bonds. It seems more likely that this is a CEC-type reaction (see p. 147), in which competition of the aluminium ions with alcian blue for binding with carboxyl groups takes place. We have found it to be a reliable technique although not infallible, and of undoubted use as a screening method. Of the various dyes specified, alcian blue is the best due to its comparative insolubility in the post-staining dehydrating alcohols. The staining solutions keep for 3–4 weeks. There are two points to note: a known positive control should be taken through with the test section; also the amount of positively-staining material may be scanty, so it is important not to over-counterstain with neutral red.

Staining solutions

0.1 g alcian blue in 100 ml of boiling 5% aqueous aluminium sulphate. Cool and filter.
0.5% aqueous neutral red

Technique

1. Sections to distilled water.
2. Drain the slide and stain with the alcian blue solution for 30 min.
3. Wash in distilled water.
4. Counterstain with the neutral red solution for 2–3 min.
5. Wash in water, dehydrate, clear and mount as desired.

Results

Sulphated mucins	blue
Nuclei	red

Carboxylated mucins will also often stain red.

37°C ('MILD') METHYLATION TECHNIQUE (Spicer 1960)

Notes

Carboxylated mucins are also identified, but by exclusion rather than positive staining, so that this technique can be placed in the 'sulphated only' group. It involves the use of methanol (plus hydrochloric acid as a catalyst for the reaction) and brings about the blockade of carboxyl groups by forming methyl esters. If alcian blue staining is applied only sulphated mucins will stain. In practice, the reactivity of the strongly sulphated mucins may also be blocked. This method, the 'mild methylation' technique, is reasonably reliable but it is important to methylate for no longer than 4h. Controls are important and are detailed. For critical work it is better, with this type of technique, to cut serial sections, numbering them so that only adjacent sections are used.

Solutions

0.1 M (0.8%) hydrochloric acid in methanol (prepare fresh)
1% alcian blue in 3% acetic acid
0.5% aqueous netural red

Technique

1. Two positive control and two test sections to distilled water.
2. Drain, treat one positive control and a test section with pre-heated reagent for 4 h at 37°C. The remaining sections are left in distilled water for the same time and at the same temperature.
3. Wash all sections well in water for 5 min or so.
4. Stain with the alcian blue solution for 5 min.
5. Wash in water. Counterstain in the neutral red solution for 2–3 min.
6. Wash in water. Dehydrate, clear and mount as desired.

Results

Sulphated mucins only (the untreated sections should show no loss of staining)	blue
Nuclei	red

METHODS FOR CARBOXYLATED MUCINS

METHYLATION-SAPONIFICATION TECHNIQUE (Spicer & Lillie 1959)

Notes

The rationale of this technique is that both carboxylated, i.e. sialomucin and hyaluronic acid, and sulphated mucins are blocked by methylation at 60°C, the former being esterified and the latter hydrolyzed. Subsequent 'saponification' in a strong alkali will break the methyl-carboxyl ester bonds allowing subsequent restoration of the alcian blue staining. The hydrolyzed sulphated mucins do not show this restoration of staining.

The technique was once popular but we find the results to be of dubious reliability. In our experience, and those of other workers, both false positive and false negative post-saponification staining can occur. There are two practical points to remember in applying the technique. Firstly, the sections tend to come off the slide during saponification. It is wise to use a section adhesive and to cover the section with celloidin (remove before staining), although according to Sorvari & Stoward (1970) section loss may be minimized by saponifying for 2 h at 4°C. Secondly, during the methylation stage phosphate groups of the nucleic acids will also be hydrolyzed so the normal nuclear basophilia will be lost. Because of this, final counterstaining in neutral red will prove difficult; we have found that eosin gives a background of acceptable contrast. Control sections are again essential and will be described.

Solutions

0.1 M hydrochloric acid in methanol
1% potassium hydroxide in 70% alcohol
1% alcian blue in 3% acetic acid
1% aqueous eosin (ws)

Technique

1. Three sections each of positive control and test material to distilled water. Label one test section and one of control material 'A', another similar pair of sections 'B' and the third pair of sections 'C'. Celloidinize all slides.
2. Place sections 'A' and 'B' in preheated methanol-hydrochloric acid for 5 h at 60°C. Place the 'C' sections in distilled water for the same time and temperature.
3. Wash all sections well in water for 5 min or so. Rinse in distilled water.
4. Treat sections 'A' with the alcoholic potassium hydroxide solution for 30 min at room temperature, leaving the 'B' and 'C' sections in 70% alcohol only for this period.
5. Wash all sections well in water for 5 min or so.
6. Remove the celloidin film from the slides and stain with the alcian blue for 5 min.
7. Wash in water. Stain with 1% aqueous eosin for 15–20 s.
8. Wash in water. Dehydrate, clear and mount as desired.

Results

Sections A	only carboxylated mucins should stain blue
Sections B	both sulphated and carboxylated mucins are blocked and there should be no alcian blue staining
Section C	all acid mucins should be stained blue
Background	pink

SIALIDASE (NEURAMINIDASE) DIGESTION FOR N-ACETYLATED SIALOMUCINS (Spicer et al 1962)

Notes

Sialidase digestion when followed by alcian blue staining gives reliable presumptive evidence of N-acetylated sialic acid moieties by loss of alcianophilia. It is a reliable technique if carefully carried out, but note that some sialomucins are sialidase-resistant (see following techniques). If the combined alcian blue-PAS technique follows digestion the sialidase-labile sialomucins, whilst losing their normal alcianophilia, will be stained red. This is because these sialomucins are PAS-positive, a feature not normally shown by the undigested material in the combined stain because they first take up alcian blue. Calcium ions, as calcium chloride, are incorporated into the enzyme solution as an activator for the reaction. Celloidinization of paraffin sections may block the action of the enzyme and is better avoided.

Solutions

Sialidase
  1 unit per 1 ml sialidase (neuraminidase) ex *Vibrio cholerae* diluted to 1 in 5 with pH 5.5 acetate buffer, with 1% calcium chloride w/v added (or may be purchased ready-diluted and activated).
1% alcian blue in 3% acetic acid
0.5% aqueous neutral red

Technique

1. Two duplicate test and two duplicate positive control sections to distilled water.
2. Treat one test and one positive control section with pre-heated buffered enzyme in a damp chamber for 16 h at 37°C. The remaining duplicate sections are treated with the buffer only for the stated time and temperature.
3. Wash all sections well in water.
4. Stain with the alcian blue solution for 5 min. Wash in water.
5. Counterstain in the 0.5% aqueous neutral red for 2–3 min.
6. Wash in water. Dehydrate, clear and mount as desired.

Results

N-acetylated (sialidase-labile) sialomucins	loss of alcianophilia
All other acid mucins	blue
Nuclei	red

BOROHYDRIDE-SAPONIFICATION-PAS TECHNIQUE FOR O-ACETYLATED SIALOMUCINS (modified from Culling et al 1975)

Notes

The N-acetyl O-acetyl form of sialomucin, in contrast to the N-acetylated, is not only resistant to the action of the enzyme sialidase but is also PAS-negative. The

PAS negativity of O-acetylated sialomucin was used by the above workers to demonstrate PAS specificity of this entity. This was done primarily for the identification of secondary colo-rectal adenocarcinomas, in which this type of mucin was considered a significant feature. The rationale of the method is that initial sodium borohydride treatment following periodic acid oxidation blocks the formed aldehydes from a wide range of normally PAS-positive substances. Alkaline hydrolysis (saponification) follows, and breaks the PAS inhibitory O-acyl bond of the resistant form of sialomucin. A subsequent periodic acid-Schiff reaction will stain magenta only the previously negative sialomucin.

There are two practical points of importance. Firstly sections may become detached from the slide during the borohydride or saponification stages. Therefore section adhesives (see p. 32) should be used and/or celloidinization of the slides. The second point to note is that glycogen staining may well still be evident at the conclusion of the technqiue. To minimize this, it is important to use an increased initial oxidation time, so that as many aldehydes as possible are blocked by the subsequent borohydride blockade. Even so, weak glycogen staining is often present in the result. Suitable positive controls are paraffin sections of normal colon or rectum.

Solutions

Sodium borohydride:

Sodium borohydride	0.1 g
Disodium hydrogen phosphate (anhyd.)	1 g
Distilled water	100 ml

Dissolve the phosphate salt in the water, followed by the sodium borohydride; the working pH should be 9.4.

Saponification solution:

Potassium hydroxide	0.5 g
70% ethanol	100 ml

1% aqueous periodic acid
Schiff reagent (see p. 135)

Technique

1. Test sections plus positive control sections to distilled water. Label one positive control and one of each test section 'A', an equivalent set 'B', and a third set 'C'.
2. Treat all sections (A, B and C) with periodic acid for 30 min.
3. Wash well in distilled water, then treat the A and B sections only with the borohydride solution for 30 min.
4. Wash well in running water, then A sections only in 70% alcohol followed by the potassium hydroxide solution for 30 min. Finally, the A sections are washed in 70% alcohol, then in several changes of distilled water followed by periodic acid treatment for 5 min.
5. Treat all sections A, B and C with Schiff reagent for 15 min.
6. Wash well in running water and counterstain with haematoxylin as per the standard PAS technique (see p. 135).

Results

Sections A only O-acetylated sialomucin stains magenta (but see Notes)
Sections B these should be negative
Sections C all normally PAS-positive substances will stain magenta.

SULPHURIC ACID HYDROLYSIS TECHNIQUE FOR SIALOMUCINS
(Lamb & Reid 1969, Allen 1970)

Notes

Both sialidase-resistant and sialidase-labile forms of sialomucin are demonstrated by this technique, which employs sulphuric acid hydrolysis to destroy their normal affinity for alcian blue. By carrying out this technique with the sialidase digestion technique, it will readily be determined whether or not a given sialomucin is in the enzyme-labile or enzyme-resistant form. It is a reliable technique but the hydrolysis tends to weaken the subsequent basophilia of acid mucins generally. Therefore minor losses of alcian blue staining should be discounted. On occasion, a sialomucin may be present that is relatively resistant to sulphuric acid hydrolysis and will need extended times of treatment before the alcianophilia is destroyed.

The original technique of Lamb & Reid called for 1 h treatment at 80°C. This drastic treatment was modified by Allen (1970) to 60°C. Section loss may occur and it is prudent to use a section adhesive and to celloidinize the sections. Due to the concomitant acid hydrolysis of the nucleic acids, nuclear type counterstains, i.e neutral red, are not successful; it is better to use a cytoplasmic dye such as eosin. The sulphuric acid solution should be pre-heated to the desired temperature in a Coplin jar placed in a water bath at the appropriate temperature.

Solutions

0.5 M sulphuric acid
1% alcian blue in 3% acetic acid
1% aqueous eosin (ws)

Technique

1. Two positive control and two test sections to distilled water.
2. Treat one of the test and one of the positive control sections (celloidinize) with the pre-heated sulphuric acid for 2 h at 60°C. The remaining test and control sections should be placed in distilled water for the time and temperature stated.
3. Wash in water for 5–10 min. Remove any celloidin films in alcohol-ether.
4. Stain with the alcian blue solution for 5 min. Wash in water.
5. Counterstain briefly (20 s or so) in 1% aqueous eosin.
6. Wash in water, dehydrate, clear and mount as desired.

Results

Sialidase-labile and sialidase-resistant sialomucins loss of alcian blue staining
All other acid mucins   blue
Background   pink

HYALURONIDASE DIGESTION FOR HYALURONIC ACID (modified from Pearse 1953)

Notes

The most easily obtainable form of the enzyme is derived from bovine testis. Using this, chondroitin sulphates A and C and hyaluronic acid are also digested, so the appropriate techniques for those entities may need to be carried out to determine exactly what has been digested. The principle of the method is that following treatment with hyaluronidase the sections are stained with alcian blue. Loss of staining, when compared to a non-treated duplicate section, establishes the presence of one or more of the three hyaluronidase-labile mucins. If only scanty deposits of mucin are present, it may be advantageous to use the more sensitive dialyzed iron-Perls technique (see p. 148). If the presence of highly sulphated mucins is suspected, a low pH alcian blue is applied. An alternative form of the enzyme is produced from bacteria such as staphylococci and pneumococci. Bacterial hyaluronidase is more selective in its action as only hyaluronic acid and hyaluronosulphate (an uncommon mucin found in cornea) are digested. Unfortunately the bacterial enzyme is difficult to obtain commercially. The optimal pH is 6.7 — this is not critical and minor deviations may be made. Following hyaluronidase digestion cell nuclei stain only weakly with neutral red, therefore staining times are extended as necessary.

Solutions

Hyaluronidase
  Dissolve 1 mg type IV testicular hyaluronidase in 1 ml of pH 6.7 phosphate buffer.
1% alcian blue in 3% acetic (1% alcian blue in 0.2 M hydrochloric acid at pH 0.5 may also be used, see Notes). Alternatively, the dialyzed iron-Perls technique may be used (see Notes).
1% aqueous neutral red

Technique

1. Two duplicate test and two duplicate positive control sections to distilled water.
2. Treat one section of test and control material with the pre-heated buffered enzyme for 3 h at 37°C. The remaining sections are placed in buffer for 3 h at 37°C.
3. Wash all sections well in water.
4. Stain with the alcian blue solution for 5 min. Wash in water.
5. Counterstain with neutral red for 10–15 min (see Notes).
6. Wash in water. Dehydrate, clear and mount as desired.

Results

Hyaluronic acid, hyaluronosulphate, chondroitin sulphates A and C	loss of alcianophilia
Other acid mucins	blue
Nuclei	pale red

GLYCOGEN

The term 'glycogen' is derived from 'glycogenic' substance and was coined by Bernard in 1849. A more contemporary synonym is 'homoglycans,' less often used than the older, more established term. Chemically it is a simple polysaccharide consisting of branched glucose chains of two types, lyoglycogen (a water-soluble form) and desmoglycogen (a water-insoluble and protein-bound form). The association of glycogen to protein is almost certainly on a physical basis, rather than a chemical one (Meyer & Jeanloz 1943). Under normal conditions glycogen is usually, but not exclusively, intracytoplasmic. It is found in cardiac and voluntary muscle, liver, hair follicles, retina, early secretory endometrium, cervical and vaginal epithelium and in cells such as megakaryocytes and leucocytes.

FIXATION AND PRESERVATION

Fixation and preservation of glycogen is important; there is general agreement that Rossman's solution, Gendre's solution (see Appendix for formulae), 10% formal-alcohol or 80% alcohol gives the most satisfactory preservation. Zenker-acetic and the Heidenhain 'Susa' fixatives are contraindicated (Manns 1958, Murgatroyd 1971). Due to the solubility of free glycogen it was traditional to avoid aqueous fixatives such as formalin. Glycogen loss in these fixatives is minimal due, probably to its close association with protein in tissue (Manns 1958). The abnormal glycogens of the glycogenoses (such as Pompe's disease) however are water-soluble, and formalin should be avoided. Fixation should be prompt and preferably carried out at 4°C. At this temperature glycogen loss is reduced and the characteristic 'streaming' or polarization effect, seen with room temperature fixation, avoided. The polarization of glycogen is absent with the freeze drying or freeze substitution techniques. The absence of glycogen polarization at low temperatures is presumably due to the slower penetration rate of the fixing fluids presenting minimal stress forces to the glycogen; therefore displacement is lessened. The type of fixative employed will affect the presentation of the glycogen in stained preparations. Alcohol and picric acid fixatives produce a coarser granule than formalin, whilst acidification of alcoholic fixatives seems to accentuate clumping of the glycogen granules.

Decalcification of calcium-containing tissue can cause loss of glycogen; in a series to determine the optimal combination of fixative and decalcifying agent, Ferrax Correa & Merzel (1966) recommended Gendre fixation followed by 5% trichloracetic acid.

In the preparation of sections for glycogen demonstration Murgatroyd (1969) recommended freeze drying for maximum preservation and preferred paraffin to frozen sections. Lake (1970) stated that unfixed cryostat sections are to be preferred when demonstrating the abnormal glycogens of the glycogenoses (celloidinization is necessary with fresh cryostat sections to prevent diffusion and loss of the glycogen). In our experience paraffin sections are usually suitable for most purposes of glycogen demonstration, although there is undoubtedly a variable loss of glycogen with paraffin processing following formalin fixation. To counter this, it will be found efficacious to secondarily fix the tissue blocks in Rossman's solution (see Appendix) for 24 h, prior to paraffin processing.

DEMONSTRATION

Besides the technique described below, the Grocott–Gomori hexamine-silver or the Langhans (1890) iodine technique can be used. The latter technique stains glycogen a dark brown colour. It is impermanent, non-specific and little used for glycogen demonstration. The main techniques for glycogen are still the PAS and Best's carmine techniques. Which of these is to be used is a matter of practical convenience. Best's carmine undoubtedly gives the more intense and selective colouration of glycogen but the staining solution does not keep well and is rather time-consuming to prepare. Unless glycogen demonstration is to be regularly carried out, it is probably simpler to use the PAS technique.

BEST'S CARMINE TECHNIQUE (Best 1906)

Notes

This once-popular, highly selective technique for glycogen stains the carbohydrate a distinctive red colour. Unfortunately it is prone to dye precipitation artefact and is time-consuming regarding reagent preparation. The rationale of the technique has been assiduously studied by several workers. They attributed the staining of glycogen by carmine to the formation of hydrogen bonds between OH groups on the glycogen and H_2 bonds on the carmine molecule (Goldstein 1962, Murgatroyd 1969).

Carmine is used in a complex solution and is obtained from extracted cochineal containing 56% by weight of carminic acid, which is the active staining ingredient. Carmine was first used in biological work as long ago as 1778, but not employed in microtechnique until 1849, and it was 1884 before pure carminic acid was used widely. The function of the potassium salts is attributed to be that of inhibiting non-specific (background) staining. This is due to ionic attraction between the negatively charged carminic acid and any available tissue cations such as the basic proteins. The ammonia in the solution appears to serve the twin functions of acting partly as a solvent for carminic acid and partly to maintain a high (10.0) pH. Below this pH level staining is less selective (Murgatroyd 1969). There are several practical points worthy of note. The dye precipitation on to the section that commonly occurs is due to evaporation of the ammonia in which the carminic acid is soluble. It is sound practice to filter the working solution and to use it only in a closed container. For similar reasons it is unwise to allow the slide to dry following staining and before washing in alcohol. Whilst Best's differentiator is often prescribed, both methanol and industrial methylated spirit can be used equally well. The staining solution fairly quickly deteriorates, even if stored at 4°C, and the staining time will need to be lengthened when it is more than 2–3 weeks old.

Of interest is the use of dyes such as alizarin and haematein, having potential hydrogen-bonding properties, to stain glycogen when used in a Best carmine-type solution. Successful results have been claimed (Murgatroyd & Horobin 1969). We have tried out the haematein variant for glycogen, but considered the results inferior to the Best's solution. Best's carmine is not specific for glycogen as fibrin and neutral mucin also stain, although more weakly (Casselman 1962, Lauren & Sorvari 1967). The latter group of workers, incidentally, were able to stain Paneth cell granules using Best's carmine, preceded by a methylation treatment for 6 h at 56°C. We have been unable to reproduce their results.

Although diastase-digested controls are not as essential with Best's technique as they are for the PAS method due to the former's high selectivity for glycogen, it is probably good practice to have such controls in mind as the Best's technique is not specific. It is important that sections of positive control material are taken through to establish the efficacy of the staining solution.

Solutions

Carmine stock solution

To 60 ml distilled water, add 2g carmine, 1g potassium carbonate and 5g potassium chloride. Boil gently in a large flask (to avoid spillage due to the resultant effervescence) for 6 min. Cool and add 20 ml concentrated ammonia. Filter and store in a dark container at 4°C where it will keep for 1–2 months.

Working solution:

Stock solution	15 ml
Conc. ammonia	12.5 ml
Methanol	12.5 ml

The staining time to be given is for the freshly prepared solution. It is worth increasing this time as the stock solution ages.

Best's differentiator:

Methanol	40 ml
Ethanol	80 ml
Distilled water	100 ml

Technique

1. Test and positive control sections to water.
2. Treat duplicate sections only of test and control material with diastase (see p. 165), subsequently washing well in water.
3. Stain the nuclei of all sections well, using one of the iron haematoxylin solutions (see p. 125). Differentiate and blue so that the background is clear.
4. Treat with the carmine solution for 10 min.
5. Without delay transfer the slides to a Coplin jar of differentiating solution (see Notes).
6. Wash in fresh alcohol, clear and mount as desired.

Results

Glycogen	bright red
Neutral mucin, mast cells, fibrin	pale red
Nuclei	blue

CHROMIC ACID-SCHIFF TECHNIQUE (CAS) (Bauer 1933)

Notes

This is the oldest of the more popular oxidant-Schiff reactions, and uses chromium trioxide as the oxidant. The colour reaction is weaker and more selective than that given by the conventional PAS technique. PAS-positive substances such as collagen, reticulin and basement membranes (basal lamina) are not stained by the method. This is due to lessened dialdehyde formation by chromic acid, as opposed to periodic acid oxidation. For this reason some workers favour the technique as giving more easily interpreted results. Lillie et al (1947) considered the technique to be unreliable as small glycogen deposits are not demonstrated. Our own feeling is that little is to be gained by using the CAS as opposed to the PAS. Diastase controls should be used, as substances of the mucin group also react.

Solutions

5% aqueous chromium trioxide
Schiff's reagent (see p. 135)

Technique

1. Test and control sections to distilled water. Diastase digest (see p. 165).
2. Wash well in water for 5–10 min. Rinse in distilled water.
3. Oxidize with the chromium trioxide solution for 1 h.
4. Wash well in several changes of distilled water.
5. Treat with Schiff's reagent for 10 min.
6. Wash in running water for 5–10min.
7. Stain with alum haematoxylin (see p. 25). Differentiate and blue.
8. Dehydrate, clear and mount as desired.

Results

Glycogen, neutral mucins, certain acidic mucins (glycogen only will be diastase-labile)	magenta
Nuclei	blue

POTASSIUM PERMANGANATE-ALCIAN BLUE TECHNIQUE
(Cook 1974)

Notes

It is well-established that certain oxidants will, unlike periodic acid, over-oxidize aldehydes formed from vic glycol-containing substances to carboxylic acids. Use is made of this in the following technique to form carboxyl groups in glycogen capable of binding electrostatically with alcian blue. Prolonged potassium permanganate oxidation is used, and the results are inferior to those of the conventional PAS technique but are sufficient to serve as practical proof of a theoretical premise. Any mucin present will stain, but diastase digestion can be applied to duplicate sections to distinguish between that and glycogen.

Solutions

1% aqueous potassium permanganate
5% aqueous oxalic acid

1% alcian blue in 3% acetic acid
1% aqueous neutral red

Technique

1. Sections to distilled water.
2. Treat with the potassium permanganate solution for 1 h.
3. Wash in water and bleach with the oxalic acid solution for 10–30 s.
4. Wash well in water for 5–10 min.
5. Stain with the alcian blue solution for 5 min. Wash in water.
6. Counterstain in the neutral red solution for 5 min.
7. Wash in water. Dehydrate, clear and mount as desired.

Results

Glycogen, mucins	blue
Nuclei	red
Background	pale blue

DIGESTION TECHNIQUES

DIASTASE/AMYLASE-PAS

Notes

Diastase digestion is often employed to render moderately selective methods for glycogen, such as PAS, highly-selective or specific in practice. According to Bernfeld (1951) the rationale hinges on the hydrolysis of the glycogen to water-soluble maltose, which dissolves in the aqueous solvent used. Malt diastase (Lillie et al 1947) or α-amylase can be used, although human saliva is equally if not more effective, if one disregards the aesthetic and safety aspects. We prefer to use a 1% diastase solution and have experienced little or no increase in section loss during treatment or subsequent staining. Any starch granules present as an incidental feature will show a PAS positivity that is also diastase-labile, although much less readily. The following points are worth noting with regard to glycogen digestion. Celloidinization of sections inhibits digestion. Using the PAS technique, post-staining digestion is not effective, unlike the Best's carmine technique where digestion of glycogen can be carried out either preceding or following staining. The fixation employed will affect the rate or the ability of the enzyme to digest glycogen. For example, it has been shown that following Gendre and glutaraldehyde fixation the digestion times may need to be increased (Byron 1970) whilst osmium tetroxide has been shown to inhibit digestion (Sasse 1965). Control sections are essential to the technique. There seems little point in using the Hotchkiss PAS as opposed to the McManus variant; again this devolves around contemporary re-thinking of glycogen fixation solubility processes. An interesting point is that only 23–24% of glycogen is oxidized by conventional periodate solutions even after prolonged treatment. It has been suggested that an increase in Schiff reaction may be obtained by incorporating an electrolyte in the iodate solution. (This would presumably result in a decreased repulsion of the negatively charged periodate ions and glycogen molecules.)

Solutions

1% aqueous malt diastase (α-amylase can also be used)
1% aqueous periodic acid
Schiff's reagent (see p. 135)

Technique

1. Two test sections and two positive control sections to distilled water.
2. Treat one of the test sections and one control section with the aqueous diastase solution for 1 h at 37°C.
3. Wash well in water for 5–10 min.
4. Treat all sections with periodic acid and Schiff's reagent and counterstain with haematoxylin in the usual way (see p. 135).
5. Dehydrate, clear and mount as desired.

Results

Glycogen (or starch)	red-staining material present in the undigested sections but absent in the digested sections
Nuclei	blue

PECTINASE

Notes

Whilst normal glycogen deposits in tissue are fairly readily digested by diastase, there occurs in the rare type IV glycogenosis (amylopectinosis) a polysaccharide that is only readily extracted by the enzyme pectinase.

Solutions

0.4% pectinase in pH 4.0 acetate buffer (see Appendix).
1% aqueous periodic acid
Schiff's reagent (see p. 135)

Technique (taken from Lillie 1965)

1. Test and control sections to water. Rinse in pH 4.0 buffer.
2. Treat a positive control section and test sections with the enzyme solution for 48 h at 37°C. Duplicate sections are treated with buffer solution only, under similar conditions.
3. Carry out the standard PAS technique (see p. 135).
4. Dehydrate, clear and mount as desired.

Results

Glycogen (both normal and abnormal) and also some mucins are rendered PAS-negative by the enzyme treatment.

Nuclei	blue

IMMUNOCYTOCHEMISTRY

Demonstrating carbohydrates by this means is not new; as long ago as 1961 bovine submandibular salivary gland mucin had been characterized using an antiserum combined with FITC, i.e. immunofluorescence. Over the years, several different antisera have been employed for a variety of moieties (Shrevel et at 1981, Magnani 1984, Battifora & Kopinski 1985, Bollinger et al 1989). Noteworthy examples are the use of anti-sulphoglycoprotein to demonstrate sulphomucins in gastrointestinal carcinoma (Hakkinen et al 1968) and the demonstration of small and large intestinal mucin antigens in a variety of pathological metaplastic lesions using the appropriate mucin antigen antisera (Ma et al 1980, De Boer et al 1981). Athough immunofluorescence is still employed to some extent, immunoperoxidase-based immunocytochemistry is more widely used. Recent developments include the use of a biotinylated binding probe for demonstrating hyaluronic acid (Azumi et al 1992). For the ultrastructural demonstration of carbohydrates, immunogold labels can be used (Ratcliff et al 1984).

The main immunocytochemical thrust in this field has been directed at the identification of the various tissue proteoglycans/glycosaminoglycans (Poole et al 1980, Mangkornkananok-Mark et al 1981, Sobue et al 1988). However, lectin histochemistry apart, where anti-lectin antisera can be used, immunocytological-type techniques for carbohydrates have made relatively little impact. This is, perhaps, surprising when one considers the usual advantages of immunocytochemistry in terms of sensitivity and specificity. Tinctorial methods are often less sensitive but, interestingly, the wider availability of antisera has not led to significant advances in carbohydrate identification. Regarding specificity of reaction, several of the standard histochemical techniques provide such reactions whilst, as is well known, specific epitopes may occur on more than one tissue site so that a specific antiserum may demonstrate several entities. The converse may arise; for example, placental hyaluronic acid epitope (Sunderland et al 1985) is placenta-specific. This means that the antiserum will be negative for pleural hyaluronic acid-producing cells (mesothelial cells) and a potential diagnostic tool for mesothelioma diagnosis is lost.

STARCH

Starch is a polysaccharide consisting of two major components: amylose and amylopectin. Starch granules are often present as contaminants from starch-containing surgical glove powders in sites of surgical operations. Occasionally these granules set up an inflammatory reaction resulting in a starch granuloma. Starch is not easily discerned in H & E preparations so its demonstration in such a lesion is important.

DEMONSTRATION

Starch granules vary from round to polyhedral in shape and are roughly 15–20 μm in size; a typical feature is the presence of a central refractile 'droplet' in each granule. Staining varies from pale pink (usually) to blue with H & E preparations, and they are PAS-positive and hexamine silver-positive (see pp 135 and 254 respectively). The granules stain blue with iodine solutions. Starch is slowly digested with diastase, and with the polarizing microscope exhibits a Maltese cross-type of birefringence.

LANGHANS IODINE TECHNIQUE (Langhans 1890)

Notes

The following slightly modified technique, whilst impermanent, gives results that are stable for a few days. After this period the blue colour of the starch reverts to the normal brown of the iodine. The production of the blue colour with iodine is the classic test for starch and involves an oxidation process by the iodine. On eventual mounting this oxidation is reversed by reduction processes. The dehydrating alcohols contain iodine to minimize its loss from the section, as the iodine is highly soluble in alcohol.

Solution

Lugol's iodine (see p. 59)

> **Technique**
>
> 1. Sections to water.
> 2. Stain with Lugol's iodine for 10 min.
> 3. Drain and blot dry.
> 4. Dehydrate rapidly in absolute alcohols that are saturated with iodine. Clear in xylene and mount in a DPX-type resin.

Results

Starch	blue
Glycogen, amyloid, cellulose	brown
Background	yellow-brown

Table 7.3   Techniques for starch, cellulose and chitin

Polysaccharide	Technique		PAS	C	B	G	AB
	E	I					
Starch	$\pm$	+	+	V	+	+	–
Cellulose	V	+	+	+	+	+	–
Chitin	+	–	+	V	$\pm$	+	–

Key: E = eosin (as in H & E); I = iodine; PAS = periodic acid-Schiff; C = Congo red; B = birefringence; G = Grocott; AB = alcian blue; V = variable reaction; + = positive reaction; $\pm$ = weak reaction; – = negative.

CELLULOSE

The demonstration of cellulose in human tissue is of little consequence in diagnostic pathology. The only occasions of importance are where the cellulose presents as undigested food particles in the lumen of an appendix. It is occasionally implicated in inflammatory lesions (for example, foreign bodies in skin, intestinal fistulae and in pulmonary tissues following inhalation of gastric contents), and then the necessity for cellulose demonstration arises.

DEMONSTRATION

Cellulose particles adopt a variety of appearances depending on origin (plant material, wood splinters etc.). A typical presentation is of fenestrated bodies or fibres. In an H & E preparation, the cellulose may be stained blue, pink or not at all. It is PAS- and hexamine silver-positive (see pp 135 and 254 respectively), stains brown with iodine, and under polarizing microscopy is birefringent. An interesting characteristic is its ability to stain with Congo red and related dyes and sometimes exhibit a green birefringence. The use of the enzyme cellulase conjugated with FITC for the specific demonstration of cellulose, has been reported by Siebert et al (1978).

CHITIN

Chitin is of the mucoprotein family and is known as homopolyaminosaccharide. Chitin is a carbohydrate and is found in combination with protein and calcium, but its physical and histochemical characteristics are such that it is usually dealt with under a separate heading. In human tissue it is of relevance only in cases of hydatid cyst formation. These cysts have a wall formed of chitin that has been laid down by the contained larvae of the dog tapeworm—*Echinococcus granulosus*. Hydatid cysts may be found in the lungs, liver or brain.

DEMONSTRATION

Chitin is a dense hyaline material which stains a bright pink in H & E preparations. It is PAS-positive, hexamine silver-positive (see pp 135 and 254 respectively), and variably Congo red-positive. As is the case in the use of a specific enzyme for the demonstration of cellulose, so too with chitin, where the enzyme chitinase has been employed conjugated with FITC.

REFERENCES

Allen M G 1970 The effect of acid hydrolysis on sialomucins at selected epithelial sites. Thesis for Fellowship of the Institute of Medical Laboratory Technology
Allison R T 1973 The effects of fixation on the subsequent demonstration of mucopolysaccharides. Medical Laboratory Technology 30: 27–31
Azumi N, Underhill C B, Kogan E, Sheibami K 1992 A novel biotinylated probe specific for hyaluronate. American Journal of Surgical Pathology 16: 116–121
Bancroft J D 1975 Histochemical techniques, 2nd edn. Butterworths, London
Battifora H, Kopinski M I 1985 Distinction of mesothelioma from adenocarcinoma. An immunohistochemical approach. Cancer 55: 1679–1685
Bauer H 1933 Microskopisch-chemischer Natwer's von Glykogen und einigen anderen Polysacharden. Zeitschrift für mikroskopische-anatomische Forschung 33: 143
Bensley S H 1952 Pinacyanol erythrosinate as a stain for mast cells. Stain Technology 27: 269
Berger C, Pizzolato P 1975 The staining of Brunner's gland and other neutral mucins by carmine, haematoxylin and orcein in alkaline solutions. Stain Technology 50: 83–86
Bernfeld P 1951 Enzymes of starch degradation and synthesis. Advance in Enzymology 12: 379

Best F 1906 Uber Karminfarbung des Glykogens unde der Kerne. Zeitschrift für wissenschaftkiche Mikroskopie und für Mikroskopische Technik 23: 319–322

Bollinger D J, Wick M R, Dehner L P, Mills S E, Swanson P E, Clarke R E 1989 Peritoneal malignant mesothelioma versus serous papillary adenocarcinoma. A histochemical and immunohistochemical comparison. American Journal of Surgical Pathology 13: 659–670

Byron F M 1970 Demonstration of glycogen in glycogenosis Types 1, 2 and 4. Journal of Medical Laboratory Technology 27: 43–48

Casselman W G B 1962 Histochemical technique, 2nd edn. Methuen, London

Charman J, Reid L 1972 The effect of decalcifying fluids on the staining of epithelial mucins by alcian blue. Stain Technology 47: 173–178

Clancy M J, Whelan W J 1967 Enzymic polymerization of monosaccharides. Archives of Biochemistry and Biophysics 118: 730–735

Cook H C 1959 A comparative evaluation of the histological demonstration of mucin. Journal of Medical Laboratory Technology 16:1–6

Cook H C 1961 A modified thionin technique for mast cells in tissue sections. Journal of Medical Laboratory Technology 18: 188–189

Cook H C 1968 Some observations on the demonstration of mucin on human tissue. Journal of Medical Laboratory Technology 25: 13–24

Cook H C 1973 A histochemical characterization of malignant tumour mucins as a possible aid in the identification of metastatic deposits. Medical Laboratory Technology 30: 217–224

Cook H C 1974 Manual of histological demonstration technique. Butterworths, London

Crow J, Gibbs D A, Cozens W, Spellacy E, Watts R W E 1983 Biochemical and histopathological studies on patients with mucopolysaccharidoses, two of whom had been treated by fibroblast transplantation. Journal of Clinical Pathology 36: 415–430

Csaba G 1969 Mechanism of the formation of mast cell granules. Acta Biologicae Academicae Scientianum Hungariae 20: 205

Culling C F A, Reid P E, Burton J D, Dunn W L 1975 A histochemical method of differentiating lower gastrointestinal tract mucin from other mucins in primary or metastatic tumours. Journal of Clinical Pathology 28: 656–658

De Boer W G R M, Ma J, Rees J W, Nayman J 1981 Inappropriate mucin production in gall bladder metaplasia and neoplasia —an immunohistological study. Histopathology 5: 295–303

Dennis J W, Laferte S, Waghorne C, Breitman M L, Kerbel R S 1987 Beta 1–6 branching of Asn-linked oligosaccharides is directly associated with metastasis. Science 236: 582–585

Dorling J 1969 Critical electrolyte concentration method in histochemistry. Journal of Medical Laboratory Technology 26: 124–130

Dorling J 1980 Localisation of sulphated glycosaminoglycans in the mucopolysaccharidoses by a simple technique using cryostat sections. Journal of Clinical Pathology 33: 897–898

Ferraz Correa A C, Merzel J 1966 Histochemical behaviour of polysaccharide methods on tissue submitted to decalcification. Acta Histochemica 25 Band, 233–238

Filipe M I 1972 The value of a study of the mucosubstances in rectal biopsies from patients with carcinoma of the rectum and lower sigmoid in the diagnosis of premalignant mucosa. Journal of Clinical Pathology 25: 123–128

Gardner D G 1968 Metachromatic cells in the gingiva in Hurler's syndrome. Journal of Oral Surgery 26: 882

Goldstein D J 1962 Correlation of size of dye particle and density of substrate with special reference to mucin staining. Stain Technology 37: 79–93

Haddock N H 1948 Alcian blue, a new phthalocyanine dyestuff. Research 15: 685–689

Hakkinen I, Järvi O, Grönroos, J 1968 Sulphoglycoprotein antigens in human alimentary canal and gastric cancer: An immunohistological study. International Journal of Cancer 3: 572

Hale C W 1946 Histochemical demonstration of acid mucopolysaccharides in animal tissues. Nature, London 157: 802

Heath I D 1961 Staining of sulphated mucopolysaccharides. Nature, London 191: 1370

Hughesdon P E 1949 Two uses of uranyl nitrate. I. Permanent metachromatic staining of mucin. Journal of the Royal Microscopical Society 69: 1–7

Hukill P B, Vidone R A 1967 Histochemistry of mucus and other polysaccharides in tumours. Laboratory investigation 16: 395–406

Kent P W, Marsden J O 1963 A sulphated sialoprotein from sheep colonic mucin. Biochemistry Journal 87: 38–39

Korhonen L, Makela V 1968 Carbohydrate-rich tissue components in lung cancer and normal bronchial tissue: a histochemical study. Histochemical Journal 1: 124–140

Lake B D 1970 The histochemical evaluation of the glycogen storage diseases. A review of techniques and their limitations. Histochemical Journal 2: 441–450

Lamb D, Reid L 1969 Histochemical types of acidic glycoprotein produced by mucous cells of the tracheobronchial glands in man. Journal of Pathology 98: 213–229

Lamb D, Reid L 1970 Histochemical and autoradiographic investigation of the serous cells of the human bronchial glands. Journal of Pathology 100: 127–138

Langhans C 1890 Ueber Glykogen in pathologischen Neubildungen unde den menschlichen Eithauten. Virchow's Archives of Pathology Anatomy and Physiology 120: 28

Lauren A P, Sorvari T E 1967 Staining of Paneth cells with Best's carmine after methylation. Stain Technology 42: 311–315

Leathem A 1990 Personal communication

Lillie R D, Laskey A, Greco J, Jacquier H 1947 Studies on the preservation and histologic demonstration of glycogen. Bulletin of the International Association of Medical Museums 27: 23

Lillie R D 1954 Histologic technic, 2nd end. McGraw-Hill, New York

Lillie R D 1965 Histopathologic technic and practical histochemistry, 3rd edn. McGraw-Hill, New York

MacManus J F A 1946 Histological demonstration of mucin after periodic acid. Nature 158: 202

Ma J, De Boer W G R M, Ward H A, Nairn R C 1980 Another oncofoetal antigen in colonic carcinoma. British Journal of Cancer 41: 325–328

Magnani L J 1984 Carbohydrate differentiation and cancer associated antigens detected by monoclonal antibodies. Biochemical Society Transactions 12: 543

Mangkornkananok-Mark M, Eisenstein R, Bahu R M 1981 Immunologic studies of bovine aortic and cartilage proteoglycans. Journal of Histochemistry and Cytochemistry 29: 547–552

Manns E 1958 The preservation and demonstration of glycogen in tissue sections. Journal of Medical Laboratory Technology 15: 1–12

Mayer P 1896 Uber Schleimfarbung. Mitteilungen aus der Zoologischen Station zu Neapel 12: 303

Meyer k H, Jeanloz R W 1943 Recherches sur Loamidon XXV. Le glycogene due muscle natif. Helvetica Chimica Acta 26: 1784

Mowry R W 1956 Observations on the use of sulphuric ether for the sulphation of hydroxyl groups in tissue sections. Journal of Histochemistry and Cytochemistry 4: 407

Murgatroyd L B 1969 Studies on the histochemical demonstration of glycogen. Thesis for Fellowship of the Institute of Medical Laboratory Technology

Murgatroyd L B 1971 Chemical and spectrometric evaluation of glycogen after routine. histological fixatives. Stain Technology 46: 111–119

Murgatroyd L B, Horobin R Q 1969 Specific staining of glycogen with haematoxylin and certain anthraquinone dyes. Stain Technology 44: 59–62

Pearse A G E 1953 Histochemistry, theoretical and applied. Churchill, London

Poole A R, Pidoux I, Reiner A, Tang L-H, Choi H, Rosenberg L 1980 Localisation of proteoglycan monomer and link protein in the matrix of bovine aortic cartilage: an immunohistochemical study. Journal of Histochemistry and Cytochemistry 28: 621

Quintarelli G, Tsuki S, Hashimoto Y, Pigman W 1960 Histochemical studies of bovine salivary glands. Biochemistry, Biophysics Research Communications 2: 423

Ratcliff A, Fryer P A, Hardingham T E 1984 The distribution of aggregating proteoglycans in articular cartilage. Journal of Histochemistry and Cytochemistry 32: 193–201

Roberts G P 1977 Histochemical detection of sialic acid residues using periodate oxidation. Histochemical Journal 9(1): 97–102

Sasse D 1965 Untersuchungen zum Cytocemischen Glykogenachweis. VII Mitteilung. Histochemie 5: 378–383

Schiff U 1866 Eine neue Reihe organischer Diamine. Justus Leibigs Annin Chem 140: 92

Scott J E, Dorling J 1965 Differential staining of acid glycosaminoglycans (mucopolysaccharides) by alcian blue in salt solutions. Histochemie 5: 22–33

Scott J E, Dorling J 1969 Periodate oxidation of acid polysaccharides (III) A PAS method for chondroitin sulphates and other glycosamino-glacuronans. Histochemie 19: 295–301

Scott J E, Dorling J, Stockwell R A 1968 Reversal of protein blocking of basophilia in salt solutions; implication in the localization of polyanions using alcian blue. Journal of Histochemistry 16: 383–386

Shrevel J, Gross D, Monsigny M 1981 Cytochemistry of cell glycoconjugates. Progress in Histochemistry and Cytochemistry 14: 1

Siebert G R, Benjaminson M A, Hoffman H 1978 A conjugate of cellulase with fluoroscein isothiocyanate: a specific stain for cellulose. Stain Technology 53: 103–106

Singh R, Gorton A E P 1989 Orcein-alcian blue staining: a new technique for demonstrating acid mucins in gastrointestinal epithelium. Journal of Clinical Pathology 42: 881–884

Sobue M, Nakashima N, Fukatsu T, Nagaska T, Katoh T, Ogura T, Takeuchi J 1988 production and characterization of monoclonal antibody to dermatan sulphate proteoglycan. Journal of Histochemistry and Cytochemistry 36: 479–485

Sorvari T E, Stoward P J 1970 Saponification of methylated mucosubstances at low temperature. Stain Technology 46: 49–52

Southgate H W 1927 Note on preparing mucicarmine. Journal of Pathology and Bacteriology 30: 729

Spicer S S 1960 A correlative study of the histochemical properties of rodent acid mucopolysaccharides. Journal of Histochemistry and Cytochemistry 8: 18–35

Spicer S S 1961 The use of cationic reagents in the histochemical differentiation of mucopolysaccharides. American Journal of Clinical Pathology 36: 393–407

Spicer S S 1965 Diamine methods for differentiating mucopolysaccharides histochemically. Journal of Histochemistry and Cytochemistry 13: 211

Spicer S S, Lillie R D 1959 Saponification as a means of selectively reversing the methylation blockade of tissue basophilia. Journal of Histochemistry and Cytochemistry 7: 123–125

Spicer S S, Meyer D B 1960 Histochemical differentiation of acid mucopolysaccharides by means of combined aldehyde fuchsin-alcian blue staining. American Journal of Clinical Pathology 33: 453–460

Spicer S S, Neubecker R D, Warren L, Henson J G 1962 Epithelial mucins in lesions of the human breast. Journal of the National Cancer Institute 29: 963–970

Steedman H F 1950 Alcian blue 8 GS; a new stain for mucin. Quarterly Journal of Microscopic Science 91: 477–479

Sunderland C A, Bulmer J N, Luscombe M, Redman C W G, Stirrat G M 1985 Immunohistochemical and biochemical evidence for a role for hyaluronic acid in the growth and development of the placenta. Journal of Reproductive immunology 8: 197–212

Wagner J C, Munday B E, Harington J S 1962 Histochemical demonstration of hyaluronic acid in pleural mesotheliomas. Journal of Pathology and Bacteriology 84: 73–78

8. Lipids

'Lipids can be defined as substances that may be extracted from the tissues by several or all of the usual fat solvents and are insoluble or only colloidally soluble in water' (Baker 1946). Lipids are normal constituents of tissues, found in adipose tissue as stored lipid for energy production, or as specialist lipid structures such as myelin. As well as carbohydrates and proteins, lipids are rarely found in a pure state in tissue sections; they are usually in combination with carbohydrates in glycolipids or with proteins in lipoproteins. This results in histochemical methods yielding less selective information than we would like. The advantage of lipid histochemistry over biochemistry is that it shows the localization of the lipid at a cytological level or sometimes an ultrastructural level. It is only recently that it has become possible to identify individual lipids with any precision as specific histochemical methods have become available.

CLASSIFICATION OF LIPIDS

The classification of lipids has been somewhat confused in the past; a detailed table is given by Bayliss-High (1990). The following Table 8.1 is a simplified working version.

Table 8.1 Simple classification of lipids

Unconjugated lipids	Conjugated lipids
Free fatty acids	*Ester lipids*
Free cholesterol	Cholesterol esters, triglycerides.
	Phospholipids
	Glycerol-based lecithins, cephalins
	(phosphoglycerides) and plasmalogens.
	Sphingosine-based
	Sphingomyelins, cerebrosides, sulphatides,
	gangliosides.

LIPID HISTOCHEMISTRY AND DIAGNOSIS

The demonstration of lipid in the routine laboratory is infrequently called for and, unless dealing with a suspected lipid storage disorder, is unlikely to require precise identification of the type present. Extraneous examples of conditions requiring lipid staining include aortic atheroma and lipid pneumonia of the lungs (due to aspiration of fatty material from the oral cavity). Certain tumours, too, contain significant quantities of fat and this can sometimes be used to advantage in their recognition. Examples of benign tumours are xanthoma of skin and thecoma of the ovary, and of malignant tumours renal adenocarcinoma, adrenal cortical adenocarcinoma and liposarcoma. In addition to these conditions are the various demyelination diseases of the CNS; these are considered in the appropriate chapter.

DEMONSTRATION OF LIPIDS

PHYSICAL PROPERTIES

The surface property of lipids is important in their demonstration. For staining purposes these are described as either '*hydrophilic lipids*'—lipids that have an affinity for absorbing water, i.e. they are water-miscible—or as '*hydrophobic lipids*—lipids that repel water which assume the typical globular shape in an aqueous environment. The hydrophobic lipids react strongly with Sudan-related dyes, whereas the hydrophilic do not and are best demonstrated by other methods, see Table 8.2.

Table 8.2   Lipids and methods for their demonstration

Method	Lipid
Bromine-Sudan black	All lipids
Sudan black, oil red O	Most lipids
Nile blue sulphate	Acidic and neutral lipids
Copper-rubeanic acid	Free fatty acids
Perchloric acid-naphthoquinone*	Free cholesterol and esters
Digitonin-PAN*	Free cholesterol and esters*
Ultraviolet Schiff	Unsaturated lipids
Osmium tetroxide	Unsaturated lipids
Calcium lipase	Triglycerides
Acid haematin	Most acidic lipids
Sodium hydroxide-acid haemaetin	Sphingomyelin
Plasmal reaction	Plasmalogen phospholipids
Modified PAS	Cerebrosides
Copper-orcinol	Gangliosides
Acriflavine-DMAB	Sulphatides

*In our hands the demonstration of cholesterol histologically is difficult and often more than one attempt is required. It is essential to include a known positive control; sections of the adrenal cortex are recommended.

FIXATION

Unfixed cryostat sections give the best results for most techniques although fixation is required in some histochemical methods to protect the lipid and the section from the reagents used. Often simple lipids are not fixed or removed by treatment with formalin. Baker's formal calcium (see p. 426) is the best routine fixative.

EXTRACTION

The definition given by Baker and quoted at the beginning of this chapter states that lipids can be removed by solvents. Lipids do show a differential solubility in organic solvents but as they are rarely found in a pure form this severely affects the results. Fixation also affects the way lipids react to a solvent, therefore extraction techniques are applied to unfixed sections. Use has been made of extraction, notably in Baker's acid haematin method, where pyridine is used specifically to remove phospholipids. It is also used as a control, when treatment in chloroform-methanol (1:1) at 56°C for 1 hour will remove all lipids.

MELTING POINT

Not all lipids are liquid at room temperature. Some hydrophobic lipids, particularly fatty acids, are crystalline at this temperature and elevated temperatures are necessary for their demonstration.

BIREFRINGENCE

A section viewed in polarized light, after staining with a Sudan dye, will show unstained crystalline lipid to be birefringent. Stained and liquid lipids do not exhibit this effect, or only weakly. It is unwise to attempt to derive too much information from the birefringent effects of lipids as their optical properties vary according to their physical state. Examining cryostat sections at room temperature usually shows monorefringent lipids such as triglycerides and free fatty acids; birefringent lipids are phospholipids, cerebrosides, sphingomyelin, free cholesterol (notched corner plates), and esterified cholesterol (Maltese cross).

Table 8.3 Surface properties of lipids

Hydrophilic	Hydrophobic
Phospholipids	Unconjugated (free fatty acids, free cholesterol)
Gangliosides	
Cerebrosides	Simple esters (triglycerides, cholesterol esters)
Sulphatides	

OIL-SOLUBLE DYES

Lipids seen in tissue as fats are normally demonstrated by Sudan dyes. Not all lipids are stained; free fatty acids and phosphoglycerides are often unstained, as is free cholesterol. Oil-soluble dyes are virtually insoluble in water and to a variable degree in alcohol. The dyes are soluble in most lipids and require a vehicle for their use. A number of solutions have been tried: 70% alcohol (Daddi 1896), also the 70% alcohol and acetone mixture of Herxheimer (1903) were used originally, but they are likely to remove small amounts of lipid. The solvents of choice are isopropyl alcohol (Lillie & Ashburn 1943), propylene glycol (Chiffelle & Putt 1951) and triethyl phosphate. We have found that 60% isopropyl alcohol or 60% triethyl phosphate gives the best results.

Oil-soluble dyes stain lipids by being more soluble in the lipids than in their solvent. Most of them are not dyes in the accepted sense, i.e. they contain no auxochromic groups but are chromogens. An exception to this is Sudan black, which contains the amino group auxochrome. This accounts for the more sensitive fat staining occurring with this dye, which is particularly apparent during staining of phospholipid-rich tissues, where some degree of salt binding occurs. The original method employed Sudan III (Daddi 1896) but was supplanted in popularity by the deeper red Sudan IV (Michaelis 1901). Other oil-soluble dyes are Sudan brown, blue or green, also oil red O, blue NA and brown D.

Counterstaining presents problems as most dyes diffuse or are bleached by aqueous mountants. For the red lipid dyes haematoxylin is used, but it tends to fade in time. The Sudans blue and black present greater problems as the normally recommended dye, carmalum, requires long staining periods and, at best, stains the nuclei only weakly. A possible alternative once suggested to us was first to carry out the Feulgen-Schiff reaction to colour the DNA before staining with Sudan black!

There are several mountants available, e.g. glycerol-jelly, Farrant's solution or Apathy's solution. There is not much to choose between them, and we usually prefer the modified Apathy mountant (see p. 111) that can be hardened by placing the mounted sections for a short period in the 37°C incubator.

SUDAN BLACK METHOD FOR LIPIDS (Lison & Dagnelie 1935, Lillie 1954, Bayliss & Adams 1972, Bayliss-High 1990)

Notes

Lillie (1954) introduced a bromination stage to depress the solubility of unsaturated lipids in organic solvents. Bayliss & Adams (1972) noted that fatty acids and phosphoglycerides were rendered insoluble in the dye bath and that crystalline cholesterol was converted to derivatives that were liquid at room temperature and hence demonstrated. Bayliss-High (1990) showed that following bromination only phospholipids will survive extraction and appear to be selectively stained. These modifications provide an easy and sensitive method for staining all lipid classes. Bayliss-High (1990) recommends it as a screening method; for morphology she advises the oil red O method that is also useful in combination with other dyes such as Baker's acid haematin. In haematology, Sudan black is a useful marker for cells of the granulocyte series, as these cells are rich in phospholipids.

STANDARD SUDAN BLACK TECHNIQUE

Solutions

Sat. solution of Sudan black in 70% ethanol
2% carmalum

Technique

1. Mount sections on to slides and allow to dry.
2. Rinse in 70% ethanol.
3. Stain in a sat. solution of Sudan black in 70% ethanol for 15 min. Filter before use.
4. Remove excess stain in 70% ethanol.
5. Stain nuclei with the carmalum solution for 5–30 min (see p. 28).
6. Wash well in water and mount in an aqueous mountant.

Results

Unsaturated lipids, cholesterol esters, triglycerides, some phospholipids	blue-black
Nuclei	pale red

BROMINATION-SUDAN BLACK

Solutions

2.5% aqueous bromine
0.5% sodium metabisulphite

Technique

1. Mount sections on to slides and allow to dry.
2. Immerse sections in the aqueous bromine solution for 30 min at room temperature in a fume cupboard.
3. Wash in water (10 min).
4. Treat with the sodium metabisulphite solution for 1 min.
5. Wash in distilled water, three changes.
6. Proceed with standard Sudan black method above.

Results

As previous method plus lecithin, free fatty
acids and free cholesterol   blue-black

BROMINATION-ACETONE-SUDAN BLACK

Technique

1. Follow steps 1–5 in previous method and allow sections to dry.
2. Treat sections with anhydrous acetone for 20 min at 4°C.
3. Follow steps 3–6 in the standard Sudan black method (see p. 176).

Results

Only phospholipids stain blue-black.

OIL RED O (French 1926, Lillie & Ashburn 1943)

Notes

The deep red staining of lipids by this method makes it one of the most popular techniques for these substances. Always use a covered container and ample amounts of solution when staining and use care in washing. Of the two alternative staining solutions presented below we prefer the isopropanol variant. Although the triethyl phosphate solution of oil red O gives brighter staining, it can also lead to a dye precipitate forming during long storage of the stained sections.

Solutions

Variant

Dissolve 0.5 g oil red O in 200 ml of isopropyl alcohol. Warm the solution in a long-necked container (2 litre volumetric flask) in a 56°C water bath for 1 h. Cool. The working solution is prepared prior to use by adding four parts of distilled water to six parts of stock solution. Mix and stand for 10 min. Filter through a fine filter paper (No. 42 Whatman).

Variant 2

Dissolve 1 g of oil red O in 100 ml of triethyl phosphate by heating in a 56°C water bath for several hours. Cool and filter (No. 1 Whatman). The working solution is prepared by adding four parts of distilled water to six parts of the stock solution. Mix well and filter through a fine filter paper as before.

Technique

1. Rinse frozen sections in water.
2. Rinse in either 60% isopropyl alcohol or 60% triethyl phosphate (both dilutions prepared with distilled water) as appropriate.
3. Stain in either dye variant for 10 min.
4. Wash briefly in 60% isopropyl alcohol or 60% triethyl phosphate. Wash well in water.
5. Stain the nuclei in Mayer's haematoxylin solution (see p. 25) for $1-1\frac{1}{2}$ min. Wash and blue.
6. Wash in water and mount in an aqueous mountant.

Results

Unsaturated hydrophobic lipids, i.e. cerebrosides, triglycerides, cholesterol esters	red
Phospholipids	pink
Nuclei	blue

NILE BLUE SULPHATE TECHNIQUE (Smith 1908)

Notes

The following technique, slightly modified from the original, gives good separation of acidic from certain non-acidic lipids. The phospholipids are stained a deeper blue than the fatty acids (Dunnigan 1968).

The Nile blue sulphate solution contains two oxazines (the salt and its free base) that stain acidic structures such as phosphate groups blue by salt linkage, and an oxazone moiety that is oil-soluble and red in colour. The staining of acidic lipids is non-specific as other acidic tissue moieties, e.g. nucleic acids, also stain. The temperature at which the reaction is carried out is important, as the various fatty acids have different melting points, so the temperature of reaction should be near or above this point. For example, the melting point of stearic acid is 70°C, palmitic 63°C and oleic acid 14°C. The recommended technique temperature is 60°C (Cain 1947). The number of unsaturated bonds in the fatty acid chains is inversely proportional to the melting point of the fatty acids.

Solution

1% aqueous Nile blue sulphate (syn. Nile blue)

The dye should be rich in oxazone to achieve good results and is tested as follows. Add a little of the powdered dye, or a few drops of the aqueous solution to 5–10 ml of xylene in a test tube and mix well. The oxazone fraction will go into solution and appear red. Should a negative or weak red colour result, the dye oxazone content may be increased by sulphuric acid oxidation as follows. Make up a 1% solution of Nile blue sulphate in 5% aqueous sulphuric acid. Boil in a reflux condenser for 1–2 h. Cool and retest in xylene; if positive, use the oxidized solution as it is.

Technique

1. Take frozen sections to distilled water.
2. Stain with the Nile blue sulphate solution for 10 min at 60°C (preheat the solution).
3. Wash in distilled water at 60°C for a few seconds.
4. Differentiate in 1% acetic acid at 60°C until the excess blue staining is removed (30 s or so).
5. Wash in tap water at room temperature and mount in an aqueous mountant.

Results

Neutral fats, cholesterol esters	red
Fatty acids, phospholipids, nuclei, some lipofuscins, acidic mucins	blue

COPPER-RUBEANIC ACID METHOD FOR FREE FATTY ACIDS
(Holczinger 1959)

Notes

Free fatty acids bind heavy metal ions to form soaps. Benda's (1900) and Holczinger's (1959) techniques use copper acetate to bind to fatty acids and rubeanic acid to demonstrate copper soaps. EDTA is used to remove non-specific absorbed copper. M HCl is employed initially to desaponify any pre-existing calcium soaps.

Solutions

0.005% cupric acetate
0.1% EDTA pH 7.0
0.1% rubeanic acid in 70% ethanol
Mayer's carmalum (see p. 28)

Technique

1. Treat duplicate sections with M HCl at 20°C for 1 h.
2. Wash well in distilled water and then air dry.
3. Treat one section with acetone at 4°C for 20 min.
4. Immerse both sections in the cupric acetate solution for 3 h.
5. Wash in the EDTA solution pH 7.0 (adjust pH with NaOH) for 10 s.

6. Repeat wash in EDTA.
7. Wash in distilled water.
8. Treat sections with the rubeanic acid solution in 70% ethanol for 10 min.
9. Rinse in 70% ethanol.
10. Counterstain nuclei in Mayer's carmalum.
11. Wash in water and mount in an aqueous mountant.

Results

Free fatty acids	dark green
Acetone-extracted section	negative
Nuclei	blue

PERCHLORIC ACID-NAPHTHOQUINONE (PAN) FOR CHOLESTEROL
(Adams 1961)

Notes

This method is more precise and sensitive than the classic Schultz method and is included here to the exclusion of the latter. In the Adams method perchloric acid is used to condense cholesterol to cholesta-3:5 diene. This is converted by 1:2 naphthoquinone to a red or blue pigment, the colour variation being due to the different physical states of the cholesterol (Bayliss-High 1990). The initial oxidation of the cholesterol is an important stage of the method and should not be omitted nor the time reduced.

Solution

1:2 naphthoquinone-4-sulphonic acid	40 mg
Ethanol	20 ml
60% perchloric acid	10 ml
Formaldehyde	1 ml
Distilled water	9 ml

Mix and use the same day.

Technique

1. Air dry sections on to slides.
2. Oxidize sections in 1% aqueous ferric chloride for 4 h.
3. Wash well in distilled water.
4. Coat sections with the naphthoquinone solution using a brush, place slide on a hot plate at 70°C, keep coating the sections with the solution until the colour develops (for 1– 5 min).
5. Rinse in 60% perchloric acid.
6. Mount in 60% perchloric acid.

Results

Cholesterol and esters	red or blue

DIGITONIN REACTION FOR CHOLESTEROL (Windaus 1909, modified)

Notes

Cholesterol forms a compound with digitonin and the resultant digitonide presents as birefringent needles or rosettes. Free cholesterol can be differentiated from its esters because the esters will be coloured by an oil-soluble dye or by using the PAN method after completing the technique. Alternatively the esters can be extracted in acetone.

Solution

0.5% digitonin in 4% ethanol

Technique

1. Dry sections on to slides.
2. Immerse in the digitonin solution for 2 h.
3. Extract esters in acetone for 1 h (optional).
4. Proceed with method of choice.

Results

Using an oil-soluble dye: no extraction

Free cholesterol	unstained
Cholesterol esters	stained

After acetone extraction and PAN technique

Free cholesterol	red or blue
Cholesterol esters	negative

After polarization and precipitation with digitonin

Free cholesterol	birefringent
(cholesterol esters are naturally birefringent and appear as Maltese crosses)	

ULTRA-VIOLET SCHIFF METHOD FOR UNSATURATED LIPIDS (Belt & Hayes 1956)

Notes

A highly selective technique in which ultraviolet light oxidizes double bonds to aldehydes, allowing subsequent Schiff staining.

Solution

Schiff's reagent (see p. 135)

Technique

1. Mount sections on to slides and expose to a source of ultraviolet light for 2 h.
2. Treat with Schiff's reagent for 15 min, with a non-irradiated control section to exclude non-lipid aldehydes.
3. Wash well in tap water and rinse in distilled water.
4. Mount sections in an aqueous mountant.

Result

Unsaturated lipids appear magenta.

SECONDARY FLUORESCENCE METHOD (Popper 1941)

Note

This is a useful screening method. The fluorochromes, being in aqueous solution, will not dissolve any lipid material.

Solution

0.1% aqueous phosphine 3R

Technique

1. Wash sections in distilled water.
2. Stain for 3 min in the aqueous phosphine 3R solution.
3. Rinse quickly in distilled water and mount in 90% glycerol.

Results

| Triglycerides, cholesterol esters, compound lipids | silvery-white fluorescence |
| Fatty acids and free cholesterol | negative |

OSMIUM TETROXIDE

Notes

The use of osmium tetroxide to demonstrate lipids is probably the oldest technique. It depends on the reduction of the osmium tetroxide to lower (black) oxides by an ethylene linkage mechanism. Some reducing substances, i.e. melanin, will also blacken (Lillie 1965). Osmium tetroxide blackens only unsaturated fatty acids and their esters, such as those of oleic acid. To demonstrate saturated fats, the tissue should be treated with alcohol following osmium tetroxide treatment, a process known as 'secondary staining'. *It is as well to remember the toxicity of osmium tetroxide vapour.*

Solution

1% aqueous osmium tetroxide

Frozen section technique

1. Fix tissue in formalin and cut frozen sections.
2. Wash in distilled water then treat with 1% aqueous osmium tetroxide for 1 h in a dark container.
3. Wash in running water.
4. Mount in an aqueous mountant.

Results

Unsaturated lipids   brown-black
Background   yellow-brown

OSMIUM TETROXIDE METHOD FOR THE DEMONSTRATION OF LIPID IN PARAFFIN SECTIONS

Notes

See previous method.

Technique

1. Fix thin slices of tissue in Flemming's fluid that contains osmium tetroxide (see Appendix 1) for 24–48 h.
2. Wash in running water for 12–16 h and paraffin process.
3. Cut sections at 5–10 μm, mount on slides and dry.
4. Remove wax with xylene and mount with a synthetic resin medium. Counterstaining, prior to mounting, with neutral red or safranin is optional.

Results

Lipids are blackened, as are other reducing substances.

CALCIUM-LIPASE FOR TRIGLYCERIDES (Adams et al 1966)

Notes

Calcium will also be stained with this method and so suitable controls are needed. Pancreatic lipase hydrolyzes triglycerides into fatty acids. In the presence of calcium ions calcium soaps are formed that are then converted to lead soaps and visualized by treatment with ammonium sulphide.

Solution

Tris buffer at pH 8.0   15 ml
2% calcium chloride   10 ml
Distilled water   ·   25 ml
Porcine pancreatic lipase   50 mg

Warm solution to 37°C and filter before use.
1% aqueous lead nitrate

Technique

1. Incubate free-floating frozen, or slide-mounted cryostat, sections in the lipase medium at 37°C for 3 h.
2. Wash sections well and mount on to slides.
3. Together with a duplicate section, not subjected to enzyme, treat with the lead nitrate solution for 15 min.
4. Wash very thoroughly in several changes of distilled water.
5. Immerse for 10 s in dilute ammonium sulphide (three drops of a commercially prepared 10% solution to a Coplin jar of distilled water).
6. Wash well, counterstain with Mayer's haematoxylin (see p. 25) for 3 min.
7. Wash in tap water, followed by a rinse in distilled water.
8. Mount sections in an aqueous mountant.

Results

Triglycerides	brown
Nuclei	blue

ACID HAEMATEIN TECHNIQUE (after Baker 1946)

Notes

The rationale of this technique is that following treatment with a dichromate solution, phospholipids and certain other acidic tissue components form a mordant-type linkage with haematoxylin that is resistant to borax-ferricyanide differentiation. If a duplicate piece of tissue is first subjected to pyridine extraction, only phospholipids are extracted and show a loss of staining (Casselman 1959). If an extracted control block is taken through, this is the most reliable technique for phospholipids.

Solutions

Picro-formal-acetic:

Saturated aqueous picric acid	50 ml
Formalin	10 ml
Acetic acid	5 ml
Distilled water	35 ml

Calcium-dichromate
   Dissolve 5 g potassium dichromate and 2 g of hydrated (1 g anhydrous) calcium chloride in 100 ml of distilled water.
Haematoxylin
   Add 0.5 g haematoxylin and 1 ml of 1% aqueous sodium iodate to 48 ml of distilled water. Bring to the boil, cool to 37°C and add 1 ml of acetic acid. This solution does not keep and should be prepared prior to use.
Differentiator
   Dissolve 0.25 g potassium ferricyanide and 0.25 g borax (sodium borate or tetraborate) in 100 ml distilled water.

Technique

1. Fix one block of the tissue in formal-calcium (1 g anhydrous calcium chloride in 10% formalin) overnight, then transfer to the calcium-dichromate solution for 18 h. Transfer the tissue to fresh calcium-dichromate solution, but at 60°C for 24 h. Wash in running water overnight then cut frozen sections. Alternatively, cut fresh frozen sections and fix in formal-calcium for 1–2 h. Wash in water briefly, then treat with the 60°C calcium-dichromate solution for 12 –16 h. Wash in several changes of distilled water for 30 min.
2. A duplicate control block or fresh frozen section is fixed in the picro-formal-acetic solution for 20 h. Wash in 70% alcohol for 1 h then in 50% alcohol for 30 min and running water for 30 min. Place in pyridine at room temperature for two changes of 1 h each, then into pyridine for 24 h at 60°C. Wash well in running water (2 h or so) then treat in a similar manner to the test block as from the room temperature calcium-dichromate stage in step 1.
3. Take all sections into water and place into the calcium-dichromate solution for 1 h at 60°C (this step may be omitted if the calcium-dichromate-treated section method has been used). Wash sections in several changes of distilled water.
4. Stain in the haematoxylin solution for 2 h at 37°C.
5. Rinse in distilled water and differentiate in the borax-ferricyanide solution for 2 h at 37°C. Wash well in water.
6. Mount in an aqueous mountant.

Results

In unextracted tissue sections, phospholipids, some cerebrosides, nuclei, acidic mucins and red blood cells stain dark blue. (In extracted sections, phospholipids have been removed and are not stained.)

SODIUM HYDROXIDE-ACID HAEMATEIN METHOD FOR SPHINGOMYELIN (Adams & Bayliss 1963)

Notes

This specific method is a development of the acid haematein method. Hydrolysis removes phosphoglycerides but leaves sphingomyelin unaffected, allowing for demonstration by the acid haematein method. Cryostat sections tend to lift from the slide.

Solutions

2 M sodium hydroxide
1% acetic acid

Technique

1. Subject free-floating frozen sections (or slide-mounted cryostat sections) to the sodium hydroxide solution for 1 h at 37°C.
2. Wash well in water and rinse in the acetic acid solution.
3. Mount sections on to slides and proceed as for the acid haematein method (see p. 184).

Results

Sphingomyelin	blue
Other tissue entities	as per previous technique

THE PLASMAL TECHNIQUE (Feulgen & Voit 1924 Terner & Hayes 1961)

Notes

Both acetal phosphatides and plasmalogens are demonstrated by this technique. Mercuric chloride hydrolysis liberates fatty aldehydes that recolour Schiff's reagent to form magenta compounds. The technique is simple but of questionable specificity. As a control, use a duplicate section and omit the mercuric chloride step. Any fixation of tissue should be short (6 h) and only in formalin. Fresh frozen (cryostat) sections are preferred as formalin-fixed tissue may form pseudo-plasmals with Schiff's reagent.

Solutions

1% aqueous mercuric chloride
Schiff's reagent (see p. 135)
2% aqueous methyl green (extracted)

Technique

1. Take either fixed frozen sections or, better, unfixed frozen sections, to distilled water.
2. Treat the test section only with mercuric chloride for 7 min.
3. Transfer all sections to Schiff's reagent for 10 min.
4. Wash in distilled water.
5. Wash in tap water for 10 min. Counterstain in the aqueous methyl green solution for 5 min.
6. Wash and mount in an aqueous mountant.

Results

Plasmals	magenta
Nuclei	green

The negative control section should show no Schiff reaction.

MODIFIED PAS FOR CEREBROSIDE (Adams & Bayliss 1963)

Notes

The chloramine T converts amino groups to carbonyls and must be handled with care as it can become explosive. Periodic acid is used to oxidize the hexose groups within cerebrosides to aldehydes. Blocking techniques are used to suppress other aldehyde reactivity.

Solutions

10% aqueous chloramine T
Performic acid:

98% formic acid	45 ml
30% (100 vol) hydrogen peroxide	4.5 ml
Conc. sulphuric acid	0.5 ml

Prepare an hour before use and stir occasionally with a glass rod, inside a fume cupboard, to release bubbles of gas from the solution.
Saturated solution of 2:4 dinitrophenylhydrazine in M HCl
0.5% periodic acid
Schiff's reagent (see p. 135)

Technique

1. Mount duplicate sections on to separate slides and extract one of these with chloroform-methanol (2:1 v/v) for 1 h at room temperature.
2. Deaminate both sections in the chloramine T solution for 1 h at 37°C.
3. Wash slides vigorously and as rapidly as possible, one at a time, in a large volume of water before transferring them immediately to performic acid for 10 min. The washing is swift, yet thorough, to prevent detachment of sections from slides.
4. Wash well in distilled water.
5. Treat in a filtered solution of 2:4 dinitrophenylhydrazine at 4°C for 2 h; this serves as a blocking step for extraneous aldehydes.
6. Wash well in water.
7. Treat with 0.5% periodic acid for 10 min.
8. Wash in distilled water.
9. Stain in Schiff's reagent for 15 min.
10. Wash in tap water for 15 min to develop colour.
11. Counterstain nuclei with an alum haematoxylin (see p. 25) if wished.
12. Wash in tap water, distilled water and finally mount sections in an aqueous mountant.

Results

Cerebrosides—magenta, indicated by the difference in staining intensity between the extracted and unextracted sections.

COPPER-ORCINOL-HCl METHOD FOR GANGLIOSIDES (Sialic Acids)
(Ravetto 1964)

Notes

The hydrochloric acid used for this method must be fresh, preferably from a newly-opened bottle. The method uses a modified Bial reagent. The resultant reaction colour is pale, but sufficient to see moderate deposits in brain. The method is unpleasant to apply and has been replaced by the BHPS method, given below, in many laboratories.

Solution

Orcinol	0.2 g
0.1 M copper sulphate	0.25 ml
Distilled water	20 ml
Conc. hydrochloric acid	80 ml

Allow the solution to mature for 4 h before use.

Technique

1. Mount frozen sections on to slides and dry thoroughly.
2. Spray the sections with orcinol solution, using a fine spray.
3. Transfer slides to a screwcap polythene container containing Hcl vapour, for 10 min at 70°C. A thin layer of concentrated Hcl is poured into the jar, which is heated to 70°C before inserting the sections.
4. Remove slides and rapidly dry them in a current of air from a compressor or cylinder.
5. Rinse in xylene and mount in Canada balsam.

Results

Gangliosides   pink

BOROHYDRIDE-PERIODATE-SCHIFF (BHPS) METHOD (from Filipe & Lake 1990)

Notes

A chloroform: methanol-extracted section should be used for comparison to exclude interference from non-lipid sialomucins. The reaction can be confirmed by comparison with a sialidase-digested control section that has been pre-treated for 18 hours at 37°C with neuraminidase, ex *Vibrio cholerae*, and diluted 1:4 with 0.1 M acetate buffer at pH 5.5, containing 0.9 mM $CaCl_2$. This digestion is not entirely satisfactory with formalin-fixed material (Bayliss-High 1990).

Solutions

0.1 M (0.38%) sodium borohydride in 1% disodium hydrogen phosphate
0.03% sodium metaperiodate
Schiff's reagent (see p. 135)
Alum haematoxylin (see p. 25)

Technique

1. Destroy existing carbonyls by reducing sections with the sodium borohydride solution for one hour at room temperature.
2. Wash thoroughly in distilled water.

3. Oxidize with the sodium metaperiodate solution for 30 minutes at room temperature.
4. Wash twice for five minutes each time in distilled water.
5. Stain with Schiff's reagent for 10 minutes.
6. Wash well in tap water and then in distilled water.
7. Counterstain with an alum haematoxylin for five minutes.
8. Blue in tap water, rinse in distilled water, then mount sections in an aqueous mountant.

Results

Gangliosides in Tay Sachs' disease	pink
Nuclei	blue

ACRIFLAVINE-DMAB FOR SULPHATIDES (Hollander 1963)

Notes

Sulphatide is stained by an acidic acriflavine solution and the reaction product converted to an insoluble red dye by using DMAB. Mast cells will also stain red.

Solutions

Acriflavine stock solution:

Acriflavine	0.1 g
Distilled water at 80°C	20 ml
Store in the dark at 4°C.	

Acriflavine working solution:

0.1 M citrate-HCl buffer pH 2.5	99 ml
Stock acriflavine solution	1 ml

DMAB solution:

p-dimethylamino-benzaldehyde	0.6 g
20% hydrochloric acid	30 ml
Isopropanol	70 ml

Technique

1. Mount frozen sections on to slides.
2. Stain for 6 min in the acriflavine solution.
3. Differentiate for 1 min in two changes of 70% isopropanol.
4. Treat with the DMAB reagent for 30–45 s.
5. Rinse in distilled water for 2–3 min.
6. Counterstain nuclei in Mayer's haemalum (see p. 25) for 3 min.
7. Blue the haemalum in tap water, rinse in distilled water and mount sections in an aqueous mountant.

Results

Sulphatides	red
Nuclei	blue

Table 8.4 Lipid storage diseases and their staining reactions. This table is based on data from Bayliss-High (1990) and other workers.

Storage disease	Lipid stored	PAS	Sudan black	Oil red O	Luxol fast blue	Toluidine blue	Feyrter thionin
Batten's	Retinoic acid	++	++	+	++	–	–
Fabry's	Ceramide trihexoside	++	++	++	++	–	–
Gaucher's	Gluco-cerebroside	+	±	±	–	–	–
Metachromatic leucodystrophy	Sulphatide	+	+	+	–	++	++
Niemann-Pick's	Sphingomyelin and cholesterol	±	++	++	–	–	–
Krabbe's	Galacto-cerebroside	++	±	±	–	–	–
Tay-Sach's	Ganglioside	++	+	+	++	(+)	++
Wolman's	Cholesterol and triglycerides	±	++	++	–	–	–

REFERENCES

Adams C W M 1961 A perchloric acid-naphthoquinone method for the histochemical localisation of cholesterol. Nature (London) 193: 331
Adams C W M, Bayliss O B 1963 Histochemical observations on the localisation and origin of sphingomyelin, cerebroside and cholesterol in normal and atherosclerotic human artery. Journal of Pathology and Bacteriology 85: 113
Adams C W M, Abdulla Y H, Bayliss O B, Weller R O 1966 Histochemical detection of triglyceride esters with specific lipases and a lead sulphide technique. Journal of Histochemistry and Cytochemistry 14: 385
Baker J R 1946 The histochemical recognition of lipine. Quarterly Journal of Microscopical Science 87: 441
Bayliss O B, Adams C W M 1972 Bromine Sudan black (BSB). A general stain for lipids including free cholesterol. Histochemical Journal 4: 505
Bayliss-High O 1990 Lipids. In: Bancroft J D, Stevens A (eds) Theory and practice of histological techniques, 3rd edn. Churchill Livingstone, Edinburgh
Belt W D, Hayes E R 1956 An ultra-violet Schiff reaction for unsaturated lipids. Stain Technology 31: 117
Benda C 1900 Eine makro-und mikrochemisch Reaction der fett Gewebsnekrose. Virchow's Archiv fur pathologische Anatomie und Physiologie und fur klinische Medizin 161: 194
Cain A J 1947 Use of Nile blue in the examination of lipids. Quarterly Journal of Microscopical Science 88: 383
Casselman W G B 1959 Histochemical techniques. Methuen, London
Chiffelle T L, Putt F A 1951 Propylene and ethylene glycol as solvents for Sudan IV and Sudan black B. Stain Technology 26: 51
Daddi L 1896 Nouvelle methode pour colorer la graisse dans les tissues. Archives Italiennes de Biologie 26: 143
Dunnigan M G 1968 The use of $NBSO_4$ in the histochemical identification of phospholipids. Stain Technology 43: 249
Feulgen R, Voit K 1924 Ueber einen Weitverbreiteten festen Aldehyd seine Entstehung aus einer Varstufe, sein mikrochemischer Nachweis unde die Wege zu seiner preparativen

Darstellung. Pflügers Archiv für die Gesamte Physiologie des Menschen unde der Tiere 206: 389

Filipe M I, Lake B D 1990 Histochemistry. In: Filipe M I, Lake B D (eds) Pathology, 2nd edn. Churchhill Livingstone, London

French R W 1926 Azure C as tissue stain. Stain Technology 1: 79

Herxheimer G W 1903 Zur Fettfürbung. Zeitbl. All. Pathologie Anatomie 14: 841

Holczinger L 1959 Histochemischer Nachweis freier Fattsäuren. Acta Histochemica 8: 167

Hollander H 1963 A staining method for cerebroside-sulphuric esters in brain tissue. Journal of Histochemistry and Cytochemistry 11: 118

Lillie R D 1954 Histopathologic technique and practical histochemistry, 2nd edn. Blakiston, New York

Lillie R D 1965 Histopathologic technique and practical histochemistry, 3rd edn. Blakiston, New York

Lillie R D, Ashburn L L 1943 Supersaturated solutions of fat stains in dilute isopropanol for demonstration of acute fatty degeneration not shown by Herxheimer's technique. Archives of Pathology 36: 432

Lison L, Dagnelie J 1935 Methodes nouvelles de colouration de la myéline. Bulletin d'Histologie Apliquée à la Physiologie et à la Pathologie et de Technique Microscopique 12: 85

Michaelis L 1901 Ueber Fett-Farbstoffe. Virchow's Archiv fur Pathologische Anatomie und fur Klinische Medizin 164: 263

Popper H 1941 Histologic distribution of vitamin A in human organs under normal and pathological conditions. Archives of Pathology 318: 766

Ravetto C 1964 Histochemical demonstration of sialic (neuraminic) acids. Journal of Histochemistry and Cytochemistry 12: 306

Smith J L 1908 On the simultaneous staining of neutral fat and fatty acids by oxazine dyes. Journal of Pathology and Bacteriology 12: 1

Terner G Y, Hayes E R 1961 Histochemistry of plasmalogens. Stain Technology 36: 265

Windaus T 1909 Ueber die quantitative Bestimmung des Cholesterins und der Cholesterinester in einigen normalen und patholgischen Nieren. Z. Phys. Chemistrie 65: 110.

9. Pigments

INTRODUCTION

Pigments dealt with in this chapter are classed as artefact and endogenous pigments; a third group, exogenous pigments, is briefly discussed. Demonstration of the latter is far from satisfactory; the histochemical methods for some metallic salts are not specific and methods do not exist for others.

Endogenous pigments are produced normally by the body; they are found in pathological conditions, when their site and quantity may be changed. There is no clear-cut classification of pigments, as minerals are also classed as pigments. The classification given below is useful but not scientifically precise. Many pigments described are shades of yellow-brown in unstained or H&E sections. The same pigment can adopt a variety of presentations and the laboratory worker should be beware of rash assumptions on an H&E section! Pigments can be divided into two groups: firstly, those that can be coloured, such as haemosiderin and lipofuscin, and secondly those that cannot be coloured, i.e. they are unreactive to dyes. These latter include formalin and carbon, but are identified by their solubility, or lack of it, in acid or alkaline solutions, or their sensitivity to bleaching solutions. Generally they are classified as:

> **Artefact:** fixation pigments (see Table 9.1).
> **Endogenous:** those produced within the tissues.
> **Exogenous:** those gaining access to the tissues—mainly minerals.

Table 9.1 Artefact pigments

Pigment	Removed by	Identified by
Formalin	Alcoholic picric acid	Dark brown to yellow granules; birefringence; site
Mercury	Alcoholic iodine	Coarse brown crystals; distribution
Chromate	Acid-alcohol	Fine yellow-brown deposits

FIXATION PIGMENTS

FORMALIN

The correct name for this birefringent pigment is acid formaldehyde haematin. Its formation is favoured by long-term fixation of highly vascular tissue in acid pH formalin, although we have also seen the formation of a formalin pigment at alkaline pH levels. The pigment may exhibit a variety of forms from a fine diffuse dark brown granule to a yellow needle-like crystal occurring in clusters. Whilst formalin pigment is usually extracellular it may occasionally be found in macrophages. It is reported to be positive with Perls method following microincineration. Unquestionably the most effective means of removing the pigment is by alcoholic picric acid, although the rationale is obscure. If preferred, treat with 0.1% sodium or potassium hydroxide in 70% alcohol, or 10 vols hydrogen peroxide but for longer periods (1–24 h). These methods are long and capricious. Formalin pigments can be largely prevented by using a buffered formalin solution with a pH over 6.5, but even in neutral-buffered formalin-fixed tissue the pigment may still occur.

Extraction solution

Saturated alcoholic picric acid.

Technique

1. Sections to alcohol.
2. Treat with the alcoholic picric acid solution for 10–30 min.
3. Wash well in water for 5 min.
4. Carry out desired staining procedure.

MERCURIC CHLORIDE

Mercuric chloride is found to a variable extent after fixation in mercuric chloride-containing fixatives. It is most pronounced with long fixation. As with formalin pigment, it varies in appearance although it is usually a large extracellular irregular brown crystal found in a birefringent form following primary fixation in formalin and secondary fixation in mercuric chloride. An interesting feature is that, on long storage of sections containing mercuric-chloride pigment, the crystal form changes to a globular one and exhibits Maltese cross-type birefringence. The universal removal technique is by forming soluble iodides and chlorides with iodine followed by hypo bleaching. The iodine treatment is attributed to both Mayer and Vigelius in 1886, whilst hypo bleaching was introduced in 1909 by Heidenhain. Lugol's iodine is used at a standard treatment time; alternatively, use a 0.5% iodine in 70% alcohol solution.

Extraction solutions

Lugol's iodine solution (see p. 59)
5% aqueous sodium thiosulphate (hypo)

Technique

1. Sections to water.
2. Treat with Lugol's iodine solution for 5 min.
3. Wash in water, bleach with 5% hypo for 10–30 s.
4. Wash well in water. Carry out proposed staining technique.

CHROMIC OXIDE

Chromic oxide is a fine yellow-brown precipitate found in tissues due to lack of washing in water following fixation in chromic acid or potassium dichromate-containing fixatives. The subsequent processing alcohols reduce the chrome salts to lower oxides, resulting in the precipitation of insoluble chromic oxides. It is rarely met with in practice and is difficult to produce intentionally. Chromic oxide pigment is monorefringent, extracellular and removed from sections by treatment with 1% acid-alcohol for 30 min.

ENDOGENOUS PIGMENTS

This is the largest group of pigments and by definition should include all those produced by the body. Here a simple classification fails, because the body also produces or utilizes iron, calcium and copper that in pathological conditions may be increased and located in abnormal situations. They are often identified separately as minerals but they are considered here as 'endogenous'. Most of these pigments are derived from blood and are called haematogenous pigments.

HAEMOGLOBIN

Haemoglobin is involved in the transport of oxygen and carbon dioxide within the blood stream. The red pigmented component is termed haem and contains ferrous iron. This cannot be demonstrated, unless it is freed from the protein by treatment with hydrogen peroxide. Other iron-containing pigments are less intensely bound to protein. Under normal conditions haemoglobin is confined to red blood cells and does not require histological demonstration.

Demonstration

There are two methods of demonstration: either the component enzyme, haemoglobin peroxidase, or the haemoglobin itself can be demonstrated. The enzyme is moderately stable and able to withstand short fixation and paraffin processing. Other peroxidase enzymes will also react. The method using patent blue is given below. Due to the basic structure of haemoglobin it is well-stained by acid dyes. Eosin, for example, stains it a vivid orange colour in a well-differentiated section; other acid dye techniques are listed in Table 9.2.

Haemoglobin is monorefringent and non-fluorescent. Fixation is best in formalin or mercuric chloride, and Drury & Wallington (1980) say that Susa preserves it poorly. The following techniques demonstrate haemoglobin well.

Table 9.2   Methods for haemoglobin

Technique	Colour	Element stained
Dunn–Thompson	Green	Haemoglobin
Amido black	Dark blue	Haemoglobin
Kiton red-almond green	Red	Haemoglobin
Leuco patent blue	Blue	Enzyme
Solochrome cyanine	Blue	Lipoprotein envelope
PTAH	Blue	Lipoprotein envelope

DUNN–THOMPSON TECHNIQUE (Dunn & Thompson 1946)

Notes

This is a modified van Gieson method with double haematoxylin staining, giving a stronger colouration to haemoglobin. Fixation in neutral formalin gives the best results.

Solutions

0.25% haematoxylin in 5% aqueous ammonium alum
4% aqueous iron alum
van Gieson (see p. 36)

Technique

1. Sections to water.
2. Stain in the haematoxylin solution for 15 min.
3. Wash in tap water.
4. Mordant in the iron alum solution for 1 min.
5. Stain in the haematoxylin solution for 10 min.
6. Rinse in tap water.
7. Stain in van Gieson's solution for 15 min.
8. Rinse in 95% alcohol for 2 min.
9. Dehydrate, clear and mount as desired.

Results

Haemoglobin casts	green
Red blood cells	greenish black
Collagen	red
Muscle	yellow

KITON RED-ALMOND GREEN TECHNIQUE (Lendrum 1949)

Notes

This highly selective technique gives colourful results after a little practice. The nuclei are strongly stained with haematoxylin to avoid subsequent masking by the green counterstain. Lendrum specified 'almond green' stain, but most contrasting anionic dyes will serve.

Solutions

Saturated brilliant kiton red B in Cellosolve
Almond green stain
   Equal parts saturated tartrazine in Cellosolve and saturated lissamine green BN200 in Cellosolve. This combined solution should be diluted 1:2 with Cellosolve before use.

Technique

1. Sections to water.
2. Stain the nuclei in an iron haematoxylin solution (see p. 37). Differentiate and blue.
3. Rinse in cellosolve. Stain with the kiton red solution for 20–30 min.
4. Differentiate in tap water. The haemoglobin will become a brighter red and the background clearer; this stage may take several minutes.
5. Drain and counterstain with the almond green solution for a few seconds only.
6. Rinse with cellosolve. Clear in xylene and mount as desired.

Results

Nuclei	blue-black
Haemoglobin (red blood cells)	red
Background	green

AMIDO BLACK TECHNIQUE (Puchtler & Sweat 1962)

Notes

Using a tannic acid-phosphomolybdic acid mordanting sequence the amido black is strongly bound by haemoglobin. It is not a capricious technique and does not require great expertise. The authors recommend Zenker-formal fixation, but this is not essential.

Solutions

5% aqueous tannic acid
1% aqueous phosphomolybdic acid
Saturated amido black 10B (syn. naphthalene black)
   In nine parts methanol to one part conc. acetic acid.
1% aqueous neutral red

Technique

1. Sections to water. The authors recommend mordanting sections overnight in Zenker-formal, should the tissue not have been fixed in this solution (see Notes).
2. Treat with the tannic acid solution for 5 min.
3. Wash well in distilled water. Treat with the phosphomolybdic acid solution for 10 min.
4. Wash well in distilled water, drain and blot dry.
5. Filter on the amido black solution and leave for 5 min.
6. Rinse in methanol-acetic (9:1) then in water.
7. Counterstain in the neutral red for 5 min. Wash, dehydrate, clear and mount as desired.

Results

Oxyhaemoglobin and methaemoglobin	dark blue
Nuclei	red

LEUCO PATENT BLUE TECHNIQUE (Lison 1938, Dunn 1946)

Notes

Patent blue is reduced to its leuco form by nascent hydrogen, and in the presence of the enzyme (haemoglobin peroxidase) it is re-colourized by hydrogen peroxide oxidation. Aniline blue may be used for the patent blue. The method is specific and reliable. Poorly fixed tissue and tissue fixed for longer than 48 h in formalin may be negative due to loss of the enzyme. A positive control section should be taken through with the test sections.

Solutions

Stock leuco patent blue
> To 100 ml of 1% aqueous patent blue V add 10 g powdered zinc and 2 ml acetic acid. Boil until the solution is a pale straw colour (approx. 10 min). Cool, filter.

Working solution
> To 10 ml stock solution add 2 ml acetic acid and 1 ml of 10 volumes hydrogen peroxide.

1% aqueous neutral red

Technique

1. Sections to distilled water.
2. Stain with the leuco patent blue solution for 3–5 min.
3. Wash well in distilled water.
4. Counterstain with the neutral red solution for 5 min. Wash.
5. Dehydrate, clear and mount as desired.

Results

Haemoglobin peroxidase (red blood cells and neutrophils)	blue
Nuclei	red

MALARIA PIGMENT

An alternative name for this pigment is 'haemozoin'. It is a blood-derived pigment found in reticulo-endothelial cells of organs such as liver, spleen and brain in cases of malaria. It is a fine, dark brown pigment and reacts histochemically like formalin precipitate in that it is birefringent and soluble in alcoholic picric acid. Unlike formalin pigment, it is invariably intracellular. Similar to haemoglobin, some of the protein-masked iron fraction of malaria pigment can be made available for the Perls reaction by treating with hydrogen peroxide. Schistosome infestation may produce a pigment histologically identical to haemozoin.

PORPHYRIN PIGMENTS

Porphyrin pigments are involved in haemoglobin synthesis and are rarely found in tissue sections. On occasion deposition occurs in familial porphyria, which is an uncommon disease in which the patient passes a port wine-coloured urine due to the presence of large amounts of porphyrins. These appear in the liver as dark brown intracellular granules. The most effective way to demonstrate the pigment is to examine fresh frozen sections with a fluorescence microscope, when a brilliant orange primary fluorescence will be seen. For details see Cripps & Scheuer (1965) and Cripps & MacEachern (1971).

BILE PIGMENTS

The breakdown process of red blood cells occurs in the reticulo-endothelial system. During the process haemoglobin is released from the red cells and iron is removed from the haem, leaving biliverdin. This is produced in phagocytic cells in the spleen and bone marrow and transported to the liver; in this form it is insoluble in water. In the liver it is reduced from biliverdin to bilirubin, which is also insoluble in water until it is conjugated with glucuronic acid. The conjugated bilirubin is passed through the liver to the gall bladder. In histological sections various stages of bile production can be present. Whilst called 'bile pigments' they are chemically different and may not react histologically and histo-chemically in the same manner. The general term 'bile pigments' is used because in the normal course of events sections of liver containing bile will invariably contain a mixture. In addition a related pigment—haematoidin, occurring in tissue—is classed as a bile pigment. This is found in old haemorrhagic areas, most often in the spleen and brain. It is thought that haem has undergone a chemical change at its site and has not been transported to the liver. The bile pigments, in summary, consist of biliverdin – bilirubin (unconjugated) – bilirubin(conjugated)–haematoidin. In liver, bilirubin and biliverdin are most often seen in association with disorders such as bile cholestasis and biliary cirrhosis.

Identification

The first step is to consider the normal localization of the substances. Biliverdin will be found in phagocytic cells in the spleen, bone marrow and lymph nodes whilst the unconjugated bilirubin is found in liver cells and the conjugated form in bile canali-culi and the gall bladder. Colour can also be used in identification, i.e. biliverdin appears as a green pigment, bilirubin as a dark brown pigment, while haematoidin is a yellow amorphous deposit.

Demonstration

Although the brown and yellow colours of bilirubin and haematoidin respectively are well-recognized in an H&E section, the green colour of biliverdin is often masked by eosin. In these instances an unstained paraffin or frozen section with a haematoxylin nuclear stain only is required. Bile pigments are not autofluorescent and are monorefringent. Their solubilities in fixed tissue sections are unhelpful, although it has been reported that haematoidin is partly soluble in fat solvents. Most techniques for demonstrating bile pigments are oxidation methods; the classic ones of Gmelin, Stein and Fouchet follow. The Schmorl reaction, van Gieson method and, on occasion, the PAS technique will also demonstrate the pigments— blue, green and magenta, respectively.

GMELIN TECHNIQUE (Tiedemann & Gmelin 1826)

Notes

Tissue containing a bile pigment treated with nitric acid produces a spectrum of colours. This colour spectrum is achieved by the oxidation of bilirubin to biliverdin, then to an admixture of biliverdin and purpurins, finally to a mixture of these plus yellow choletins. The method is capricious and impermanent; it gives the best results with large bile pigment deposits.

Solution

Conc. nitric acid

Technique

1. Sections to distilled water and place a coverslip on the sections.
2. Place one or two drops of concentrated nitric acid to one side of the coverslip and draw under the coverslip by a piece of blotting paper placed at the opposite side.
3. Wipe off excess solution and examine immediately.

Results

In the presence of bile pigment the following colour spectrum will gradually appear:

green–blue–purple–red–yellow

STEIN TECHNIQUE (Stein 1935)

Notes

Bilirubin is oxidized by iodine to form green biliverdin, although in practice this is not readily observed. Bile pigments take up iodine and stain a dark brown. Although the method is slow and non-specific it clearly demonstrates even small bile pigment granules. A method similar in principle to Stein's is the use of pH 2.2 potassium dichromate to achieve oxidation of bilirubin to green biliverdin (Glenner 1957). The final dehydration is carried out in acetone as ethanol will extract the iodine colouration.

Solutions

Lugol's iodine (see p. 59)
Tincture of iodine:

Iodine	2.5 g
Potassium iodide	2.5 g
Distilled water	25 ml
Absolute alcohol	75 ml

Mix 3 parts of Lugol's iodine with 1 part of the tincture of iodine.
5% aqueous sodium thiosulphate (hypo)
1% aqueous neutral red

Technique

1. Sections to water.
2. Stain with the iodine solution for 6–12 h.
3. Wash in water and differentiate in the hypo for 15–30 s.
4. Wash in water and counterstain lightly with neutral red for 1–2 min. Wash.

Results

Bile pigments	green (or brown)
Any amyloid or glycogen present	brown
Nuclei	red

FOUCHET TECHNIQUE (Fouchet 1917)

Notes

In the presence of trichloracetic acid, bile pigments are oxidized by ferric chloride to form a mixture of green bilirubin and blue cholecyanin. The technique is quick and simple and demonstrates both coarse and fine pigment deposits. We consider it to be the method of choice. While counterstains such as neutral red are suitable, van Gieson's solution seems to accentuate the green-blue reaction product.

Solution

Fouchet's reagent:

25% aqueous trichloracetic acid	100 ml
10% aqueous ferric chloride	100 ml

van Gieson's solution (see p. 36)

Technique

1. Sections to distilled water.
2. Stain with Fouchet's reagent for 5 min.
3. Rinse in distilled water.
4. Counterstain with van Gieson's solution for 2–3 min.
5. Rinse in distilled water, or drain and wash in alcohol. Dehydrate, clear and mount as desired.

Results

Bile pigments	blue-green
Collagen	red
Muscle	yellow

LIPOFUSCINS

These pigments are produced from the process of oxidation of lipids and lipoproteins. They have a variable structure differing with distribution in the body. The oxidation of the lipid material is progressive and accounts for the variable staining reactions and the different colours, shape and size of the pigments. Lipofuscin is normally laid down during the ageing process. It is also seen in vitamin E deficiency and, not uncommonly, as an unexpected pigment in unlikely situations (e.g. cervix, omentum).

These pigments are seen in many tissues: the more common are liver, cardiac muscle cells, the inner layer of the adrenal cortex, the interstitial cells of the testis and the cytoplasm of neurones. During progressive oxidation, the first produced lipofuscins are only partly oxidized, including ceroid. This and other 'early lipofuscins' retain some of the staining characteristics of lipids but may fail to stain by other methods. The histochemical reactions vary by the amount of oxidation that has occurred. The further the oxidation, the stronger the reaction seen with the reduction methods. It is necessary to use more than one method to demonstrate lipofuscin—other pigments are also capable of reducing solutions, including melanin. Lipofuscins are mainly formed from lysosomes but also mitochondria (Lambert 1980).

Demonstration

There are many staining techniques for lipofuscins. The two most precise depend upon the lipid content staining with Sudan dyes (sudanophilia) and acid-fastness with the Ziehl–Neelsen technique. The more oxidized lipofuscins give a strong result with the Schmorl reaction due to their increased reducing ability. Some of the early lipofuscins are PAS-positive although the reason for this is not known. Other methods are shown in Table 9.3.

Table 9.3   Methods for lipofuscins

Method	Colour/reaction
Long ZN	Magenta
Sudan black	Black
Schmorl	Dark blue
Masson–Fontana	Black
PAS	Magenta
Giemsa	Greenish
Aldehyde fuchsin	Purple
Basic dyes	According to dye
Thionin pH 3.0	Dark green
Primary fluorescence	Yellow
Bleaching	Removal

Melanosis coli pigment

This is a misleading term as the pigment is a lipofuscin rather than melanin. It is found in macrophages in the lamina propria of the colon and rectum and is associated with long-term ingestion of phenolic laxatives. It is Schmorl-and PAS-positive.

SUDAN BLACK TECHNIQUE

Solution

Saturated Sudan black B in 70% alcohol

Technique

1. Paraffin sections to 70% alcohol.
2. Stain overnight at room temperature in the Sudan black B solution (filter the desired quantity into a Coplin jar).
3. Wash and differentiate out the excess background dye in 70% alcohol.
4. Wash in water and mount in an aqueous mountant such as Apathy's mountant.

Results

Lipofuscin pigment, red blood cells	black
Background	weak grey

LONG ZIEHL–NEELSEN TECHNIQUE (PEARSE 1960)

Notes

Victoria blue may be used to advantage for basic fuchsin in the staining solution.

Solutions

Carbol fuchsin (see p. 245)
0.2% aqueous methylene blue

Technique

1. Sections to water.
2. Stain in filtered carbol fuchsin for 3 h at 56°C.
3. Wash well in water.
4. Differentiate in 1% acid-alcohol until the excess background staining is lost (1–3 min).
5. Wash in water, counterstain in the aqueous methylene blue solution for $\frac{1}{2}$–1 min. Wash.
6. Dehydrate and differentiate the counterstain in alcohol. Clear and mount as desired.

Results

Lipofuscin	bright magenta
Nuclei	blue
Background	pale magenta to pale blue

SCHMORL TECHNIQUE (taken from Golodetz & Unna 1909)

Notes

There are two often-quoted rationales for the Schmorl technique. Potassium ferricyanide is reduced to ferrous salt, which in the presence of the ferric ions forms Prussian blue. Alternatively the ferric chloride is reduced to the ferrous salt that reacts with potassium ferricyanide to form Turnbull blue. The result is than an insoluble blue pigment is formed by the reducing agents in situ. The time of reaction depends on the substance to be demonstrated; for lipofuscin 5 or 6 min is usually sufficient. Melanin requires a shorter incubation time (2–3 min). Ferric sulphate may be used in place of the ferric chloride and seems to result in a lighter background to the sections. A control section is taken through with the test sections. It is important to wash thoroughly in water before counterstaining with neutral red, otherwise staining will be weak and show precipitation of the dye.

Staining solutions

1% aqueous potassium ferricyanide (prepare fresh) with equal parts 1% aqueous ferric chloride or 1% aqueous ferric sulphate. Use within 30 min of mixing.
1% aqueous neutral red

Technique

1. Sections to distilled water.
2. Treat with the reagent mixture for 30 s to 10 min (see Notes).
3. Wash well in tap water for several minutes.
4. Counterstain in the neutral red solution for 5 min.
5. Wash, dehydrate, clear and mount in a synthetic resin.

Results

Argentaffin (enterochromaffin) cells, chromaffin cells, melanin, some lipofuscins, thyroid colloid, sulphydryl groups	dark blue
Nuclei	red

CONTROLLED pH THIONIN TECHNIQUE (Lillie 1954)

Notes

At a pH of 3.0 thionin will selectively stain lipofuscin, the blue dye combining with the brown pigment to give a dark green colouration.

Staining solution

0.25% thionin in pH 3.0 buffer (see Buffer Tables)

Technique

1. Sections to distilled water.
2. Stain with the thionin solution for 3 min.
3. Wash in distilled water, blot dry, clear and mount in a DPX-type mountant.

Results

Lipofuscin	dark green
Nuclei	blue

MELANIN

Melanin is an intracellular pigment varying in colour from light brown to black, the colouration depending upon the amount of melanin at the site. It is normally located in skin, retina, substantia nigra of the brain, and hair shafts. Melanin is produced from tyrosine (see p. 91) and the active sites of melanin production are well-demonstrated by the DOPA oxidase reaction (see p. 320). The melanins are bound to proteins and these complexes are located within cells that, in skin, are known as melanophores. The main importance of this pigment lies in its identification in secondary deposits of malignant melanoma.

Demonstration

Melanin can be identified by methods using its reducing capabilities with silver (Masson–Fontana) and ferricyanide (Schmorl). The active sites can be demonstrated by enzyme methods as described above. The solubility of melanin in strong alkali is used, as is the bleaching effect with potassium permanganate. Fluorescence can be produced by the treatment of melanin precursor cells with formaldehyde—formaldehyde-induced fluorescence (FIF). See Table 9.4.

Table 9.4 Methods for melanin

Method	Type of method	Colour	Comments
Masson–Fontana	Silver reduction	Black	Other substances will react
Schmorl	Ferricyanide reduction	Blue	Other substances will react
DOPA reaction	Enzyme	Brown	Specific
Potassium permanganate	Bleaching	Colourless	Selective
Sodium hydroxide	Solubility	Removed	Selective
FIF	Fluorescence	Yellow	Selective

Bleaching technique

Bleaching of melanin pigment in tissue sections is required either to confirm its identity, or to more easily study the cell picture in a heavily pigmented lesion. This most often arises in melanotic tumours of animals. With regard to the former situation it should be borne in mind that lipofuscin pigment is also similarly bleached, although at a much slower rate. In practical terms, the technique times given are those at which only melanin pigment should be bleached.

Notes

As well as the simple potassium permanganate solution given below it is possible to use the permanganate-sulphuric acid solution employed in silver techniques for reticulin. This is quicker in action (5 min or so) but more likely to cause the section to become detached from the slide. Whatever solution is used it is prudent to use a section adhesive when the slides are prepared. Following the permanganate treatment, it will be found that staining by H&E is, to some extent, inhibited. This is particularly noticeable regarding weak eosin staining.

Technique

1. Take sections to water. These should include positive control sections if a precise pigment identification is being essayed.
2. Treat with 1% aqueous potassium permanganate solution for 10 – 30 min.
3. Wash briefly in water then treat with 5% aqueous oxalic acid until the sections are colourless (approximately 1 min.).
4. Wash well in running water for several minutes then apply the appropriate demonstration technique.

MASSON–FONTANA TECHNIQUE (Fontana 1912, Masson 1914)

Notes

Masson's technique using Fontana's silver solution does not employ a reducing bath and only demonstrates substances capable of silver-salt reduction. It is simple and the success, or otherwise, of the technique devolves on the preparation of the ammoniacal silver solution. A positive control section should be taken through with the test. We prefer the longer room-temperature treatment for more precise results.

Solutions

Silver solution

Add concentrated ammonia drop by drop to 20 ml of 10% aqueous silver nitrate, mixing well between each drop, until the formed precipitate almost re-dissolves. A faint opalescence will be evident when the end-point is reached. Should the ammonia addition be overshot, add 10% aqueous silver nitrate drop by drop with constant mixing, until a faint opalescence is obtained. Finally, add 20 ml of distilled water, mix and filter. Store in a dark container. The solution may be used repeatedly for up to 1 month, although a fresher solution gives better results for lipofuscin and argentaffin granules.

0.5% aqueous sodium thiosulphate (hypo)
1% aqueous neutral red

Technique

1. Sections to distilled water.
2. Treat with ammoniacal silver solution in a dark container (e.g. a Coplin jar painted black) for either 20–40 min at 56°C or overnight at room temperature.
3. Wash well in several changes of distilled water.
4. Treat with 0.5% hypo for 2 min (a stronger solution tends to bleach the reduced silver).
5. Wash, counterstain in the neutral red solution for 3–5 min.
6. Wash, dehydrate, clear and mount as desired.

Results

Melanin, argentaffin (enterochromaffin) cells, chromaffin, some lipofuscin pigment	black
Nuclei	red

FORMALDEHYDE-INDUCED FLUORESCENCE (Eranko 1955)

Notes

Certain aromatic amines—e.g. dopamine, catecholamines, 5HT—when exposed to formaldehyde form non-fluorescent isocarboline derivatives that after spontaneous dehydrogenation become fluorescent. Mast cells, enterochromaffin cells, adrenal chromaffin cells, C cells of thyroid and melanin-producing cells fixed in formalin or formaldehyde vapour, exhibit a yellow primary fluorescence. This is useful when demonstrating a secondary amelanotic melanoma. This type of lesion can be difficult to diagnose and yields a negative melanin reaction, but as melanoma cells contain dopamine they are capable of showing the formalin-induced fluorescence for identification.

The best results are achieved using freeze-dried slightly humid paraformaldehyde vapour-fixed material but the following technique gives acceptable results using formalin-fixed frozen sections. Paraffin-processed material may also be used, though with inferior results. Also note (Corrodi et al 1964) that the FIF of biogenic amines but *not* that of other autofluorescent substances can be destroyed by treating the aldehyde-fixed sections (before microscopy) with 0.5% sodium borohydride for 30 min.

Technique

1. Deparaffinize formalin-fixed paraffin sections in xylene. Frozen sections are rinsed in distilled water.
2. Rinse the paraffin sections in clean xylene and mount in a DPX-type mountant (avoid Canada balsam as this is autofluorescent), or mount the frozen sections in 50% glycerol.
3. Examine the sections using a mercury vapour ultraviolet emission lamp incorporating a red suppression filter (e.g. BG 38), ultraviolet exciter filter (e.g. UG1) and colourless barrier filter (e.g. K430).

Results

Melanin-precursor cells	weak yellow fluorescence
Other naturally fluorescing material, e.g. elastin	silver-white

Alternatively (Hoyt et al 1979)

Prepare a solution of 6% paraformaldehyde in pH 7.2 phosphate buffer at 90°C. Cool and filter. Fix blocks for 1–3 days and then section. Results as before.

IRON AND HAEMOSIDERIN

Iron is absorbed from the gastro-intestinal tract and combines with a protein molecule for its transportation to the bone marrow where it is incorporated into the haemoglobin molecule. Iron is also stored in the bone marrow and spleen in its ferric state as haemosiderin when it is loosely combined with protein. When haemoglobin is broken down in tissue haemosiderin is produced. The fine golden brown pigment in tissue sections is usually derived from damaged red cells and occurs in macrophages. It consists of hydrated ferric oxide formed by the intracellular degradation of ferritin (Richter 1978). Haemochromatosis and haemosiderosis are two conditions where there is a heavy deposition of haemosiderin in the liver.

Demonstration

Not all iron in tissues can be demonstrated. On occasions metallic iron introduced into the tissues by industrial exposure will fail to react with the usual methods. Iron firmly bound with protein, as in haemoglobin, will also fail to react unless released from the protein by treatment with hydrogen peroxide. It is rarely necessary to demonstrate this type of iron in the routine laboratory.

Perls reaction is used to demonstrate ferric iron (ferritin is also demonstrated) and is one of the classic histochemical methods, being introduced by Perls in 1867. The Schmeltzer technique (1933) will demonstrate both ferric and ferrous iron, although the latter is rarely found in tissues.

PERLS TECHNIQUE (Perls 1867)

Notes

Hydrochloric acid splits the bound protein, allowing potassium ferrocyanide to combine specifically with ferric iron to form ferric ferrocyanide (Prussian blue). Weak solutions used for a lengthy period give more precise results; Bunting (1949) found that 2% solutions were best. Whilst stronger results are produced by carrying out the reaction at a raised temperature (e.g. 56°C), false positive results can be obtained and it is recommended that room temperature is used. A control section of positive material should always be taken through with the test material.

Following reaction with ferrocyanide-hydrochloric acid the sections should be well washed in water; otherwise, with a neutral red counterstain, a heavy dye precipitate will be formed on the section. Mounting should be in a DPX-type mountant to prevent the eventual fading of the Prussian blue that occurs in mountants such as Canada balsam. In this technique a common artefact is the presence of blue granules, either on or around the section, following treatment with the hydrochloric-ferrocyanide mixture. In our experience this may be due to either an old deteriorated potassium ferrocyanide solution or iron contaminants in the floating-out water (rust, etc.) during sectioning. The simplest remedy is to have a suitably sized beaker containing distilled water to one side of the bath. The distilled water is maintained at the correct temperature and it is a simple matter to float out sections to be stained by the Perls reaction.

Solutions

2% aqueous potassium ferrocyanide
2% hydrochloric acid
1% aqueous neutral red

Technique

1. Test sections and a control section to distilled water.

2. Mix equal parts of the hydrochloric acid and potassium ferrocyanide solutions and filter on to the sections. Leave for 30 min at room temperature, changing to a fresh solution after 15 min.
3. Wash for several minutes in water.
4. Stain with the neutral red solution for 5 min. Wash in water.
5. Dehydrate and differentiate in alcohol. Clear and mount in a DPX-type mountant.

Results

Haemosiderin (ferric iron salts)	blue
Nuclei	red
Background	pale red

QUINKE TECHNIQUE (Quinke 1880)

Both ferric and ferrous iron salts are converted to a black ferrous sulphide by treating with yellow ammonium sulphide. This method is not specific for iron salts as both silver and lead deposits are also blackened.

TIRMANN TECHNIQUE (Tirmann 1898)

This is similar in principle to the Perls reaction, but the ferrous iron haemosiderin is converted to ferrous ferricyanide (Turnbull blue) by potassium ferricyanide. Hydrochloric acid is used to split the remaining protein moiety from the iron. The method is regarded as specific.

SCHMELTZER TECHNIQUE (Schmeltzer 1933)

Schmeltzer utilized ammonium sulphide treatment to convert the ferric iron to ferrous iron and, by subsequently carrying out the Tirmann reaction, simultaneously demostrated both ferric and ferrous iron. There seems to be considerable discrepancy in the literature about the concentrations of the reagents used, which usually means that it is of little real significance in practice! Celloidinization of sections is advisable, mainly due to the action of ammonium sulphide. Any silver or lead present will be seen as black deposits.

Solutions

Undiluted yellow ammonium sulphide solution (usually 10% of H_2S w/v)
20% aqueous potassium ferricyanide
2% hydrochloric acid
1% aqueous neutral red

Technique

1. Test and control sections to distilled water.
2. Treat with the ammonium sulphide solution for 1–3 h.
3. Wash well in several changes of distilled water over several minutes.

4. Mix equal parts of the hydrochloric acid and potassium ferricyanide solutions and filter on to the sections. Leave for 15 – 20 min.
5. Wash well in water for several minutes.
6. Stain with the neutral red solution for 5 min. Wash in water.
7. Dehydrate and differentiate in alcohol. Clear and mount in a DPX-type mountant.

Results

Ferric and ferrous iron	blue
Nuclei	red
Background	pale red

CALCIUM

Insoluble inorganic calcium salts, normally found in bone and teeth, can be shown by several techniques (see also crystals identification, p. 416). Calcium circulates in the blood in free ionic form, which is not demonstrable histochemically. Abnormally, calcium is formed in tissue in hyperparathyroidism, necrosis (e.g. tuberculous caseation) and in association with some tumours such as myeloma.

Demonstration

Various types of calcium salt can be demonstrated but those most commonly occurring are calcium phosphate and carbonate. Calcium salts are usually monorefringent (see p. 416).

H&E appearance

Calcium salts are purple-blue in colour but on occasion may not stain. The haematoxylin staining is attributed to trace elements of iron in the calcium salts and is not diagnostic for calcium per se.

Chemical test to differentiate between phosphate and carbonate radicals

To identify more positively a given calcium salt, two paraffin sections are taken to distilled water and a coverslip placed on each. A small drop of conc. hydrochloric acid is drawn under the coverslips and the effect noted microscopically. If the salt consists of calcium carbonate it will dissolve, liberating bubbles of carbon dioxide. If the salt is that of calcium phosphate the salt will dissolve without effervescence.

Staining with dyes

Various dyes react with calcium salts in a variety of ways. Alizarin, purpurin, naphthochrome green B and nuclear fast red act by forming chelate complexes with the metallic calcium whereas alcian blue stains by salt linkage with the phosphate radical. These methods stain only the larger deposits of calcium salts well, the smaller deposits weakly. None of these stains is specific for calcium.

VON KOSSA TECHNIQUE

The technique and principle of this method are given on page 410. Calcium as such is not demonstrated (only the phosphate or carbonate radicals). It demonstrates both large and small deposits of calcium. Although not specific (melanin also tends to blacken) it remains the method of choice. For the reduction of silver using light or ultraviolet rays, it is possible to use 0.5% aqueous hydroquinone for 5 min following silver nitrate treatment for 10–20 min in the dark (Gomori 1952). Unfortunately, this variant results in a rather granular background and is not widely used. As a rule, non-acidic fixation of tissue should be used, such as formalin or alcohol.

ALIZARIN RED S METHOD FOR CALCIUM (McGee-Russell 1958)

Notes

Calcium forms an orange-red dye lake with alizarin red S. The staining time is dependent upon the amount of calcium in the sections and should be microscopically controlled until the deposits are orange-red in colour but not too diffuse. The calcium deposits stained with alizarin red S are birefringent. The dye lake is specific for calcium at pH 4.2.

Solution

2% alizarin red S (aqueous) pH adjusted to 4.2 with 10% ammonium hydroxide.

Technique

1. Sections to water.
2. Rinse in distilled water.
3. Transfer sections to alizarin red S solution for 1–5 min (see Notes).
4. Blot, rinse in acetone for 30 s.
5. Treat with acetone-xylene 1:1 for 15 s.
6. Rinse in fresh xylene and mount as desired.

Results

Calcium deposits   orange-red

PURPURIN TECHNIQUE (from Lillie 1965)

Notes

Purpurin demonstrates only the larger aggregates of calcium salts and does so by forming a mordant lake with the metal. Counterstaining should be light as the purpurin staining is easily masked. The post-staining treatment with sodium chloride presumably acts to stabilize the stain compound formed.

Solutions

Saturated alcoholic purpurin (syn. 1:2:4-trihydroxyanthraquinone)
0.75% aqueous sodium chloride

Technique

1. Sections to alcohol.
2. Place in a Coplin jar of the alcoholic purpurin solution for 10 min.
3. Treat with the sodium chloride solution for 3 min. Wash in water.
4. Counterstain, if desired, with Mayer's haematoxylin solution (see p. 25) for $1\frac{1}{2}$ min. Wash in water and blue.
5. Wash in water. Dehydrate, clear and mount as desired.

Results

Calcium	red
Nuclei	blue

CALCIUM-PRUSSIAN BLUE TECHNIQUE (Hurst et al 1951)

Notes

Calcium ammonium ferrocyanide is precipitated by the reaction of calcium salts with a potassium ferrocyanide-ammonium acetate solution. This precipitate, when treated with ferric chloride, forms Prussian blue. This is an ingenious method for demonstrating calcium salts in tissue, but unfortunately, only the large deposits react well. Following treatment with the ferrocyanide-ammonium acetate the section is rinsed in 40% alcohol. This rinsing must be minimal or the reaction will be weakened. The final colour product is not strong, so that counterstaining should be light. Any magnesium salts present in the tissue will also react but this is unlikely, in practice, to cause confusion.

Solutions

Ferrocyanide-ammonium acetate
Dissolve 10 g ammonium acetate in 100 ml of 40% alcohol, add 1 g potassium ferrocyanide. Dissolve by placing in the 56°C oven. Cool before use.
10% aqueous ferric chloride
0.5% aqueous neutral red

Technique

1. Sections to alcohol and rinse in 40% alcohol.
2. Treat with the ferrocyanide-ammonium acetate solution for 30 s.
3. Rinse quickly in two baths of 40% alcohol, then in distilled water.
4. Treat with the ferric chloride solution for 5 min.
5. Wash in water, if desired stain lightly with the neutral red solution ($\frac{1}{2}$–1 min).
6. Dehydrate, clear and mount in a DPX-type mountant.

Results

Calcium salts	blue
Background	pale blue or colourless
Nuclei	red

FLUORESCENT MORIN TECHNIQUE (from Pearse 1960)

Notes

Most metallic salts are demonstrated by this method. As in many fluorescence techniques there is a gradual loss of fluorescent staining on storage of the sections. A control section treated with weak hydrochloric acid is also taken through; any dissolved morin-positive crystals can be regarded as calcium salts.

Solutions

1% hydrochloric acid
0.2 g morin (syn. pentahydroxyflavone) dissolved in a solution consisting of 0.5% acetic acid in 85% alcohol.

Technique

1. Two duplicate sections to distilled water. Treat one only with the hydrochloric acid solution for 10 min.
2. Wash well in water, then in alcohol.
3. Treat both sections with the morin reagent for 3 min.
4. Wash and dehydrate in alcohol, clear and mount in a DPX-type mountant.

Results

Using a fluorescence microscope with a mercury vapour lamp and a BG 12 exciter and K 530 (yellow) barrier filter:

Calcium, aluminium, barium, zirconium (also red blood cells)	bright yellow-green
Background	dull green
Calcium salts	not stained in the extracted section

COPPER

Copper is a normal constituent of many tissues but histochemical methods are not sensitive enough to demonstrate it at normal body levels, only in increased amounts in liver, for example in Wilson's disease and primary biliary cirrhosis.

Demonstration

There are four main methods available for showing copper: the dye lake method of Mallory & Parker (1939) using non-ripened alkaline haematoxylin, the DMABR method of Howell (1959), and the rhodanine technique (Jain et al 1978), as well as the standard method of Uzman (1956) using rubeanic acid; the latter two are described below. It should also be noted that copper may be indirectly demonstrated by the Shikata orcein technique (see p. 258) for copper-associated protein. According to Davies et al (1989) this is the more reliable approach to the diagnosis of Wilson's disease.

RUBEANIC ACID TECHNIQUE (from Okamoto & Utamura 1938)

Notes

Rubeanic acid (dithio-oxamide) forms a coloured copper rubeanate compound with copper. The technique is not sensitive but gives clear results. Fixation is important in that formalin should be used but mercuric chloride is contra-indicated. A positive control section should always be taken through with test sections. Sections are prone to lift from the slide in this technique. It is prudent to use a section adhesive (see p. 32) and to celloidinize the slide.

Solutions

0.1% rubeanic acid in 5 ml absolute alcohol to which is added 10% aqueous sodium acetate 100 ml.
0.5% aqueous neutral red

Technique

1. Sections to distilled water.
2. Place in a Coplin jar filled with the rubeanic-acetate solution for 8–16 h at 37°C, i.e. overnight for convenience.
3. Wash briefly in distilled water and blot dry. Counterstain briefly (1–2 min) in the neutral red solution.
4. Dehydrate, clear and mount as desired.

Results

Copper rubeanate	greenish black
Nuclei	red

RHODANINE TECHNIQUE (Lindquist 1969, Jain et al 1978)

Notes

This is a reliable method for copper, also the positive red colour is considered by many to be more easily discerned than the dark green of the rubeanic acid technique. A further advantage is that sections are less readily detached from the slide. The rationale is that rhodanine forms chelate bonds with copper.

Solutions

Stock solution
 Dissolve 2 g rhodanine* in 100 ml ethanol (shake well before use).
Working solution
 Stock solution 3 ml and distilled water 47 ml.
Borax solution
 0.5% aqueous sodium borate.
Mayer's haematoxylin (see p. 25)

---

* obtainable as p-Dimethylaminobenzylidine rhodanine (Merck)

> **Technique**
>
> 1. Test and control sections to distilled water.
> 2. Treat with rhodanine solution for 3 h at 56°C (pre-heat).
> 3. Wash well in water and stain the nuclei with Mayer's haematoxylin for 1–2 min.
> 4. Wash in several changes of distilled water then in the borax solution for 2–3 s.
> 5. Wash in water, dehydrate, clear and mount as desired.

Results

Copper	red granules
Nuclei	blue

EXOGENOUS PIGMENTS AND MINERALS

These pigments are usually found in the body due to industrial exposure. Their most likely sites are lungs and skin (see Table 9.5). Techniques will be given for metallic salts in tissue, but for laboratories possessing the necessary equipment, electron probe microanalysis is the definitive means by which metals may be identified.

CARBON

This is found in the lungs (except the newborn) and in lymph nodes. It is an inert and unreactive element and lacks methods for its demonstration, and is moreover resistant to bleaching and to solution in strong acids. It is easily identified because of its blackness, localization and irregular shape.

Table 9.5 Exogenous pigments

Pigment	Usual site	Method
Carbon	Lungs, lymph nodes	None available
Silica	Lungs	None available but birefringent
Asbestos	Lungs	Perls, birefringent if recent (and therefore uncoated)
Lead	Kidney, bone	See below
Beryllium	Lungs, skin	See below
Aluminium	Lungs, skin	See below
Silver	Skin, nasal mucosa, gum	Rhodanine method, see Bancroft & Stevens (1990)
Gold	Gum, skin	See below

SILICA

Tiny particles are found abnormally in fibrous tissue of lungs and lymph nodes. It is an inert substance for which there is no definitive technique; the particles show birefringence.

ASBESTOS

It is seen as long beaded fibres that cause a fibrous reaction. Prolonged exposure leads to the disease asbestosis. Initially the fibres show birefringence; after the fibrous reaction the fibres become coated in protein and develop their characteristic morphology. The protein sheath contains haemosiderin, giving a positive reaction with the Perls method. The asbestos fibre with its coated protein sheath is known as an asbestos body, and is easily seen in an H&E preparation and the Perls reaction.

ALUMINIUM AND BERYLLIUM

The appearance of aluminium in an H&E preparation varies from a fine brown granule to small crystalline plates staining a pale pink colour. Besides the technique described, aluminium will exhibit a secondary fluorescence in the morin technique (see p. 213). Beryllium deposits are usually seen in lung tissue and often present as calcified conchoidal (shell-like) bodies that are typical of, but not specific to, beryllium. These beryllium conchoidal bodies usually give positive reactions for haemosiderin (Perls technique, see p. 208). The naphthochrome green B method can also be employed but is less selective than the solochrome azurine, as other metallic dye lakes may be formed.

SOLOCHROME AZURINE TECHNIQUE (Pearse 1957)

Notes

Beryllium and aluminium form a deep blue complex with the chelating agent solochrome azurine. The technique is simple and can be applied to conventionally fixed, paraffin-processed material. Both aluminium and beryllium stain with the solochrome azurine in aqueous solution, but at an alkaline pH aluminium will fail to react. We have found that the method works well. Positive control sections should be taken through if available, with untreated duplicate sections to serve as negative controls.

Solutions

Solution A
   0.2% aqueous solochrome azurine (syn. pure blue B).
Solution B
   0.2% solochrome azurine in molar sodium hydroxide.
1% aqueous neutral red

Technique

1. Three duplicate sections of test and positive control material to distilled water.
2. Stain one section in solution A, one in B for 20 min, and treat one in distilled water only.
3. Wash in water. Counterstain all sections in the neutral red solution for 3–5 min.
4. Wash in water. Dehydrate, clear and mount as desired.

Results

Solution A: aluminium and beryllium	blue
Solution B: beryllium only	blue-black

| Distilled water only | no reaction |
| Nuclei | red |

LEAD

Deposits of lead may uncommonly appear in tissues such as kidney and the skin, usually as a result of industrial disease. Two techniques will be presented: one precise and one less so, but which has the advantage of not requiring specialized reagents. As with any metallic salt demonstration in tissue, it is wise to avoid fixatives containing metals as these may produce non-specific reactions; formalin or alcohol is preferred. If possible, positive control material should also be taken through.

UNRIPENED HAEMATOXYLIN TECHNIQUE (Mallory 1938)

Notes

The rationale of the method depends on the use of fresh, i.e. unripened, and un-mordanted haematoxylin to stain lead deposits by forming a mordant-type linkage. As might be expected, other metals may also react but it makes for a useful screening technique. It is essential that the stain solution be prepared fresh, just before use.

Solution

Dissolve 0.05 g haematoxylin in 1 ml ethanol. Add 100 ml of filtered saturated aqueous calcium carbonate solution.

Technique

1. Sections to water.
2. Stain with the haematoxylin solution for 2–3 h at 56°C.
3. Wash in running tap water for at least 10 min.
4. Dehydrate, clear and mount as desired.

Results

| Lead | blue-grey to black |

RHODIZONATE TECHNIQUE (taken from Bancroft & Stevens 1990)

Notes

This is a more precise method than the Mallory and employs rhodizonic acid that forms a metal chelate with lead and its salts.

Solutions

Rhodizonate solution:

| Rhodizonic acid sodium salt | 0.2 g |

Distilled water	99 ml
Glacial acetic acid	1 ml

0.1% light green in 1% acetic acid

Technique

1. Sections to distilled water.
2. Treat with rhodizonate solution for 1 h.
3. Wash well in tap water.
4. Counterstain with the light green solution for 2 min.
5. Wash in water and mount in an aqueous mountant.

Results

Lead	red
Background	green

GOLD

Notes

On rare occasions it is necessary to demonstrate gold or its salts in tissue, either as gum lesions from fillings in teeth, or as in experimental studies involving gold uptake in tissue during therapy (Doré & Vernon-Roberts 1976). The rationale is of photochemical binding of silver ions by gold, which is subsequently reduced to a black reduced silver compound. Selectivity of demonstration is achieved by pre-treating a duplicate section with a hydrolysis-potassium cyanide sequence that specifically removes gold. This confirms that what appears black in the non-hydrolyzed section is gold, as distinct from other metals. Potassium cyanide is a highly poisonous substance and should be handled and stored with great care. As with all silver techniques scrupulous attention to distilled washing of slides and glassware is important if background deposition is to be avoided. In this context celloidinization of the slides is specified in the method; this is partly to keep the sections on the slide, but also to prevent untoward background silver deposition.

THE SILVER METHOD FOR GOLD

Solutions

1% hydrochloric acid
0.1% aqueous potassium cyanide
Silver solution (prepare fresh)
  To 20 ml well-filtered 15% aqueous gum arabic (acacia) add 30 ml distilled water.
  Mix well and add 7 ml saturated aqueous sodium sulphite. Mix well and add 5 ml
  10% aqueous silver nitrate—mixing until the solution is a clear straw colour.
Developer
  Dilute 1 part of commercial photographic developer with 7 parts distilled water
  (any high contrast fine grain developer will serve).
5% aqueous sodium thiosulphate (hypo)

Technique (Doré 1974)

1. Duplicate sections of test and positive control material (if available) to distilled water.
2. Treat one section of each pair with the hydrochloric acid for 10 min at 60°C (pre-heat), wash well in distilled water then treat with the potassium cyanide for 20 min.
3. Rinse all sections in alcohol and celloidinize. Rinse well in distilled water.
4. Place all sections in a Coplin jar filled with the silver solution and illuminate the jar for 15 min using a 75 watt tungsten bulb set at a distance of between 10 and 15 cm.
5. Wash well in several changes of distilled water over 10 min.
6. Treat with developer under dark room conditions for 10 min. Wash in distilled water.
7. Treat with the hypo solution for 2 min then wash in running water.
8. Remove the celloidin film in the usual way with alcohol and ether, and counterstain as desired, e.g. with neutral red, eosin or van Gieson.
9. Dehydrate, clear and mount as desired.

Results

Gold deposits	black granules
Background	according to counterstain
Hydrolyzed section	negative

SILVER

This is not often seen in tissue sections, occurring most commonly in skin or dental amalgam lesions of gum; the latter gives a positive Schmorl reaction. A bleaching technique for silver granules in tissue is to treat sections for up to 5 min with a solution of 5% aqueous sodium thiosulphate 32 ml and 0.5% aqueous potassium ferricyanide 8 ml in a Coplin jar. H&E staining is applied and the final treated and stained section compared to the original. In dental amalgam deposits, there may be only a partial loss of pigment as amalgams vary in their metallic composition, and silver salts may be only one of the constituents.

REFERENCES

Bancroft J D, Stevens A 1990 Theory and practice of histological techniques, 3rd edn. Churchill Livingstone, Edinburgh
Bunting H 1949 Histochemical detection of iron in tissues. Stain Technology 24: 109
Corrodi H, Hillarp N A, Jonasson C 1964 Fluorescence methods for the demonstration of monoamines. 3. Sodium borohydride reduction of the fluorescent compounds as a specificity test. Journal of Histochemistry and Cytochemistry 12: 582
Cripps D J, MacEachern W N 1971 Hepatic and erythropoietic protoporphyria. Archives of Pathology 91: 497
Cripps D J, Scheuer P 1965 Hepatobiliary changes in erythropoietic protoporphyria. Archives of Pathology 80: 500
Davies S E, Williams R, Portmann B 1989 Hepatic morphology and histochemistry of Wilson's disease presenting as fulminant hepatic failure: a study of 11 cases. Histopathology 15: 385–394

Doré J L 1974 A study of the demonstration and distribution of gold in tissue sections. Thesis for FIMLS (Dip. Med. Tech.)

Doré J L, Vernon-Roberts B 1976 A method for the selective demonstration of gold in tissue sections. Medical Laboratory Sciences 33: 209–214

Drury R A B, Wallington E A 1980 Carleton's histological technique, 5th edn. Oxford University Press, Oxford

Dunn R C 1946 Haemoglobin stain for histologic use based on cyanol-haemoglobin reaction. Archives of Pathology 41: 476

Dunn R C, Thompson 1946 A simplified stain for haemoglobin in tissue and smears using patent blue. Stain Technology 21: 65

Eranko O 1955 Distribution of adrenaline and noradrenaline in the adrenal medulla. Nature 175: 88

Fontana A 1912 Verfahren zur intensiven und reschen Farbung des Treponema pallidum and anderer Spirochäten. Dermalologische Wocehnschrift 55: 1003

Fouchet A 1917 Methode nouvelle de recherche et de dosage des pigments biliares dans le serum sanguin. Comptes Rendus de Seances de la Societe de Biologie et de ses Filiales 80: 826

Glenner G 1957 Simultaneous demonstration of bilirubin, haemosiderin and lipofuschin pigments in tissue sections. American Journal of Clinical Pathology 27: 1

Golodetz L, Unna P C 1909 Zur chemie der Haut III. Das Reduktionsvermögen der histologischen Element der Haut. Mh. Prakt, Dermatologie 48: 149

Gomori G 1952 Microscopic histochemistry. Chicago, Chicago University Press

Howell J S 1959 Histochemical demonstration of copper in copper fed rats and in the hepatolenticular degeneration. Journal of Pathology and Bacteriology 77: 423

Hoyt R F, Sorokin S P, Bartlett 1979 A simple fluorescence method for serotonin-containing endocrine cells in plastic embedded lung, gut and thyroid gland. Journal of Histochemistry and Cytochemistry 27: 721

Hurst V, Hutton W E, Nycholls J 1951 A new histochemical reaction for calcium. Journal of Dental Research 30: 489

Jain S, Scheuer P J, Archer B, Newman S P, Sherlock S 1978 Histological demonstration of copper and copper associated protein in chronic liver diseases. Journal of Clinical Pathology 31: 784

Lambert J R 1980 Brown bowel syndrome in Crohn's disease. Archives of Pathology and Laboratory Medicine 104: 201–205

Lendrum A C 1949 Staining of erythrocytes in tissue sections: a new method and observations on some of the modified Mallory connective tissue stains. Journal of Pathology and Bacteriology 61: 443

Lillie R D 1954 Histopathologic technique and practical histochemistry. McGraw-Hill, New York

Lillie R D 1965 Histopathologic technique and practical histochemisty, 3rd end. McGraw-Hill, New York

Lindquist R S 1969 Studies on the pathogenesis of hepatolenticular degeneration. II Cytochemical methods for the localisation of copper. Archives of Pathology 87: 370–379

Lison L 1938 Zur Frage der Ausscheidung and Speicherung des Hämoglobins in der Amphibienniere. Beitrage zur Pathologichen Anatomie and sur Allgemeinen Pathologie 101: 94

McGee-Russell S M 1958 Histochemical methods for calcium. Journal of Histochemistry and Cytochemistry 6: 22

Mallory F B 1938 Pathological technique. Philadelphia, Saunders

Mallory F B, Parker F 1939 Fixing and staining methods for lead and copper in tissues. American Journal of Pathology 16: 517

Masson P 1914 La glande endocrine de l'intestine chez l'homme. Comptes Rendus Hebdomadaires des Seances de l'Academie des Science 158: 59

Okamoto K, Utamura M 1938 Biologische Untersuchen des Kepfers uber die histochemische Kupfernachweiss Methode. Acta Scholae Medicinalis Universitatis Imperialis in Kisto 20: 573

Pearse A G E 1957 Solochrome dyes in histochemistry with particular reference to nuclear staining. Acta Histochemica 4: 95

Pearse A G E 1960 Histochemistry, theoretical and applied, 2nd edn. Churchill, London

Perls M 1867 Nachweis von Eisenoxyd in geweissen Pigmentation. Virchow's Archive fur Pathologische Anatomie und Physiologie und fur Kliniche Medizin 39: 42

Puchtler H, Sweat F 1962 Amido black as a stain for haemoglobin. Archives of Pathology 73: 245

Quinke H I 1880 Zur Pathologie des Blutes. Dtsch. Archive Lkin. Medicine 25: 567

Richter G W 1978 The iron-loaded cell—the cytopathology of iron storage. American Journal of Pathology 91: 363–412

Schmeltzer W 1933 Der mikrochemische Nachweiss von Eissen in Gewebselmentenmitels Rhodenswasserstoffsaure und die Konservierung der Reaktionin Paroffinol. Zietschrift fur Wissenschaftliche Mikroscopie 50: 99

Stein J 1935 Reaction histochemique stable de detection de la bilirubine. Comptes rendus de seances de la Societe de Biologie et de ses Filiales 120: 1136

Tiedemann F, Gmelin P J 1826 Die Verdauung nach Versuchen, Bol. 1. K Gross Heidelberg

Tirmann J 1898 Ueber den Uebergang des Eisens in die Milch. Gorbersdorfer Veroffentt 2: 101

Uzman L L 1956 Histochemical localisation of copper with rubeanic acid. Laboratory Investigation 5: 299

10. The diffuse endocrine system

The 'APUD system' was the name applied to groups of cells containing cytoplasmic neurosecretory granules. The title was coined by Pearse (1968) due to the biochemical ability of the cells — they have a high amine content and are able to take up and decarboxylate amine precursors, hence 'Amine Precursor Uptake and Decarboxylation' (APUD).

The concept of this cell system was thought by Pearse to have originated with Nonidez (1932), who demonstrated that thyroid parafollicular cells contained argyrophil granules, and were involved in an endocrine secretion. Later, after work by many people, it was demonstrated that calcitonin was produced by these cells: the hormone is involved in controlling blood calcium levels in the body. As a result Pearse and his co-workers called the thyroid parafollicular cells 'C' cells. The cytochemistry and electron microscopy of these and similar amine-containing cells were thoroughly investigated by these workers and others between 1964 and 1970. In the 1968 concept, three sets of characteristics were discussed: the cytochemical and morphological features and origins of the cells. Current thinking is that a more appropriate term to describe this group of cells is the 'Diffuse Endocrine System (DES)'. In this chapter we are concerned with the cytochemical reactions including the immunological reactivity, the morphological features and diagnostic applications.

CYTOCHEMICAL FEATURES

DES cells:
1. contain an amine or can secondarily take it up,
2. contain an amino acid decarboxylase,
3. contain α-glycerophosphate dehydrogenase,
4. contain non-specific esterase or cholinesterase,
5. contain sufficient concentrations of side chain carboxyl groups to enable them to be seen by masked metachromasia,
6. contain immunocytochemically demonstrable amine constituents.

MORPHOLOGICAL FEATURES

1. Electron-dense, fixation-labile mitochondria.
2. High content of free ribosomes.
3. High levels of smooth endoplasmic reticulum.
4. Low levels of rough endoplasmic reticulin.
5. Secretory vesicles.
6. Prominent microtubules and centrosomes.

According to Gould (1978), most protein-secreting cells exhibit the features discussed above to some degree, and it has been shown that polypeptide hormone-producing cells have the same cytochemical and ultrastructural characteristics. These cells, together with the thyroid 'C' cells, form the DES (Diffuse Endocrine System). In sites such as the pancreatic islets, adrenal medulla and the anterior pituitary, the polypeptide hormone-producing cells are clumped together to form a recognizable endocrine gland. Elsewhere, and particularly in the gastrointestinal tract they are scattered throughout the mucosa to form a diffuse system.

Table 10.1 indicates the major groups of cells of the DES system. It is not intended to be complete, and additions are constantly being made. The information is drawn from Pearse (1968), Dawson (1976, 1982), Gould (1978) and Wilson & Chalk (1990).

Table 10.1   The diffuse endocrine system

	Name of cells	Polypeptide	Amine stored
Thyroid	C	Calcitonin	5HT
Pituitary	Corticotroph	ACTH	
	Melanotroph	MSH	
	Somatotroph	Somatrophin	Tryptophan
	Mammotroph	Prolactin	
Pancreatic islets	$A(\alpha^2)$	Glucagon	
	$B(\beta)$	Insulin	
	$D(\alpha^1)$	Somatostatin	
	S	Secretin	
	D	GIP	
Duodenum small bowel	EG	Enteroglucagon	5HT
	EC	—	
	H	VIP	
	D	Somatostatin	
	G	Gastrin	5HT or dopamine
	A	Enteroglucagon	
Stomach	D	Somatostatin	
	EC	Serotonin	5HT
GI tract	EC (Kultschitsky)		5HT
Adrenal gland	A	—	Adrenaline
	NA	—	Noradrenaline

DEMONSTRATION OF DES CELLS

It is important that aldehyde fixation is used for the cells of the DES system which store an amine. The reaction between the amine and the aldehyde produces, for 5HT, a carboline derivative and this is the reducing agent for the various reagents used in the demonstration of these cells.

In H&E-stained sections, most DES cells have the same characteristics: they are oblong or triangular in shape with a broad base abutting the basement membrane and the underlying vascular supply (Dawson 1982). The variable number of secretory granules they contain are difficult to see without using specialized techniques.

The different types of methods for the demonstration of DES cells are listed below. It is worth noting that the β cells of the pancreas do not conform to the guidelines laid down for DES cells with histochemical techniques. They are usually identified by their sulphur amino acid content, using aldehyde fuchsin.

Chromaffin cells

These cells are associated with the sympathetic nervous system. They are found in the adrenal medulla, sympathetic ganglia and paraganglia. In the adrenal medulla the cells are divided into A cells, which produce adrenaline, and NA cells, which secrete noradrenaline. These substances will precipitate chrome salts, resulting in the chromaffin reaction. Chromate oxidation rapidly produces the brown pigment seen in adrenaline- and noradrenaline-containing cells. Iodates can also be used as an oxidizing agent and are employed to distinguish between the two substances as they oxidize noradrenaline far more rapidly than adrenaline. Chromaffin granules will reduce ammoniacal silver and ferricyanide, showing the argentaffin reaction (see below) and a positive Schmorl's reaction respectively, providing that chromate fixation was employed. Note that secondary chromate fixation following primary formalin fixation is not as effective. These techniques may be used to demonstrate the rare tumour of the adrenal medulla — the phaeochromocytoma.

Table 10.2   Effects of fixation

Cells	Fixation	Result
Chromaffin cells	Dichromate	Brown granules
Chromaffin cells	Formaldehyde	Unstained granules
Chromaffin cells	Formaldehyde postfixed in dichromate	Weak yellow-brown
Argentaffin cells	Formaldehyde	FIF, silver reduction
Argentaffin cells	Formaldehyde postfixed in dichromate	Weak chromaffin reaction
Argentaffin cells	Dichromate	Variable chromaffin reaction

Enterochromaffin cells (Kultschitsky cells)

Scattered cells in the gastric mucosa of various animals were identified as yellow coloured cells following fixation in dichromate (Heidenhain 1870). Kultschitsky (1897) described them as containing fine oxyphil granules whilst Schmidt (1905) recognized them in the human duodenum and called them 'chromaffin cells'. Ciaccio (1907) attributed their chromaffin reaction to adrenaline and called the chromaffin cells found in gastric mucosa 'enterochromaffin cells' (EC). Masson (1914) showed that the cells produced the argentaffin reaction (see below). Erspamer & Asero (1952) identified the amine as 5-hydroxytryptamine (5HT). The cells that are scattered throughout the intestinal tract comprise the major part of the 'diffuse' endocrine system and today the term enterochromaffin is unsuitable for these cells as only a few of these will demonstrate the chromaffin reaction. A far better title is 'endocrine cells of the gastrointestinal tract' that then can be divided into suitable subgroups depending upon the hormone they secrete. The subgrouping of cells in relation to their staining reactions is still viable and a brief description is given below.

Argentaffin cells

These cells can be found in almost all areas of the gastrointestinal tract. They also occur in the pancreas, gall bladder and genitourinary tract. There are many argentaffin cells in the ileum, appendix and in the crypts of Lieberkuhn but few are seen in the stomach as these are mainly argyrophil cells. Argentaffin cells are usually pear-shaped and they have an eosinophilic cytoplasm. The granules they contain lie between the nucleus and basement membrane. Following formalin fixation these granules will directly reduce silver (argentaffin reaction), couple with diazonium salts and reduce ferric ferricyanide (Schmorl technique). They exhibit a bright autofluorescence. They have an affinity for osmium tetroxide and will also show the argyrophil reaction. Argentaffin cells will show the chromaffin reaction but differ from the adrenal medulla cells in showing the reaction after formaldehyde fixation. The consensus is that they produce 5-hydroxytryptamine (5HT).

Argyrophil cells

These are found in the gastrointestinal mucosa in similar locations to argentaffin cells but in much larger numbers. Many are found in stomach mucosa, a rare site for argentaffin cells. They can also be located in the pancreas. Argyrophil cells can be impregnated with silver but a reducing agent is required to produce the deposit of metallic silver. The main difference between argentaffin and argyrophil cells is the greater amount of reducing substance to be found in the argentaffin cells.

The argyrophil cells can be demonstrated by the Bodian and Grimelius silver, and lead haematoxylin methods; specific argyrophil cells such as α_1 and α_2 cells of the pancreas are best demonstrated by the Hellerström & Hellman and Grimelius methods respectively.

Argentaffin reaction

Cells that have the ability to directly reduce silver solutions, producing an insoluble black metallic silver precipitate, are termed argentaffin cells. Aldehyde fixation is mandatory for this reaction so that β-carboline reducing groups are formed.

Table 10.3 Recommended staining methods

Chromaffin cells	Chromaffin reaction, iodate reaction (NA cells), formalin-induced fluorescence, Giemsa, Schmorl, Masson–Fontana, lead haematoxylin
DES argentaffin cells	Alkaline diazo, Schmorl, Singh, lead haematoxylin, Masson–Fontana
DES argyrophil cells	Bodian, Grimelius (α_2 cells of pancreas), Pascual, Hellerström & Hellman (α_1 cells of pancreas), lead haematoxylin

All argyrophil methods will also demonstrate argentaffin cells.

Argyrophil reaction

These cell granules will also react with silver solutions. They differ from argentaffin cells because argyrophil cells require an additional reducing agent (usually hydroquinone or formalin) before they can reduce silver solution to metallic silver. There are many more of them than argentaffin cells. All argentaffin cells will show argyrophilia, but the argentaffin reaction will not be seen in argyrophil cells.

TYPES OF TECHNIQUE

1. Basic dyes, including metachromatic dyes.
2. Silver methods.
3. Amine identification.
4. Polypeptide identification.
5. Electron microscopy.
6. Immunocytochemistry.

BASIC DYES

Cationic dyes react with carboxyl groups in polypeptides, but are not specific as they are unable to demonstrate hormones. Metachromatic dyes are frequently used with prior acid hydrolysis in 0.2 M HC1; this unmasks further side chain carboxyls (Solcia et al 1968). In our opinion and that of Dawson (1982) better results are obtained by using haematoxylin combined with a stabilized lead solution. The staining mechanism is the same, the lead imparting a stronger colouration to the DES cells. Both methods are given below.

METACHROMATIC DYES AFTER ACID HYDROLYSIS (after Solcia et al 1968)

Notes

Cationic dyes react with carboxyl, sulphate and phosphate groups of polypetides and the results can be improved by prior hydrolysis that removes the reactive groups in nucleotides, and unmasks protein side chain carboxyls.

Solutions

Either *Azure solution*
   0.01% azure A in distilled water.
or *Toluidine blue solution*
   0.01% toluidine blue in distilled water, buffered to pH 5 with McIlvaine's buffer.
Acid solution for hydrolysis
   0.2 M hydrochloric acid.

Technique

1. Sections to water.
2. Place in acid hydrolysis solution (0.2.M HC1) for 3–4 h at 60–65°C for formalin, paraformaldehyde and Bouin fixed tissue; 12 h for glutaraldehyde or Helly fixed tissue.
3. Wash well in water.
4. Stain in either:
   a. Azure A solution for 6 h.
   b. Toluidine blue solution for 6 h.

5. Either rinse in water and mount in an aqueous mountant, or blot dry, soak in absolute isopropanol for 1 min, clear and mount as desired.

Results

DES granules	purple-red
Background	blue

LEAD HAEMATOXYLIN TECHNIQUE (Solcia et al 1969)

Note

It is thought that there is a carboxyl group linkage with lead haematoxylin. An optional satisfactory counterstain is tartrazine in Cellosolve.

Solutions

Stabilized lead solution:

5% aqueous lead nitrate	50 ml
Saturated aqueous ammonium acetate	50 ml

Filter, then add 2 ml of conc. formalin. Saturation point of ammonium acetate in water is approximately 120%.

Lead haematoxylin staining solution:

Stabilized lead solution	10 ml
0.2 g haematoxylin in 1.4 ml 95% ethanol	1.5 ml
Distilled water	10 ml

Mix in the above order with repeated stirring. Stand the mixture for 30 min, filter and make up the filtrate to 75 ml with distilled water.

Technique

1. Sections to water.
2. Stain in lead haematoxylin solution for 2–3 h at 37°C or 1–2 h at 45°C.
3. Wash in distilled water, dehydrate, clear and mount as desired.

Results

Carcinoid tumours, endocrine and DES cell granules   dark blue-black

Other structures, e.g. muscle, nerves, nuclei may also stain blue-black.

ARGYROPHILIC SILVER METHODS

Silver methods that employ a reducing agent (argyrophilic) will demonstrate some DES cells. These methods, according to Dawson (1982), are semi-specific and are of value for screening purposes. By using the methods given below it is possible to identify and separate A (α_2) cells and D (α_1) cells of the pancreas.

GRIMELIUS SILVER METHOD FOR ARGYROPHIL CELLS, ESPECIALLY A CELLS OF THE PANCREAS (Grimelius 1968)

Notes

A silver reduction method, for which Bouin-fixed material gives best results. To increase the impregnation following reduction, wash well in distilled water and return to the silver bath at 60°C for 5–10 min. Drain the slide and repeat the reduction step. Repeat this sequence until the positive material is a strong brown/black colour and the background yellow.

Solutions

Silver solution:

Acetate buffer (pH 5.6)	10 ml
Distilled water	87 ml
1% silver nitrate (aqueous), fresh	3 ml

Reducing solution:

Hydroquinone	1 g
Sodium sulphite	5 g
Distilled water	100 ml

Technique

1. Sections to distilled water.
2. Transfer sections to silver solution at 60°C for 3 h.
3. Drain silver solution from slides.
4. Place sections in freshly prepared reducing solution at 45°C for 1 min.
5. Rinse sections in distilled water.
6. Counterstain if required (e.g. neutral red).
7. Wash in tap water.
8. Dehydrate in graded alcohols.
9. Clear and mount as desired.

Results

Carcinoid tumours, A cells of the pancreas	positive (brown-black)
B and D cells of the pancreas	negative
Many other argyrophil cells	positive (brown-black)

ALCOHOLIC SILVER NITRATE METHOD FOR ARGYROPHIL CELLS, ESPECIALLY D CELLS OF THE PANCREAS (Hellerström & Hellman 1960)

Note

This is an alcoholic silver reduction method. Bouin fixation is necessary, either as a primary or secondary step.

Solutions

Silver solution:

Silver nitrate	10 g
Distilled water	10 ml
95% alcohol	90 ml
M nitric acid	0.1 ml

Before use the pH of the solution is adjusted to 5.0 with conc. ammonium hydroxide (ammonia).

Developing solution:

Pyrogallic acid	5 g
95% alcohol	95 ml
Conc. formalin	5 ml

Technique

1. Sections to tap water, 1 h.
2. Dehydrate to 95% alcohol.
3. Place sections in silver solution at 37°C overnight and protect from light.
4. Rinse rapidly in 95% alcohol — no longer than 10 s.
5. Transfer sections to developing solution for 1 min.
6. Rinse in three changes of 95% alcohol for 1 min.
7. Rinse in absolute alcohol for 1 min each.
8. Clear and mount as desired.

Results

D cell granules of the pancreas	positive (brown-black)
A and B cells of the pancreas	negative
Some other argyrophil cells	positive

BODIAN PROTARGOL TECHNIQUE (Bodian 1936)

Notes

The protargol method gives strong argyrophilic demonstration of most tissue entities, nerve fibres, melanin, A and D cells of the pancreas and argyrophil cells. Sections are treated with protargol (a compound formed of gelatine and silver nitrate) in the presence of metallic copper. It is thought that the role of the copper is to produce nitric acid which leads to a fall in pH of the solution producing a slowing down of the reaction, with consequent lessened risk of over-impregnation.

Following copper-protargol treatment, the sections are progressively reduced in a hydroquinone-gold chloride-oxalic acid treatment. Background precipitation is not uncommon in this technique, and thorough washing between the various treatments will reduce this.

Solutions

Copper-protargol solution
   Prepare fresh 50 ml of 1% aqueous protargol (silver proteinate BDH) to which
   are added (in a Coplin jar) 2 g of clean copper foil cut into small pieces.
Primary reducer
   Hydroquinone 1 g; sodium sulphite 5 g; in 100 ml distilled water. Prepare fresh
   (the sodium sulphite acts as a stabilizer allowing the solution to be kept for up to
   2 days at 4°C).

1% aqueous gold chloride
2% aqueous oxalic acid
5% sodium thiosulphate (hypo)
1% aqueous netural red

Technique

1. Sections to distilled water.
2. Treat with the copper-protargol solution overnight at 37°C (exact time
   is not critical but no longer than 48 h).
3. Wash in several changes of distilled water and reduce in the
   hydroquinone solution for 10 min.
4. Wash well in distilled water. Thorough washing at this stage is most
   important; rinse first in distilled water, then in tap water for several
   minutes and finally in distilled water again.
5. Treat with the yellow gold chloride solution for 5 min.
6. Wash well in several changes of distilled water.
7. Treat with the oxalic acid solution for 5 min (only at this stage should
   silver blackening be evident).
8. Fix in the hypo solution.
9. Wash well in distilled water.
10. Rinse in tap water.
11. Counterstain in the neutral red solution.
12. Rinse in tap water.
13. Dehydrate, clear and mount as desired.

Results

A and D cells of the pancreas, carcinoid tumours   black
Argyrophil cells   black

REDUCING SILVER METHOD FOR ARGYROPHIL CELLS (Pascual 1976)

Notes

Silver methods using a reducing agent will blacken argyrophil and argentaffin cells.
The Bodian (1936) method using protargol and hydroquinone reduction has been
widely used and most silver techniques, such as that of Grimelius (1968) for

argyrophil cells, have been developed for the identification of different argyrophil cells of the DES system. The double silver impregnation modification of Pascual (1976) gives good contrast of the argyrophil cells without background impregnation. As indicated, argentaffin cells also stain. For comparison a direct silver reduction method should also be used.

Solutions

Bodian's reducing solution:

Anhydrous sodium sulphite	5 g
Hydroquinone	1 g
Distilled water	100 ml

Silver solution
  0.5% aqueous silver nitrate.
1% aqueous neutral red

Technique

1. Sections to water.
2. Place in freshly prepared silver nitrate solution for 2 h at 60°C or overnight at room temperature.
3. Rinse in distilled water.
4. Transfer sections to freshly prepared Bodian's reducing solution, heated to 60°C, for 5 min.
5. Wash in tap water for 3 min and rinse in distilled water.
6. Re-impregnate in the same silver solution at 60°C for 10 min.
7. Rinse in distilled water.
8. Repeat the reducing solution as in steps 4 and 5.
9. Counterstain in neutral red for 3 min.
10. Rinse in tap water, dehydrate, clear and mount as desired.

Results

Argyrophil cells	black
Nuclei	red

AMINE DETECTION

The capacity of DES cells to produce and store amines by taking up their precursor substance is their most important feature. Some also take up dihydroxyphenylalanine (DOPA) and decarboxylate it to its respective amine. Amines combine with aldehydes to produce specific fluorescent compounds. Most amines diffuse rapidly from their cells, so for their demonstration the technique of freeze drying and formaldehyde vapour is required. As shown in Table 10.1, 5-hydroxytryptamine (5HT) and dopamine are the most important amines and these diffuse slowly from their granules. They combine with paraformaldehyde and aqueous formaldehyde to produce a yellow fluorescence. This is known as formaldehyde-induced fluorescence (FIF) and is a good method for demonstrating 5HT (see p. 207). The combi-

Table 10.4 Histochemical features of normal endocrine cells of pancreas and GI tract (compiled from Dawson 1976)

Cell type	Secretion	Argentaffin	Diazo	Hell+ Hell.	Grimelius	Bodian	Tol. Blue	Acid hydrol.	Lead haem.	PTAH	DMAB nitrite	Alde. Fuch.
Pancreas												
A(α_2)	Glucagon	–	–	–	+	+	±	+	+	+	+	–
B	Insulin	–	–	–	–	–	–	–	–	–	–	+
D(α_1)	Somatostatin	–	–	+	+	+	+	+	+	+	+	–
GI tract												
EC	5HT	+	+	+	+	+	+	+	+	0	0	0
EG	Glucagon	–	–	+	+	+	±	+	+	0	0	0
G	Gastrin	–	–	±	±	–	–	±	+	0	0	0
S	Secretin	–	–	0	±	0	0	0	+	0	+	0
VIP	VIP	–	–	0	0	0	0	0	±	±	0	0
GIP	GIP	–	–	0	+	0	0	0	+	0	0	0

Key: + = positive staining; ± = doubtful or faint staining; – = no staining; 0 = no reliable observations available.

nation of 5HT and formaldehyde produces β-carboline and as well as being fluorescent it is a reducing agent. It can reduce silver salts to metallic silver (argentaffin), ferricyanide to ferrocyanide (Schmorl reaction) and will couple with a diazonium salt (Fast red B) to produce an insoluble coloured azo dye. Three standard methods for argentaffin cells are available: the Masson–Fontana method (see p. 206), the Singh silver reduction method and the alkaline diazo method of Gomori; these can be used to identify argentaffin carcinoid tumours.

SINGH'S MODIFICATION OF THE MASSON–HAMPERL ARGENTAFFIN TECHNIQUE (Singh 1964)

Notes

This is a direct silver reduction method. Some workers prefer to leave the sections overnight in the silver solution at room temperature in a light-tight container.

Solutions

Incubating solution

To 10% aqueous silver nitrate add conc. ammonia (0.880) until the precipitate formed just dissolves. To this clear solution add 10% aqueous silver nitrate drop by drop until a fine persistent opalescence is obtained. To each 1 ml of silver solution add 9 ml of distilled water.

1% aqueous sodium thiosulphate

Technique

1. Sections to water.
2. Wash well in several changes of distilled water.
3. Place in pre-warmed silver solution at 60°C for 15–30 min.
4. Rinse in distilled water.
5. Fix in the sodium thiosulphate solution for 1 min.
6. Wash in distilled water.
7. Dehydrate, clear and mount as desired.

Results

Argentaffin cells   contain black discrete granules

ALKALINE DIAZO TECHNIQUE (Gomori 1952)

Notes

Argentaffin cells reduce diazonium salts to produce an insoluble coloured azo dye. Fresh tissue fixed in formaldehyde is best but rarely works on post-mortem material. Should the reaction not work on well-fixed tissue it is often profitable to obtain different sources of diazonium salt. There appears to be a variation in batches sold and the salts also have a limited shelf-life. When preparing the fast red solution, thoroughly shake the dry reagent before adding the distilled water.

Solution

Staining solution:

1% aqueous fast red B	5 ml
Saturated lithium carbonate (aqueous)	2 ml

Keep solutions at 4°C before mixing, then use immediately.

Technique

1. Sections to water.
2. Transfer sections to incubating solution at 4°C for 1–4 min.
3. Wash well in tap water.
4. Lightly stain nuclei in alum haematoxylin (see p. 25).
5. Wash well in tap water.
6. Dehydrate, clear and mount as desired.

Results

Argentaffin cell granules	orange
Nuclei	blue
Background	yellow

CHROMAFFIN REACTION

Notes

Originally the chromaffin reaction was used to identify adrenal medulla. It has long been known that if adrenal was fixed in chrome salts then medullary cells could be seen by their brown colour. Other chromaffin cells in the gastrointestinal tract and some enterochromaffin cells will show the same reaction. The adrenaline and noradrenaline produced by these cells are oxidized by chrome salts to produce a melanoid pigment. Iodate oxidation is thought to demonstrate NA (noradrenaline)-producing cells more intensely than A (adrenaline) cells. It was reported by Coupland & Hopwood (1966) that initial fixation of the adrenal medulla in glutaraldehyde (pH 7.4) followed by fixation in chrome salts produced a strong chromaffin reaction in the NA cells, and that the A cells (adrenaline-storing) were negative. The following fixatives give acceptable results: Orth's, Muller's or Regaud's.

Technique

1. Fix for 2 days.
2. Wash in tap water.
3. Process tissue and embed in paraffin wax.
4. Section (5 μm) and dewax in xylene.
5. Dehydrate, clear and mount sections as desired.

Results

Chromaffin cells	yellow-brown

THE IODATE METHOD FOR NORADRENALINE (Hillarp & Hökfelt 1955)

Notes

This method depends upon the more rapid oxidation by iodate of noradrenaline than adrenaline.

Technique

1. Place thin (0.5 mm) blocks of fresh adrenal in 10% aqueous potassium iodate. Leave for 16 h at room temperature. Do not exceed the time.
2. Place in 10% formalin for 2 h.
3. Cut frozen sections 10–20 μm thick.
4. Wash in distilled water.
5. Sections may be counterstained and then dehydrated, cleared and mounted as desired.

Results

Noradrenaline   brown

MODIFIED GIEMSA FOR CHROMAFFIN CELL GRANULES

Notes

The best results with this method are obtained if fixation is carried out in a dichromate-containing fixative. If this is not possible then secondary fixation, of either tissue or section, in dichromate gives an acceptable result. Sections should be as thin as possible.

Solutions

Staining solution:

Standard Giemsa stain	2 ml
Buffered distilled water (pH 6.8)	48 ml

0.5% acetic acid

Technique

1. Sections to water.
2. Rinse in distilled water.
3. Stain in the dilute Giemsa stain overnight.
4. Rinse in distilled water.
5. Wash in the acetic acid until the section becomes pink (about 2 min).
6. Wash in tap water.
7. Dehydrate rapidly through graded alcohols to xylene.
8. Mount in synthetic resin.

Results

Chromaffin cell granules stain greenish-yellow or bottle green, depending upon fixation used.

ELECTRON MICROSCOPY

Tissue processed for electron microscopy will show the presence of intracellular dense neurosecretory granules. The standard immunoperoxidase reaction can be adopted for electron immunocytochemistry.

RELEVANT IMMUNOCYTOCHEMISTRY

The component cells of the diffuse endocrine system produce specific amines and peptides so that immunocytochemistry affords a precise means for the identification of normal or tumour cells by the employment of specific antisera. Pituitary thyrotropic cells can be demonstrated by anti-TSH suitably labelled, G cells of the pylorus with anti-gastrin, D cells of the pancreatic islets with anti-somatostatin, and so on.

In a similar fashion it is possible to identify carcinoid tumours by their content of serotonin by employing anti-5HT immunocytochemistry. A more practical approach is to use antisera that have a pan-endocrine cell affinity so that a broad spectrum demonstration is afforded. Table 10.5 illustrates the more popular antisera in use for carcinoid tumour identification.

Which one is chosen is a matter of personal preference but it is worth keeping in mind that chromogranin is a protein associated with the cell cytoplasmic granules. This means that poorly granulated cells are likely to be weakly reactive or negative and will not, therefore, be of greater material assistance than the conventional, i.e. non-immunocytochemical, methods such as the Grimelius.

NSE and PGP 9.5, on the other hand, are more likely to yield a positive result where all else has failed, with the latter gaining in popularity for a number of reasons: these include the reaction of NSE with non-DES elements and its higher cost.

Table 10.5   General markers for carcinoid tumours

Antiserum	Poly/monoclonal	Enzyme pre-treatment (with paraffin sections)
Neurone-specific enolase (NSE)	Poly	No
Protein gene product (PGP 9.5)	Poly	No
Chromogranin	Mono	No

DIAGNOSTIC APPLICATIONS

Some of the tumours of the diffuse endocrine system (popularly known as 'apudomas') are common and include the carcinoid tumours of the gastrointestinal tract and bronchus, also the small cell ('oat cell') carcinoma of the lung with, less frequently, the medullary carcinoma of thyroid (derived from the parafollicular cells).

Other, less common, tumours include the paragangliomas, carotid body tumours and those arising from the pancreatic islets (e.g. insulinomas and glucagonomas). Most carcinoid tumours have a reasonably characteristic morphology, as seen by

H&E, consisting of nests or cords of small uniform cells so that the special techniques are used in a confirmatory context. Occasionally, the more aggressive tumours may present a picture indistinguishable from a poorly differentiated carcinoma, so that the use of special techniques is important.

Apart from the carcinoid tumours, the usual means of confirming the H&E picture is by immunocytochemistry. The appropriate antiserum is applied—anti-insulin, anti-calcitonin for example—although ectopic, i.e. inappropriate, hormone production by neoplastic endocrine cells is not uncommon, making precise identification difficult. Some small cell tumours of the lung will be positive with the general immunocytochemical antisera such as NSE and PGP 9.5; this forms a useful diagnostic confirmation of the H&E picture, which is a reasonably characteristic one.

Another useful diagnostic correlate, this relating to medullary tumours of the thyroid, is the presence of stromal amyloid deposits that will show a Congo red positivity.

Carcinoid tumours may be argentaffin, argyrophil or histochemically unreactive (sometimes there are elements of each in an argentaffin tumour). *Argentaffin tumours* are largely confined to the appendix, caecum and ileum, and in the H&E show cells with prominent fine eosinophilic cytoplasmic granules. Positive reactions are normally obtained with the Masson–Fontana type of silver method plus immunocytochemical reactions using the general antisera. The *argyrophil tumours* (e.g. stomach and bronchus) do not react with Masson–Fontana or diazo techniques, but are positive with the Grimelius and Bodian techniques and the general antisera using immunocytochemistry. The *unreactive tumours* (e.g. some colorectal and the more aggressive, i.e invasive, tumours) can only be demonstrated immunocytochemically using antisera such as NSE and PGP 9.5. On occasion, however, even this approach may be unrewarding.

REFERENCES

Bodian D 1936 A new method for staining nerve fibres and nerve endings in mounted paraffin sections. Anatomy Records 65: 89

Ciaccio C 1907 Sopra speciali cellule granulose della mucosa intestinale. Archives Its. Anat. Embriol 6: 482

Coupland R E, Hopwood D 1966 The mechanism of the differential staining reaction for adrenaline and noradrenaline storing granules in tissue fixed in glutaraldehyde. Journal of Anatomy (London) 100: 227

Dawson I M P 1976 The endocrine cells of the gastrointestinal tract and the neoplasms which arise from them. Current Topics in Pathology 63: 221

Dawson I M P 1982 In: Bancroft J D, Stevens A (eds) Theory and practice of histological techniques, 2nd edn. Churchill Livingstone, Edinburgh

Erspamer V, Asero B 1952 Identification of Enteramine, the specific hormone of the enterochromaffin cell system as 5-hydroxytryptamine. Nature (London) 169: 800

Gomori G 1952 Microscopic histochemistry. Chicago University Press, Chicago

Gould R P 1978 In: Anthony P P, Woolf N (eds) Recent advances in histopathology. Churchill Livingstone, Edinburgh

Grimelius L 1968 A silver nitrate stain for α_2 cells in human pancreatic islets. Acta Societa Medical Uppsala 73: 243

Heidenhain R 1870 Untersuchungen über den Bau der Labdrüsen. Archives Mikrosk Anatomica 6: 368

Hellerström C, Hellman B 1960 Some aspects of silver impregnation of the islets of Langerhans in the rat. Acta Endocrinologica 35: 518

Hillarp N A, Hökfelt B 1955 Histochemical demonstration of noradrenaline and adrenaline in the adrenal medulla. Journal of Histochemistry and Cytochemistry 3: 1

Kultchistky N 1897 Zur Frage über den Bau des Darmkanals. Archives Mikrosk Anatomica 49: 7

Masson P 1914 La glande endocrein de l'intestine chez l'homme. C.R. Acad. Sciences, Paris 158: 159

Nonidez J F 1932 The origin of the parafollicular cell, a second epithelial component of the thyroid gland of the dog. American Journal of Anatomy 49: 479

Pascual J S F 1976 A new method for easy demonstration of argyrophil cells. Stain Technology 51: 231

Pearse A G E 1968 Common cytochemical and ultrastructural characteristics of cells producing polypeptide hormones (the APUD series) and their relevance to thyroid and ultimobranchial C cells and calcitonin. Proceedings of the Royal Society B. 170: 1

Schmidt J E 1905 Beiträge zur normalen und patholigischen Histologie einiger Zellarten der Schleimhaut des menshclichen Darmakanales. Archives Mikrosk Anatomica 66: 12

Singh I 1964 A modification of the Masson-Hamperl method for staining argentaffin cells. Anatomische Anzeiger 115: 81

Solcia E, Vassallo G, Capella C 1968 Selective staining of endocrine cells by basic dyes after acid hydrolysis. Stain Technology 43: 267

Solcia E, Capella C, Vassalo G 1969 Lead haematoxylin as a stain for endocrine cells. Significance of staining and comparison with other selective methods. Histochemie 20: 116

Wilson P O G, Chalk B T C 1990 In: Bancroft J D, Stevens A (eds) Theory and practice of histological techniques, 3rd edn. Churchill Livingstone, Edinburgh

11. Infective agents in tissue

ORGANISMS

There can be few laboratory workers not familiar with the method devised by Gram over a century ago. With many modifications, it has remained the standard technique for demonstrating organisms in pathology. On occasion tissues show a non-specific inflammatory reaction and by demonstrating micro-organisms, a definitive diagnosis can be made, often not possible with an H & E preparation.

The rationale of the method is that certain blue cationic dyes stain the nucleic acids of organisms (the background tissue also stains). Sections are treated with iodine and differentiated in a suitable dye solvent, alcohol, aniline or acetone. The tissue background and some types of organism lose their blue staining and take up a cationic dye of contrasting colour (usually red) subsequently applied. Blue-stained organisms are termed 'Gram-positive' and those stained with the counterstain (red) 'Gram-negative'. The result is that not only are organisms demonstrated, but different strains are shown in differing colours, affording an arbitrary division into two main groups and thus aiding their identification.

The means by which some organisms retain the blue primary dye and others lose it upon differentiation is due to the action of iodine. The exact way in which iodine influences dye fastness to differentiation is not clear. The traditional view is that iodine combines with the dye and Gram-positive organisms as a type of mordant or trapping agent to form a solvent-resistant dye complex. This viewpoint is undoubtedly over-simplified and consideration is given to the role played by iodine in dye penetration or isoelectric point deviation. Gram-positive organisms have a thicker wall than the Gram-negative (Rogers et al 1980) and this is important in the retention of the blue dye/iodine complex. Interestingly, fibrin will remain largely Gram-positive in the absence of the iodine treatment. In Gram staining, non-viable Gram-positive organisms will often stain Gram-negative. A few Gram variants are given with specialized techniques for organisms such as the mycobacteria, legionella, helicobacter and spirochaetes. Other techniques that demonstrate organisms are Giemsa (see p. 70) and methyl green-pyronin (see p. 98).

Organisms in clumps stain a weak blue colour in H&E preparations and are seen fairly readily, but an individual organism is difficult to visualize and special stains are necessary. Fixation is not important but initial freshness of tissue and the use of positive controls are, so that should the test section be negative it is an indicator that the solutions and the skill of the operator are beyond reproach!

GRAM TECHNIQUE (Gram 1884)

Notes

Both Gram-positive and negative bacteria are demonstrated in the following technique. Although overdifferentiation with the acetone is possible, it is the method of choice for consistently good results. The technique for smears is similar in principle to that for sections and the points to remember are that they should either be heat-dried on a hot plate before staining, or wet-fixed for 20–30 min in 95% alcohol; before staining it is not necessary to take the smears through xylene and alcohols. The potassium iodide in the iodine will facilitate solution of the insoluble iodine in the aqueous solvent. Tissue which has been decalcified in strong acids (or too long in weak acids) will give inconsistent staining.

Solutions

Crystal violet
   0.5% crystal violet in 25% alcohol (74 OP industrial methylated spirit).
Gram's and Lugol's iodine
   Add 1 g iodine to 2 g potassium iodide plus a few ml of distilled water in a mortar. Grind until dissolved and make up to a 300 ml volume for Gram's and 100 ml volume for Lugol's variant, with distilled water. The former solution is usually satisfactory for the technique.
1% aqueous neutral red

Technique

1. Sections to water.
2. Stain with the crystal violet solution for 2 min.
3. Wash in water. Treat with an iodine solution for 2 min.
4. Wash in water and differentiate in acetone for 1 or 2 s only. Wash in water.
5. Counterstain with 1% aqueous neutral red for 3 min.
6. Wash, dehydrate quickly, clear and mount in a DPX-type mountant.

Results

Gram-positive organisms, fibrin, some fungi, Paneth cell granules, keratohyalin, keratin	blue
Gram-negative organisms, cell nuclei	red

MODIFIED GRAM TECHNIQUE (Gram 1884)

Notes

Although only Gram-positive organisms are demonstrated by this technique, brilliant staining is afforded. The method is capricious, as it is not always possible to extract fully background crystal violet staining using the aniline-xylene differentiator. This is compensated for by the fact that it is virtually impossible to overdifferentiate.

Solutions

5% aqueous eosin ws yellowish
Crystal violet solution (see Gram's technique, above)
Gram's iodine solution (see Gram's technique, above)
Aniline-xylene mixture (equal parts)

Technique

1. Sections to water.
2. Stain with the eosin solution for 5 min. Wash briefly in water.
.3. Stain with the crystal violet solution for 2 min. Wash in water.
4. Treat with Gram's iodine solution for 2 min.
5. Wash briefly in water and blot dry.
6. After initial agitation of the section, leave in a Coplin jar of aniline-xylene for 5 min.
7. Rinse in xylene and mount in a DPX-type mountant.

Results

Gram-positive organisms, keratohyalin, keratin   blue
Background   pink to red

Table 11.1   Significant organisms and their Gram reactivity

Type	Form	Gram staining
Actinomyces	Filaments	Positive filament/negative clubs
Anthracis	Large straight bacilli	Positive
Bacteroides	Bacilli or coccobacilli	Negative
Clostridia	Large bacilli	Positive
Escherichia coli	Bacilli	Negative
Haemophilus	Coccobacilli	Negative
Klebsiella	Bacilli	Negative
Lactobacillus	Bacilli	Positive
Mycobacterium	Bacilli	Positive
Neisseria	Diplococci	Negative
Pneumococcus	Diplococci	Positive
Proteus	Bacilli	Negative
Pseudomonas	Bacilli	Negative
Salmonella	Bacilli	Negative
Shigella	Bacilli	Negative
Staphylococcus	Cocci (in clusters)	Positive
Streptococci	Cocci (in chains)	Positive

GRAM–TWORT TECHNIQUE (Twort 1924, Ollett 1947)

Notes

This technique is time-consuming and under- or over-differentiation can occur. Even so, a good preparation gives exceptional colour distinction of organisms from tissue background. Before differentiating, it is important that the slide is completely dry (warming over a lighted lamp bulb for 10 min, following blotting, is useful).

Solutions

Crystal violet solution (see Gram's technique, above)
Gram's iodine solution (see Gram's technique, above)
2% acetic acid in ethanol
Stock neutral red-fast green stain:

0.2% neutral red in ethanol	90 ml
0.2% fast green FCF in ethanol	10 ml

Before use, dilute 1 part stock solution with 3 parts distilled water.

Technique

1. Sections to water.
2. Stain with the crystal violet solution for 3 min. Wash in water.
3. Treat with the Gram's iodine solution for 3 min. Wash in water and blot dry (see Notes).
4. Differentiate in preheated acetic-alcohol at 56°C until the section is a 'dirty-straw' colour (15 min will usually suffice).
5. Wash briefly in distilled water.
6. Counterstain in the neutral red-fast green stain solution for 5 min.
7. Wash in distilled water. Differentiate in acetic-alcohol at room temperature for approximately 10 s until no more red colour diffuses out.
8. Rinse in alcohol. Clear and mount in a DPX-type mountant.

Results

Gram-positive organisms, fibrin, some fungi, keratohyalin, Paneth cell granules, keratin	blue
Gram-negative organisms, cell nuclei	red
Cell cytoplasms, collagen, red blood cells, etc.	green

ZIEHL–NEELSEN (ZN) TECHNIQUE FOR TUBERCLE BACILLI (Ziehl 1882, Neelsen 1883)

Notes

Mycobacteria such as tubercle bacilli have a lipid-rich cell wall capable of taking up strong phenol-dye solutions so that they retain the dye upon subsequent differentiation in acid or alcohol, i.e. they are acid- and alcohol-fast. Most other organisms lose the dye and take up the counterstain. It has been shown (Harada 1976) that acid-fastness of mycobacteria stained with carbol fuchsin is due to the presence of carboxyl and hydroxyl groups on unsaturated lipids present in bacterial cells.

The technique is not specific for tubercle bacilli, there being a tap water contaminant that stains similarly and is equally fast to differentiators. Fortunately, the acid- and alcohol-fast organisms of tap water usually present as clumps sitting on the tissue, i.e. in a different focal plane, and are readily distinguishable. Whichever ZN variant is used, it is important to take through a positive control section as the carbol fuchsin solutions deteriorate with age (and newly prepared solutions may not work!). Counterstaining should be light, otherwise the bacilli may be masked; some workers prefer to counterstain with an alum haematoxylin solution as opposed to methylene blue. In our experience methylene blue provides a slightly better contrast to the carbol fuchsin-stained organisms and is given in the following techniques.

The histological appearance in tuberculosis is usually (but not always) typical; even so, the demonstration of tubercle bacilli is a useful confirmatory procedure. Tissue which has the obvious histological characteristics of tuberculosis quite often will contain few or no stainable organisms. This may be traced to the fact that the patient has been treated with the usual anti-tuberculous drugs, which results in non-staining organisms. Additionally, tissue from unsuspected tuberculosis cases, i.e. untreated, may still contain only few bacilli; for example, bone lesions usually contain far fewer organisms compared to lung. Basic fuchsin is the usual dye in the technique but other dyes, e.g. Victoria blue, may be used instead. The phenol in the staining solution probably acts as a surface tension depressant to allow the dye ions to enter the lipid envelope of the tubercle bacilli more easily. Avoid decalcification of tissue in strong acids as acid-fastness may be lost; formic acid solutions are preferred (Wong & Wu 1979). Heating carbol fuchsin solution with naked flames is potentially hazardous and an alternative course of action is to use a Coplin jar containing the dye in a 56°C incubator. A Ziehl–Neelsen-type method that employs a room temperature stain bath is that of Kinyouin, which is given below. If desired, this 'cold' carbol fuchsin can be used to good effect in place of the conventional solution in the following technique; the acid-alcohol differentiation time is reduced to 1 min.

An opportunistic organism *Mycobacterium avium intracellulare* associated with AIDS infection is being increasingly encountered and stains positively with ZN techniques.

If potentially tuberculous unfixed material for cryostat sectioning is received, full aseptic procedures should be adopted, i.e. use of gloves, gowns, etc. Following sectioning the slides should be fixed in 10% formalin for at least 10 min before staining, and all equipment including the cryostat interior should be thoroughly sterilized in either formalin or a glutaraldehyde solution. The 'Howie' 1978 Code of Practice handbook should be consulted for full details. Hooklets of the dog tapeworm *E. granulosus* are weakly ZN-positive. It is necessary to use 1% sulphuric acid as the differentiator; the differentiation time is shorter and should be stopped when the hooklets are stained and the background is reasonably clear.

Solutions

Carbol fuchsin solution
Dissolve 1 g basic fuchsin (use the coarse granule, not the more purified type specified for Schiff's reagent) in 10 ml ethanol. Dissolve 5 g of phenol in 100 ml of distilled water. Mix the two solutions together. Filter.
0.2% aqueous methylene blue

Technique

1. Sections to water.
2. Filter on the carbol fuchsin and heat three times until the 'steam rises' (over a period of 10 min), or heat in a Coplin jar at 56°C for 30 min. Alternatively, use the Kinyouin solution (see p. 243) for 10 min at room temperature.

3. Wash well in water. Differentiate in 1% acid-alcohol for 1 or 10 min (see Notes). Wash in water for 5–10 min.
4. Counterstain with the methylene blue solution for 30 s. Wash in water.
5. Differentiate and dehydrate in alcohol until the sections are a weak blue. Clear and mount in a DPX-type mountant.

Results

Tubercle bacilli, hair shafts, and (to a lesser degree) red blood cells, clubs of actinomycotic filaments and spermatozoa heads	magenta
Background	weak blue

ALTERNATIVE ZN-TYPE TECHNIQUE (Poltz et al 1964)

Notes

With this variant of the ZN technique a combined differentiator and counterstain is used. This works quite well but the malachite green tends to fade, sometimes after a short time.

Solutions

Carbol fuchsin solution, see ZN technique above
Differentiator-counterstain:

2% aqueous malachite green	100 ml
Acetic acid	15 ml
Glycerol	25 ml

There is usually no need to filter the solution.

Technique

1. Sections to water and stain with the heated carbol fuchsin (as for the standard ZN technique).
2. Wash in water.
3. Counterstain in a Coplin jar of the acidified malachite green solution for 4 min.
4. Wash, blot, dehydrate, clear and mount in a DPX-type mountant.

Results

Tubercle bacilli (see results for standard ZN technique)	magenta
Background	pale blue-green

MODIFIED COLD ZN TECHNIQUE (Kinyouin 1915)

Notes

No heating of the carbol fuchsin is required in this technique which employs a stronger solution of the dye. The dye solution is an aqueous one, unlike the traditional solution, and is difficult to prepare; for good results it is important that full solubility of the dye in the solvent is achieved.

Solutions

Carbol fuchsin solution
Dissolve, with the aid of heat, 4 g of basic fuchsin in 20 ml forf distilled water. Melt some phenol crystals in a flask, under a hot tap, and add 8 ml of the melted phenol to 100 ml of distilled water. Add the two solutions together, mix and filter.
0.2% aqueous methylene blue

Technique

1. Sections to water.
2. Filter on the carbol fuchsin solution for 4 min. Do not heat.
3. Wash. Differentiate in 1% acid-alcohol for 1 min.
4. Wash and counterstain as for the standard ZN technique.
5. Dehydrate, clear and mount in a DPX-type mountant.

Results

Tubercle bacilli, etc. (see results for standard ZN technique)	magenta
Background	pale blue

MODIFIED ZN TECHNIQUE FOR LEPROSY BACILLI (Faraco 1938, Fite et al 1947)

Notes

Compared with tubercle bacilli, the leprosy bacilli are much less acid- and alcohol-fast and their lipid envelope is more easily affected by fat solvents, diminishing the staining reaction. In this modification of the standard ZN technique, differentiation with alcohol and acid is minimal. Initial dewaxing is done in a mixture of a vegetable oil and xylene. It is important not to over-stain with the methylene blue, as it will not be possible to remove the excess dye in alcohol.

Solutions

As for standard ZN technique.

Technique

1. Warm the sections and de-paraffinize by placing in a mixture of two parts xylene to one part vegetable oil (clove and origanum oils are suitable). Leave for at least 10 min.
2. Blot dry and wash in water. This step may be repeated, should any xylene-oil remain on the section.
3. Filter on the carbol fuchsin solution for 20 min. Do not heat.
4. Wash. Differentiate in 1% acid-alcohol for 1 min.

5. Wash well in water and counterstain in weak (0.2%) methylene blue for 5–10 s.
6. Wash, blot, dry and clear in xylene. Repeat the blotting-xylene treatment until the section is clear.
7. Mount in a DPX-type mountant.

Results

Leprosy bacilli, hair shafts and (to a lesser degree) red blood cells   magenta
Background   pale blue

FLUORESCENCE TECHNIQUE FOR TUBERCLE BACILLI AND LEPROSY BACILLI (Silver et al 1966)

Notes

It is a curious fact that most workers agree that the fluorescence demonstration of the tubercle bacilli (particularly) is superior to the ZN-type technique, and yet few use it! (This may be due to the inherent problems of fluorescence microscopy, the relative impermanence of preparations, and the fact that expertise is necessary to initially visualize the section without too great a time consumption.) On the other hand, an important advantage is that screening of sections for tubercle bacilli is much quicker, as isolated bacilli are more easily seen.

Background tissue fluorescence is masked by the potassium permanganate treatment. To stain for leprosy bacilli, avoid alcohol dehydration at the conclusion of the technique and de-wax initially in a vegetable oil-xylene mixture (see above). Sections stained by the ZN technique can be de-stained by lengthy 1% acid-alcohol treatment if so wished, and re-stained using the following fluorescence technique. The converse gives unsatisfactory results.

Solutions

Auramine-rhodamine solution
Add 1.5 g of auramine O and 0.75 g rhodamine B to 50 ml of distilled water and 75 ml glycerol. Mix and add 10 ml phenol liquefied by melting at 56°C. The solution will keep for up to 2 months.
0.5% hydrochloric acid in 70% alcohol (for tubercle bacilli) *or*
0.5% aqueous hydrochloric acid (for leprosy bacilli)
0.5% aqueous potassium permanganate

Technique

1. Sections to water.
2. Mix the auramine-rhodamine solution and filter. Treat the section for 10 min at 60°C (the stain should be pre-heated).
3. Wash in water for 2 min.
4. Differentiate in either of the hydrochloric acid solutions for 2–3 min as appropriate.
5. Wash in water for 2 min.
6. Treat with the potassium permanganate solution for 1 min.

7. Wash in water for 2 min. Blot dry.
8. Dehydrate (omit for leprosy bacilli), clear and mount in a DPX-type mountant.

Results

Using the fluorescence microscope with a yellow K530 barrier filter:

| Tubercle or leprosy bacilli | golden-yellow |
| Background tissue | dark green |

THE DEMONSTRATION OF *Legionella pneumophila*

In 1976 attention was focused on a type of pneumonia having a high mortality; at an American Legion convention in Philadelphia, USA 182 cases were reported, of which there were 29 deaths. In 1977 the causative organism was identified as a small Gram-negative coccobacillus and was named *Legionella pneumophila*. From a histological point of view it is a difficult organism to demonstrate. It stains poorly by the conventional Gram technique and in our hands is not stained by methyl green-pyronin, although it does stain weakly with the Giemsa technique. The Dieterle silver technique, although originally described for the demonstration of spirochaetes, has proved to be a useful method for these organisms in routine histological sections and is described below.

DIETERLE TECHNIQUE FOR *Legionella pneumophila* (Dieterle 1927)

Notes

The gum mastic solution gives best results if used immediately after the 3 days needed for its preparation and it is important to ensure its thorough solution in the alcohol. It is also important for the reaction that the temperatures are strictly adhered to. Formalin-fixed frozen and celloidin sections may be 'stained' as well as paraffin.

The uranyl nitrate step serves to prevent argyrophilic background material such as nerve fibres from being impregnated, and the gum as a diffusion vehicle for the silver particles to give even impregnation. Otherwise the rationale is as for most silver techniques, i.e. reduction of bound silver nitrate to a black reduced silver salt. As with most silver techniques, the main disadvantages are that practice is required for consistent results and that other background elements exhibit silver blackening to a varying degree, e.g. connective tissue fibres and various pigment granules. Note that other commonly occurring organisms are also argyrophilic by this method.

Solutions

0.5% uranyl nitrate in 70% alcohol
10% gum mastic in absolute alcohol (stand for 3 days before use)
1% aqueous silver nitrate
Reducer:

| Hydroquinone | 1.5 g |

Sodium sulphite	0.25 g
Conc. formalin	10 ml
Acetone	10 ml
Pyridine	10 ml

Add distilled water to a final volume of 90 ml, mix and dissolve, then add 10 ml of the alcoholic gum mastic solution (the solution appears 'milky').

Technique

1. Sections to distilled water.
2. Treat with the uranyl nitrate solution for 30 min at 55°C.
3. Wash briefly in distilled water then in 95% alcohol.
4. Treat with the gum mastic solution for 30 s.
5. Rinse in 95% alcohol for 1 s only, then transfer to distilled water.
6. Treat with the silver nitrate solution for 1–6 h in the dark (take through several sections and remove at intervals until the optimal time is determined).
7. Wash in distilled water for 1 s only.
8. Place in reducer for 8 min.
9. Wash in distilled water for 1 s then 96% alcohol followed by acetone.
10. Clear and mount as desired.

Results

Organisms including *L. pneumophila*, also melanin	black
Background	yellow

THE DEMONSTRATION OF HELICOBACTER

Helicobacter pylori (formerly assigned to the Campylobacter group of organisms) is an organism that, since its recognition in 1984, has been firmly linked to gastritis and duodenal ulceration. It is a Gram-negative bacillus having the distinctive morphology of a stumpy curved rod.

It can be readily shown in conventional paraffin sections, but the actual demonstration calls for some thought. Staining by the conventional Gram technique gives indifferent results in histological materials and some workers find that, with experience, *H. pylori* can be identified satisfactorily using haematoxylin and eosin. However, for the less experienced, special stains are helpful and an effective and popular technique is the Warthin & Starry (see p. 252). This is a time-consuming method and one that requires some expertise for best results; some workers prefer to use a Giemsa technique—often in a modified form. Our preference is for staining with cresyl fast violet which we find simple and effective. The technique is essentially that for the demonstration of sex chromatin (see p. 332) accepting that there is no need to celloidinize the sections; aim to under-differentiate the cresyl fast violet. The helicobacter should appear a dark purple colour against a lighter purple background.

In gastric biopsies the organisms are normally found on the epithelial surface or in the mucosal glandular folds. It is recommended that a positive control slide is taken through, if possible, so that the relative colour balance of organisms to background can be assessed.

SPIROCHAETES

In tissue the most common spirochaete is *Treponema pallidum*, the causative organism of syphilis. Another less commonly seen spirochaete is the leptospira found in Weil's disease, which may be transmitted from rats, also the spirochaetes of Borrelia that are found in the tick-borne Lyme disease. These organisms are not seen in routine preparations, and special techniques are necessary. The Giemsa technique will stain the spirochaetes purple-red but visualization is not easy. The most successful methods employ silver impregnation and these will be described. Formalin fixation gives the best results.

BLOCK IMPREGNATION TECHNIQUE (Bertarelli & Volpino 1906)

Notes

This is a modification of the Levaditi method and gives, in our experience, superior results. Block impregnation techniques tend in general to be less erratic than those designed for sections, but naturally suffer from the drawback of needing unprocessed tissue that may well not be available.

For reasons that are not clear, the reducing solution should be at least 3 months old, so it is advisable to keep some ready for use on the shelf. The addition of acetic acid, and use of a lower pH silver solution seems to give a clearer background than the Levaditi method.

Solutions

Silver solution
   1.5 g silver nitrate in 50 ml ethanol and 50 ml distilled water.
Reducer:

Tannic acid	3 g
Pyrogallic acid	5 g
Anhydrous sodium acetate	10 g
Distilled water	350 ml

The solution should be at least 3 months old before use.

Technique

1. Take a 2 mm piece of formalin-fixed tissue and, if available, a similar block of positive control material, and wash well in several changes of distilled water over 1–3 h.
2. Place in the silver solution for 24 h at 37°C in the dark.
3. Add 0.25 ml glacial acetic acid for every 100 ml volume of the silver solution and leave for a further 4 days at 37°C in the dark.
4. Wash in several changes of distilled water over 1–3 h.
5. Reduce for 2–3 days at room temperature in the dark.
6. Wash in several changes of distilled water over 3 h.
7. Paraffin process and cut sections. It is wise to cut one section from the periphery of the block and one nearer the centre and thus obtain different degrees of silver impregnation. Mount on slides, dry, deparaffinize in xylene and mount as desired.

Results

Spirochaetes (plus some organisms and fungi)	black
Background	yellow

PARAFFIN SECTION TECHNIQUE (Warthin & Starry 1920)

Notes

This is the standard, although time-consuming, silver technique for spiro-chaetes in paraffin sections. A degree of expertise is needed to obtain a reasonable result due to the variation in the development of the silver; over-development yields heavily impregnated spirochaetes against a dark and granular background, whilst under-development shows weakly impregnated spirochaetes against a pale background. The temperature of the developer is all-important for successful results for which, in place of Scotch glue, gelatin can be used. As with the Dieterle silver method most of the common organisms are also blackened.

Solutions

Prepare a litre of Walpole acetate-acetic buffer pH 3.6 (see p. 431) and use in the preparation of the following solutions.

Silver solution
  1% silver nitrate in pH 3.6 buffer.

Developer
  Add 0.3 g hydroquinone to 10 ml of buffer. Take 1 ml and add 15 ml of warmed 5% Scotch glue (or gelatin); mix and maintain at 40°C. Take 3 ml of 2% silver nitrate in pH 3.6 buffer and maintain at 55°C. The two solutions are mixed immediately before use.

Technique

1. Sections to water and rinse in pH 3.6 buffer (celloidinize the section to minimize background precipitation).
2. Stain with the pre-heated silver solution for $1\frac{1}{2} - 1\frac{3}{4}$ h at 55–60°C. During this period prepare the developer, which should also be pre-heated (use a water bath).
3. Treat with developer for $3\frac{1}{2}$ min at 55°C (the sections should turn a golden-brown).
4. Pour off the developer and rinse in tap water for several minutes at 55–60°C then in room temperature buffer. Tone if desired in 0.2% aqueous gold chloride.
5. Dehydrate, clear and mount as desired.

Results

Spirochaetes, also the Gram-negative organisms of cat scratch disease and Helicobacter organisms	black
Background	yellow-brown

MODIFIED DIETERLE TECHNIQUE FOR SPIROCHAETES (Burns 1982)

This modified technique seems to give better results than the Warthin & Starry method for spirochaetes in paraffin sections. Because a somewhat 'dirty' background is given, we have found this modified technique, though better than the original for demonstrating spirochaetes, less satisfactory for demonstrating *L. pneumophila*. The temperatures specified for the various solutions are important and should be adhered to for good results.

Solutions

5% uranyl nitrate in 70% alcohol
The other solutions are as for the non-modified technique (see p. 249).

Technique

1. Sections to distilled water.
2. Treat with pre-heated uranyl nitrate solution for 1 h at 60°C.
3. Treat with the gum mastic solution for 3 min.
4. Rinse in 95% alcohol.
5. Rinse in distilled water for 1 min and allow to drain until almost dry (approx. 10 min).
6. Place in pre-heated silver nitrate solution overnight at 40°C.
7. Rinse in distilled water.
8. Place in reducer for 3–5 min (until pale yellow to tan).
9. Rinse in distilled water, then in 95% alcohol followed by acetone.
10. Clear and mount as desired.

Results

Spirochaetes	black
Background	yellow-brown

FUNGI

The usual fungi to be encountered in tissue are *Aspergillus fumigatus*, *Candida albicans* and, less commonly, *Cryptococcus neoformans* and *Histoplasma capsulatum*. The latter two fungi are found as mucoencapsulated yeasts, whilst the former exhibit both yeast forms and mycelia. Fungal mycelia, if plentiful, can often be seen in H & E preparations but the yeast forms only with difficulty. Special stains are of value for fungal demonstration and there is a reasonably wide choice of techniques. These include PAS (see p. 135), Gram (see p. 242), Best's carmine (see p. 162), Southgate's mucicarmine (see p. 140), alcian blue (see p. 146), and the two described below—the Grocott variant of Gomori's hexamine silver and Gridley's technique. In demonstrating cryptococci by the PAS or Grocott techniques, the organism itself is coloured; using the Southgate mucicarmine or alcian blue techniques only the capsule is stained. It will be seen from Table 11.2 that there are significant differences in results for fungi using staining techniques. Formalin fixation is recommended for fungi demonstration. *Candida albicans* and

Pneumocystis carinii infections are important AIDS-related opportunistic features and are becoming more widely encountered.

GROCOTT HEXAMINE (METHENAMINE)-SILVER TECHNIQUE
(Gomori 1946, Grocott 1955)

Notes

This is the method of choice for demonstrating fungi and *Pneumocystis carinii* (which is now considered to be a type of fungus). Chromic acid-formed aldehydes from certain structures reduce a hexamine-silver mixture at an alkaline pH, and are selectively blackened. The method is not specific for fungi and is time-consuming, but rarely fails to demonstrate any fungi present in tissue. A control should always be taken through to establish the efficacy of the reagents employed.

Over-impregnation results in connective tissues being blackened, making fungal identification more difficult. Terminate treatment with the hexamine-silver when the fungi appear a dark brown colour and the background is still clear, i.e. aim at slightly under-impregnating. The inclusion of the borate gives a final pH of approximately 8.0.

Solutions

5% aqueous chromium trioxide (chromic acid)
1% aqueous sodium metabisulphite
Stock hexamine-silver solution
   To 100 ml of 3% aqueous hexamine add 5 ml of 5% aqueous silver nitrate. A white precipitate will form that dissolves on shaking. The solution keeps for 1–2 months at 4°C.
Working solution
   Dilute 2 ml of freshly prepared 5% aqueous sodium tetraborate solution with 25 ml of distilled water.
   Mix and add 25 ml of stock hexamine-silver. Mix.
0.1% aqueous gold chloride
5% aqueous sodium thiosulphate (hypo)
0.2% light green in 0.2% acetic acid

Technique

1. Test and control sections to water.
2. Treat with the chromic acid solution for 1 h. Wash in water.
3. Bleach in the metabisulphite solution for 1 min.
4. Wash in tap water 5–10 min, then in several changes of distilled water.
5. The working hexamine solution should have been pre-heated to 56°C using a Coplin jar in a water bath. Treat the section in this solution at 56°C and examine after 10–20 min and after that at 3 min intervals until the fungi are blackened (see Notes) but the background is clear.
6. Wash in 3 changes of distilled water and tone in 0.1% aqueous gold chloride for 3 min.
7. Wash in water, fix in sodium thiosulphate for 5 min. Wash again.

8. Counterstain in light green for 1–2 min. Wash in water.
9. Dehydrate, clear and mount as desired.

Results

Cellulose, *P. carinii*, fungi, chitin, amoebae, some mucins, melanin, glycogen, starch	black
Background	green

GRIDLEY'S TECHNIQUE (Gridley 1953)

Notes

This technique is the Bauer–Schiff and aldehyde fuchsin techniques in combination. Whilst some workers feel that the Gridley technique reveals more of the internal structure of fungi than other methods, the types of fungus demonstrated are paralleled by the much simpler PAS technique. Another point to remember is that elastic fibres and some connective tissue mucins stain purple, making fungus demonstration more difficult in tissues such as skin.

Solutions

4% aqueous chromium trioxide (chromic acid)
Schiff's reagent (see p. 135)
Aldehyde fuchsin solution (see p. 58)
Saturated tartrazine in Cellosolve
Sulphurous acid rinse:

10% aqueous sodium metabisulphite	6 ml
Molar hydrochloric acid	5 ml
Distilled water to	100 ml

Technique

1. Sections to water.
2. Treat with the chromic acid solution for 1 h. Wash in tap water, then in distilled water.
3. Treat with Schiff's reagent for 15 min.
4. Treat with the sulphurous acid solution for 3 changes over 6 min.
5. Wash in water for 10 min.
6. Treat with the aldehyde fuchsin solution for 20–30 min.
7. Wash in 50% alcohol then in water.
8. Wash in absolute alcohol and stain with the tartrazine solution for $\frac{1}{2}$–1 min.
9. Wash in Cellosolve, dehydrate, clear and mount in a DPX-type mountant.

Results

Fungi, elastin, some mucins	purple
Background	yellow

Table 11.2   Staining reactions of fungi

Organism	HE	Gram	PAS	CAS+	Gridley	Reticulin	Grocott	Alcian blue	Mucicarmine	Best's carmine
Candida albicans	±	+	+	+	−	+	±	−	+	
Aspergillus fumigatus (pulm.)	+	−	+	+	±	+	+	−	−	±
A.fumigatus (plug)	±	−	±	+	+	+	+	−	−	−
Cryptococcus neoformans	−	±	+	+	+	+	+	+	+	+
Histoplasma capsulatum	−	−	+	+	+	+	+	±	±	+
Sporothrix schenckii	−	+	+	+	+	+	+	+	−	+
Blastomyces dermatitidis	−	−	+	+	+	+	+	−	−	+
Epidermaphyton floccosum	−	−	±	±	±	±	+	−	−	+
Trichophyton rubrum	−	−	±	±	±	+	+	−	−	+
T. verrucosum	−	−	+	+	+	+	+	−	−	+
Actinomyces bovis*	±	+	±	+	+	+	+	−	−	±

*Not a true fungus; +CAS, chromic acid-Schiff (Bauer technique).

VIRUSES AND THEIR INCLUSION BODIES

Except for the hepatitis B surface antigen, viruses are not easily identified or visualized by light microscopy with, or without, the use of special stains. In certain viral conditions intracellular aggregates form and these can be demonstrated in conventional tissue sections; they are known as virus inclusion bodies. They are invariably globular in shape and vary, not only in size, but in their location in that they may be intranuclear (e.g. cytomegalovirus and herpes simplex), intracytoplasmic (e.g. rabies and measles) or both (e.g. viral warts of skin). The inclusion bodies vary greatly in their composition and can contain DNA or RNA.

The presence of either of the nucleic acids means that techniques such as the Feulgen for DNA (see p. 96) or methyl green-pyronin for RNA (see p. 98) can be successfully employed. The protein moiety imparts acidophilia to virus inclusion bodies, enabling them to be seen to a lesser or greater extent in routine H&E preparations. Special stains are of a definite advantage in showing these structures although much depends on the type of virus inclusion present as to which method is of greater value. For example, herpes and cytomegalic virus inclusion bodies are readily seen in conventional H & E preparations, also Papanicolaou-stained material, whilst those of rabies, measles and Rickettsia stain better using techniques such as Giemsa (see p. 70), Mann's methyl blue-eosin (see p. 80) or phloxine-tartrazine (see p. 71); the latter method stains Negri bodies of rabies brilliantly but inconsistently. Virus inclusions of the skin condition molluscum contagiosum are often only well shown by the Macchiavello technique, and those of rabies (Negri bodies) by the phosphotungstic acid-eosin techniques. Both specialized virus inclusion techniques will be described, with a modified orcein technique for virus hepatitis antigen. Whilst formalin fixation is adequate for these techniques, better results are given for virus inclusion bodies if mercuric chloride or potassium dichromate-containing solutions are used.

Non-viable virus protein may not stain, and specialized methods, such as in-situ hybridization employing suitable labelled probes, are indicated.

MACCHIAVELLO TECHNIQUE FOR VIRUS INCLUSION BODIES
(Macchiavello 1937)

Notes

This technique, which is like a modified ZN stain, will demonstrate most inclusion bodies. Negri bodies are sometimes seen with this simple technique, which requires some expertise to obtain a good result. A permanganate bleach stage is optional, and our experience with the method leads us to suspect that it is superfluous.

Solutions

0.5% basic fuchsin in pH 7.2 phosphate buffer (see Buffer Tables, Appendix 3)
0.5% aqueous citric acid
0.2% aqueous methylene blue
Acidified potassium permanganate solution (see p. 49)
5% aqueous oxalic acid

Technique

1. Sections to water.
2. Treat with the acidified potassium permanganate solution for 5 min. Wash and bleach with 5% aqueous oxalic acid (see Notes). Wash well in water.
3. Stain with the basic fuchsin solution for 5 min. Wash in water.
4. Differentiate in citric acid until only the virus inclusion bodies are left stained (3–6 min). Wash in water.
5. Counterstain lightly in the methylene blue solution for 10–20 s.
6. Wash, dehydrate, clear and mount as desired.

Results

Virus inclusion bodies	magenta
Background	pale blue

PHOSPHOTUNGSTIC-EOSIN TECHNIQUE FOR NEGRI BODIES
(Massignani & Malferrari 1961)

Notes

Whilst techniques such as Giemsa, Mann's or Macchiavello's purport to stain the typical formation of rabies, first described by Negri in 1903, they do not always give clear-cut demonstrations; an H&E preparation will often be as informative. Phloxine-tartrazine can yield good results, but can prove unhelpful. The phosphotungstic acid-eosin technique is undoubtedly the best technique now available. The solution is rather time-consuming to prepare but the results are consistently good.

According to the authors, the role of the phosphotungstic acid with eosin is that of dye-mordant formation rather than one of lowering the pH to give an acid eosin. An alternative mechanism to be considered is that the phosphotungstic acid, acting as a colourless dye, enters most of the tissue pores (intermicellar spaces), excepting those of fine porosity such as the virus inclusion bodies and red blood cells. The eosin is largely excluded from all but these two entities. When staining the nuclei with haematoxylin, it is important to differentiate well so that the background is left unstained.

Staining solution

Grind together 1 g eosin ws yellowish and 0.7 g phosphotungstic acid. Add 10 ml of distilled water and mix. Bring the total volume to 200 ml with ethanol. Add two drops of saturated aqueous lithium carbonate and stir continuously for 10 min. Restore to the original 200 ml volume with ethanol and filter. The solution keeps well under room temperature storage conditions.

Technique

1. Sections to water.
2. Stain the nuclei with one of the alum haematoxylin solutions (see p. 25). Differentiate well and blue. Wash in water then in ethanol.
3. Stain in the phosphotungstic-eosin solution for 8 min.
4. Wash in water briefly then differentiate by giving short dips in 50%, 70%, 80% and 90% alcohol and longer dips in 95% and absolute alcohol. (Give two or more changes of absolute alcohol of 4 min each.)
5. Clear in xylene and mount in a DPX-type mountant.

Results

Negri bodies	bright pink
Red blood cells	pink
Background	pale pink or colourless
Nuclei	blue

MODIFIED ORCEIN TECHNIQUE FOR HEPATITIS B SURFACE ANTIGEN (Shikata et al 1974)

Notes

In this type of viral hepatitis the affected hepatocytes show a typical cytoplasmic ground glass appearance, and the contained HBs (Australia) antigen can be demonstrated by orcein with prior oxidation by potassium permanganate. The rationale is that of sulphur-containing proteins being oxidized to form reactive sulphonate residues which react with orcein. In a similar way, using a pre-oxidation step, both aldehyde fuchsin and alcian blue will stain the HBs antigen. The definitive demonstration of HBs antigen is by immunocytochemistry, but the Shikata orcein technique is still popular in many routine laboratories, together with the oxidation-aldehyde fuchsin technique. Non-immunocytochemical techniques are not specific for HBs antigen and although elastic fibres are easily distinguishable from the viral antigen deposits, a potential source of error arises if copper-associated protein is present in the hepatocytes. The success or failure of the technique devolves around the batch of orcein employed. Most workers employ synthetic orcein, and some advocate the need for freshly prepared solutions, but in our experience the important point is to obtain initially a batch of orcein that works. It is important to take through a positive control slide in sequence with the test slides.

Solutions

Acidified potassium permanganate:

0.25% aqueous potassium permanganate	95 ml
3% aqueous sulphuric acid	5 ml

5% aqueous oxalic acid
Orcein solution:

Orcein (synthetic)	1 g
70% ethanol	100 ml
Conc. hydrochloric acid	1 ml

Saturated tartrazine in Cellosolve (2-ethoxy-ethanol)

Technique

1. Sections to water.
2. Treat with acidified potassium permanganate for 5 min.
3. Wash briefly in water.
4. Bleach sections with the oxalic acid solution for $\frac{1}{2}$ to 1 min.
5. Wash well in water (5 min or so).
6. Rinse in 70% alcohol.
7. Stain in preheated orcein for 1.5 h at 37°C (use Coplin jar).
8. Rinse in 70% alcohol and examine microscopically, and if the positive control is stained satisfactorily, proceed.
9. Rinse in Cellosolve, and stain with tartrazine for 2 min.
10. Rinse in Cellosolve, clear and mount as desired.

Results

HBs antigen, elastic fibres, hair shafts and copper-associated protein	dark brown
Background	yellow

TISSUE PARASITES DEMONSTRATION

There are many types of parasitic infestation of tissue, although in human tissue from the colder-climate countries these tend to be uncommon. It is a specialist subject and no attempt will be made here to provide comprehensive coverage. An H &E preparation is usually perfectly adequate, and this may be supplemented by using Giemsa (see p. 70) or the iron haematoxylin techniques (see p. 86). Two techniques are described: one a multicoloured technique designed to illustrate the variegated structure of helminths and protozoa, and one that is particularly useful for demonstrating the smaller parasites, such as Leishman–Donovan bodies. A useful reference book for parasites is Piekarski (1962). The PAS technique is always worth doing for the larger parasites as it will demonstrate any chitinous ectoskeleton.

MODIFIED LEISHMAN TECHNIQUE FOR *Leishmania donovani* (from Leishman 1901)

Notes

A fairly lengthy staining time is used in this method with a lower-than-usual pH dye solution to give reasonably clear-cut demonstration of Leishman–Donovan bodies.

These particular parasites are minute and not easily seen in H&E and conventional Romanowsky-type staining of tissue sections. They are also positive with the Warthin–Starry silver technique.

Solution

Leishman stain (available commercially from most laboratory suppliers) diluted 1 part: 4 parts of pH 4.7 buffer (see Buffer Tables, Appendix 3).

Technique

1. Take sections to distilled water.
2. Treat with the diluted Leishman stain for 1–11–2 hours.
3. Rinse in distilled water and differentiate in weak (1 in 10 000) acetic acid until the desired colour balance is achieved.
4. Rinse in distilled water and blot dry. Dehydrate quickly, clear and mount as desired.

Results

Leishman–Donovan bodies	pale blue
Collagen, red blood cells	pale pink
Nuclei	blue-purple

POLYCHROMATIC TECHNIQUE (Vetterling & Thompson 1972)

Notes

Although the staining solutions are time-consuming to prepare, the technique is relatively simple in execution and, with practice, seems to give good demonstration of the different parasite structures in contrasting colours. Helly fixation is recommended, although other routine fixatives can be used.

Solutions

Haematoxylin solution
   Dissolve 0.5 g haematoxylin and 1 g of ferric ammonium sulphate in a mixture of 50 ml 0.6% sulphuric acid and 50 ml 95% alcohol. Filter and allow to ripen for 4–8 weeks before use.
Biebrich scarlet-orange G solution
   Dissolve 0.25 g Biebrich scarlet ws, 0.25 g orange G, 0.54 g phosphotungstic acid and 0.5 g phosphomolybdic acid in a mixture of 50 ml distilled water and 50 ml 95% alcohol.
Fast green solution
   Dissolve 0.5 g fast green FCF in 100 ml of 95% alcohol.
Acid-alcohol solution:

   0.5 M sulphuric acid   10 ml

Distilled water	50 ml
95% alcohol	40 ml

Sodium bicarbonate solution:

Sodium bicarbonate	0.5 g
Distilled water	50 ml
95% alcohol	40 ml

Technique

1. Sections to alcohol.
2. Treat with the haematoxylin solution for 15–30 min.
3. Wash in water. Differentiate in the acid-alcohol solution for a few s.
4. Treat with the sodium bicarbonate solution for 2 min.
5. Stain with Biebrich scarlet-orange G solution for 15–30 minutes. Wash in 95% alcohol.
6. Stain with the fast green solution for 15 s.
7. Wash and dehydrate in alcohol, clear and mount as desired.

Results

Nuclei, nucleoli, mitochondria	blue-black
Nuclear histones, nematode cuticle, coelomocyte granules	red
Red blood cells, refractile bodies of coccidia, trematode cuticular spines and granules, refractile bodies of nematode excretory glands	yellow
Background	green

IMMUNOCYTOCHEMISTRY

Significant numbers of infective agents can now be demonstrated by immunocyto-chemistry using conventional formalin-fixed paraffin sections. Whether one needs to employ this type of method largely depends on two considerations. Firstly, are there already in existence satisfactory, conventional, i.e. non-immunocytochemical techniques? Secondly, given that immunocytochemistry is a more sensitive technique which is specific for a particular epitope, does the number of investigations justify keeping the antisera in the laboratory? The answer to the latter is relatively easily answered if the laboratory in question is a reference, or specialist one, dealing with potentially infected material. Such a laboratory would be found where organ transplants are performed, or where AIDS cases are referred. In these situations antisera against, for example, cytomegalovirus, *P. carinii* and the different hepatitis B antigens may well prove invaluable.

To answer the first question is less easy as it is a more subjective scenario. Most organisms and fungi are easily and satisfactorily demonstrated by non-immunocytochemical methods, and one would be hard-put to justify the use of, for example, anti-mycobacteria or anti-Candida in the routine laboratory. However, some infective agents such as *L. pneumophila* and Toxoplasma—even, perhaps, Helicobacter—are less easily demonstrated in tissue, and immunocytochemistry undoubtedly facilitates the diagnosis.

REFERENCES

Bertarelli G, Volpino G 1906 Weitere Untersuchungen über die Gegenwart der Spirochaete pallida in den Schnitten primärer sekundärer und tertiärer Syphilis. Zentralblatt für Bakteriologie, Parasitenkunde, Infektionskrankheiten und Hygiene 41: 74

Burns P A 1982 Staining intestinal spirochaetes. Journal of Medical Laboratory Sciences 39: 75

Dieterle R R 1927 Method for the demonstration of spirochaete pallida in single microscopic sections. Archives of Neurology and Psychiatry 18: 73

Faraco J 1938 Bacillos de Mansen e cortes de paraffina; Methodo complementar para a pesquiza de bacillos de Mansen e Cortes de material incluido el paraffina. Revista Brasileira de Leprologia 6: 177

Fite G L, Cambre P J, Turner M H 1947 Procedure for demonstrating lepra bacilli in paraffin sections. Archives of Pathology 43: 624 ,

Gomori G 1946 A new histochemical test for glycogen and mucin. American Journal of Clinical Pathology 16: 177

Gram C 1884 Ueber die isolierte Farbung der Schizomyceten in Schnitt und Trocnenpräparäten. Fortsch Med 2: 185

Gridley M G 1953 A stain for fungi in tissue sections. American Journal of Clinical Pathology 23: 303

Grocott R G 1955 A stain for fungi in tissue sections and smears. American Journal of Clinical Pathology 25: 975

Harada I T 1976 The nature of mycobacterial acid-fastness. Stain Technology 51: 255

Kinyouin J J 1915 A note on Uhlenhuth's method for sputum examination for tubercle. bacilli. American Journal of Public Health 5: 867

Leishman W B 1901 Note on a simple and rapid method of producing Romanowsky staining in malarial and other blood films. British Medical Journal 2: 757

Macchiavello A 1937 Richettsia. Revista Chill Hig. Med. Pre. 1: 5

Massignani A M, Malferrari R 1961 Phosphotungstic acid-eosin combined with haematoxylin as a stain for Negri bodies in paraffin sections. Stain Technology 36: 5

Neelsen F 1883 Zentralblatt für die Medizinischen Wissenschaftern 21: 497

Ollett W S 1947 A method for staining both Gram positive and Gram negative bacteria in sections. Journal of Pathology and Bacteriology 59: 357

Piekarski G 1962 Medical parasitology. Leverkusen-Bayerwerk Farenfabriken Bayer

Poltz G, Rampey J H, Furmandeau B 1964 A method for staining acid-fast bacilli in smears and sections of tissue. American Journal of Clinical Pathology 42: 552

Rogers H J, Perkins H R, Ward B J 1980 Microbial cells walls and membranes. Chapman & Hall

Shikata T, Uzawa T, Yashiware N, Akatsura R, Yamazari S 1974 Staining methods of Australia antigen in paraffin sections—detection of cytoplasmic inclusion bodies. Japanese Journal of Experimental Medicine 44: 25

Silver A, Sonnerwirth A C, Alex N 1966 Modifications in the fluorescence microscopy technique as applied to identification of acid-fast bacilli in tissue and bacteriological material. Journal of Clinical Pathology 19: 583

Twort F W 1924 An improved neutral red, light green doublestain for staining animal parasites, microorganisms and tissue. Journal of State Medicine 32: 351

Vetterling J M, Thompson D E 1972 A polychromatic stain for use in parasitology. Stain Technology 47: 164.

Warthin A S, Starry A C 1920 A more rapid and improved method of demonstrating spirochaetes in tissues. American Journal of Syphilis, Gonorrhea and Venereal Diseases 4: 97

Wong F T S, Wu P C 1979 The influence of decalcifying fluids on the demonstration of Mycobacterium tuberculosis in paraffin sections. Medical Laboratory Sciences 36: 153–157

Ziehl F 1882 Zur Farbung des Tuberkelbacillus. Deutsche Medizinische Wochenschrift 8: 0451

12. Immunocytochemistry

The significantly developing aspect of histology in recent years is immunocyto-chemistry, the science of which is applied to the relationship between tissue structure and composition and the chemical activities of the immunoglobulin molecule. It is necessary at this stage to give some definitions to allow the reader, possibly new to the subject, to understand what follows.

Antigen (Ag) (immunogens)

This term is applied to substances which cause the formation of antibodies. They are substances of different chemical types (usually proteins and glycoproteins) capable of stimulating the immune system of an animal to produce a response specifically directed at the inducing substance and not other related substances. The antigen produces a mutual specificity with the antibody it causes (Weir 1973).

Antibodies (Ab)

These are complex protein molecules produced by plasma cells and certain lymphocytes. The producing cells can be found in the germinal centres of lymph nodes, follicles of the spleen and other sites. Antibodies are produced in response to an antigenic stimulus and are known as immunoglobulins. Polyclonal (rabbit or goat) and monoclonal (mouse or rat) antibodies are available for antigen identification. When choosing an antibody it is necessary to confirm that the antibody-antigen reaction will withstand the fixation and processing in use.

Immunoglobulins (Ig)

These are glycoproteins consisting of two heavy and two light polypeptide chains linked by disulphide bonds. Splitting produces two univalent fragments capable of binding antigen (Fab) and a third fragment without this capacity (Fc). There are five classes of human immunoglobulins, called IgA, IgD, IgE, IgG and IgM:

IgA is the main immunoglobulin in sero-mucous secretions in respiratory and gastrointestinal tracts, where it defends surfaces by inhibiting adhesion of organisms to the epithelium. It comprises 13% of the total immunoglobulins.

IgD is present on lymphocyte surfaces.

IgE is present in activated mast cells and is involved in hypersensitivity reactions.

IgG is the immunoglobulin of internal body fluids. It crosses the placental barrier and is the major immunoglobulin in the neonate. It combats microorganisms and their toxins and forms approximately 80% of the total immunoglobulins.

IgM is largely restricted to plasma. It is a very effective agglutinator, produced early in the immune response and it is the first line of defence, forming 6% of the total immunoglobulins.

Monoclonal antibodies

Monoclonal antibodies are consistent while the same clone remains available; they are a single immunoglobulin subclass and have a defined specificity to one epitope of the antigen molecule. A disadvantage is that an epitope may not resist formalin fixation and paraffin embedding and may be present in more than one tissue substance. Monoclonal antibodies as a tissue culture medium can usually be diluted 10–100 times.

Polyclonal antibodies

Polyclonal antisera consist of a mixed population of antibodies that will be immunoreactive with a variety of epitopes on the antigen molecule. They survive fixation well to react with the antibody and, though lacking true specificity, show increased sensitivity compared to monoclonal antisera.

IMMUNOCYTOCHEMICAL METHODS

DIRECT METHOD

This is a single layer method using a labelled primary antibody. It is simple to use but the method is not sensitive enough to give good contrast with enzyme labels. Fluorescent labels are normally used, i.e. fluorescein-labelled anti-human immunoglobulins and complement which can be applied to cryostat sections (fresh or acetone-fixed) of kidney and skin biopsies. Possible non-specific binding sites (Fc receptors, hydrophobic and electrostatic binding sites) are blocked with a layer of normal rabbit serum before application of the primary rabbit antibody. The direct method has applications at the electron microscope level where a gold-labelled antibody can be used (see p. 277).

INDIRECT METHOD

This method is far more sensitive than the direct method. Non-specific binding sites in the tissue sections are blocked before applying the primary antibody with a layer of normal serum but from the species providing the second, labelled antibody. The increase in sensitivity is related to the hyperimmunity of the second layer antisera, according to Sternberger & Sternberger (1986). The method has the advantage that most unlabelled primary antibodies raised in the same species can be detected with just one labelled antibody ot the immunoglobulins of that species. In general, broad spectrum anti-immunoglobulins are used, reactive with IgG, IgA and IgM, so that the immunoglobulin type of the primary does not matter. On occasion it is advantageous to use a more restricted second antibody, e.g. to the IgG subtype of a primary monoclonal antibody. This provides a more efficient labelled antibody and could eliminate some background staining (Van Noorden 1990).

UNLABELLED ANTIBODY ENZYME COMPLEX METHODS (PAP and APAAP)

The original immunoenzyme bridge method using enzyme-specific antibody (Mason et al 1969, Sternberger 1969), discussed in the earlier book in this series has been superseded by the technique using a soluble peroxidase anti-peroxidase complex (PAP) (Sternberger et al 1970). These complexes are formed from three peroxidase molecules and two anti-peroxidase antibodies and are used as a third layer in the staining method. They are bound to the unconjugated primary antibody (e.g. rabbit anti-human IgG) by a second layer of 'bridging' antibody (e.g. swine anti-rabbit immunoglobulin). This is applied in excess so that one of its two identical binding sites binds to the primary antibody (e.g. swine anti-rabbit immunoglobulin), and the other to the (rabbit) PAP complex. Sternberger et al (1970) reported that the method is 100–1000 times more sensitive than indirect methods using either fluorescein or peroxidase-conjugated antisera, and a total of 20 anti-peroxidase antibody and peroxidase tracers can be applied as separate solutions. In practice, this potential large increase in sensitivity is not always evident (Heyderman 1986), but the technique is generally accepted as being clean and sensitive.

Alkaline phosphatase antibodies raised in the mouse can, by the same principle, be used to form alkaline phosphatase anti-alkaline phosphatase complexes (APAAP). These have similar uses and advantages to the PAP complexes (Cordell et al 1984) and are particularly useful when studying tissue containing pre-existing brown pigments, e.g. melanin. The red colour of the APAAP contrasts well.

UNLABELLED ANTIBODY ENZYME METHOD USING IMMUNOGOLD SILVER STAINING (IGSS)

The use of colloidal gold as a marker system for immunocytochemistry was introduced by Faulk & Taylor (1971) and it is used in direct and indirect methods, particularly at the electron microscope level. Its application at the light microscope level was introduced by Holgate et al (1983a, b). In this method, the gold particles are enhanced by layers of metallic silver. To produce metallic silver with a tolerance for natural light, the technique uses silver lactate as the ion supplier and hydroquinone as the reducing agent in a protective colloid of gum arabic at pH 3.5. Sometimes pre-treatment of the section with Lugol's iodine and sodium thiosulphate may be required to increase the intensity of staining. The silver enhancement technique is given following the gold methods. The method has greater sensitivity than the PAP technique, and modifications to the original technique have been reviewed by De Mey & Moeremans (1986). The two methods given are from Robinson et al (1990) with minor modifications.

AVIDIN-BIOTIN METHODS

These methods rely on the affinity of glycoprotein avidin for biotin. Avidin is present in egg white and is composed of four subunits which form a tertiary structure possessing four biotin-binding hydrophobic pockets. The oligosaccharide residues present in egg white avidin, and its charge properties, appear to give it some affinity for tissue components, particularly lectin-like proteins, which results in non-specific binding. A similar molecule, Streptavidin (mol. wt. 60 kd) is extracted from the culture broth of the bacterium *Streptomyces avidinii*. The lack of oligosac-charide residues and its neutral isoelectric point give Streptavidin some advantages, and it is becoming widely used.

Three methods have been described using avidin-biotin that use biotin-labelling of the primary (direct) or secondary (indirect) antibody. In the labelled avidin method the tracer is attached directly to the avidin molecule (Guesdon et al 1979). In the Avidin-Biotin Complex (ABC) method (Hsu et al 1981), a complex of avidin and biotinylated tracer, which contains free avidin-binding sites, is applied to the biotinylated antibody. In these techniques, as most biotin molecules can be attached to a single antibody, a high tracer to antibody ratio may be achieved. This gives high sensitivity, allowing a high dilution of the primary antiserum to be used. The avidin-biotin technique has every indication of becoming the standard labora-tory immunocytochemical method employing peroxidase.

LABELS

Immunocytochemical reactions are made visible by the incorporation of a suitable label into the reaction. Fluorescent molecules, enzymes, biotin (not a true coloured label) and colloidal gold with, or without, silver nitrate are most commonly used. Primary antibodies may be labelled for the direct method (see below) but it is more usual to label the antibodies of the second stage. In the unlabelled antibody-enzyme methods the label is not chemically conjugated to the antibody but acts as an antigen, bound in a complex to the antibody.

ENZYME LABELS

Horseradish peroxidase is the most widely used enzyme label although alkaline phosphatase, glucose oxidase and β-D-galactosidase have increasing applications. An enzyme label must produce a coloured end-product in the final step of the procedure and attention should be given to the correct pH, substrate and chromogen concentrations for the incubation.

PEROXIDASE

This most useful reaction product is derived from the oxidative polymerization of 3,3',-diaminobenzidine tetrahydrochloride (DAB). The action of antibody-bound peroxidase on hydrogen peroxide produces oxidation of the DAB and the reaction product is localized on the site of the antigen-antibody reaction as a dark brown and insoluble deposit giving good contrast with the unreactive parts of the section. Alternative chromogens are 4-chloro-1-naphthol, which gives a blue-grey colour, and 3-amino-9-ethylcarbazole, also a potential carcinogen, which gives a reddish-brown colour. These alternatives give final reaction products that are soluble in alcohol, so the preparations are mounted in aqueous mountants.

Blocking endogenous peroxidase

If there is active peroxidase present in the tissue to be incubated, it is blocked before the peroxidase-labelled antibody is applied in order to confirm whether the end-product is endogenous or antibody-associated enzyme. This is important if smears of fresh material or frozen sections are being used, but even in paraffin-processed material the 'peroxidase' (catalase) in the red blood cells remains active and can produce an intrusive reaction. Blocking is usually carried out before application of the primary antibody, but can be done at a later stage provided that it precedes the peroxidase-labelled reagent. For paraffin sections the blocking agent is usually hydrogen peroxide-methanol, which must be reasonably fresh. Frozen sections may be detached from slides by this, but less violent blocking is provided by substituting the methanol, itself a partial inhibitor of peroxidase, for distilled water. Even so, a solution of this strength may injure the immunoreactivity of some antigens. If endogenous peroxidase in paraffin sections is particularly strong and cannot be removed by the above means, stronger hydrogen peroxide can be used for a short time, followed by periodic acid (Heyderman & Monaghan 1979). These two steps are followed by treatment with borohydride solution which converts any aldehydes in the tissue to less 'sticky' alcohol groups. This treatment results in clean preparations but may prevent a few antigens from reacting (e.g. leukocyte common antigen).

ALKALINE PHOSPHATASE

This enzyme gives a bright blue colour with naphthol AS-MX phosphate and the diazonium salt fast blue BB, and a bright red colour with fast red TR. Both of these reaction products are alcohol-soluble. Alternatively an insoluble blue-brown reaction product can be produced from 5-bromo-4-chloro-3-indolyl phosphate and nitro BT. Endogenous alkaline phosphatase is not a problem in paraffin sections since its activity, except for intestinal activity, is destroyed by paraffin processing. In frozen sections it is inhibited at the enzyme development stage by adding an inhibitor to the incubating medium. Alkaline phosphatase as a label is not suitable for use on frozen or paraffin sections of intestinal material because of pre-existing alkaline phosphatase in the mucosa. By using a non-brown label, there are fewer interpretation problems with melanin-containing cells.

GLUCOSE OXIDASE

This is a plant enzyme, absent from animal tissues, so that no precautions are necessary. The enzyme reacts with nitro BT and glucose to produce a dark blue deposit that can be mounted in DPX (Suffin et al 1979).

β-D-GALACTOSIDASE

The enzyme used for labelling is derived from bacteria and acts optimally at a different pH from the mammalian variety—consequently it is not a suitable label for identifying bacterial antigens. This indigogenic method gives a turquoise blue, insoluble reaction product.

BIOTIN

This is a non-enzymic label that is used in immunocytochemistry in combination with avidin. Many molecules of biotin can be conjugated to the Fc portion of one immunoglobulin molecule and, since biotin combines tightly with avidin, avidin that is labelled with enzyme labels can be used to reveal the site of the antigen-antibody reaction. One avidin molecule can combine with four biotin molecules and a labelled avidin-biotin complex (ABC) can also be prepared.

METHODOLOGY

FIXATION

Fixation affects the activity of antigens with the choice of fixative depending upon the antigen or hormone to be detected. In general, formaldehyde gives acceptable results and so does formaldehyde freshly generated from paraformaldehyde powder. The routine histology laboratory has to rely on formalin-fixed paraffin sections that are, on occasion, not ideal for this purpose. The antigenic sites of some substances are immunologically inactive following routine formalin fixation and there is a need for prior enzyme (trypsin) treatment (q.v.). Cell surface markers of lymphocytes, for example, require specialized fixatives if optimal staining is to be achieved (Holgate et al 1986, Pollard et al 1987). Cryostat sections post-fixed in methanol, acetone, or acetone mixed with chloroform are satisfactory for the preservation of some of the labile substances and give improved tissue structure. A useful general fixation procedure for fresh cryostat sections and smears is acetone 10 min, followed by thorough drying.

Other substances require a mild cross-linking fixative such as formalin; without it they are soluble and are lost from the tissue during incubation. Cytokeratin intermediate filaments of the cytoskeleton of epithelial cells can be stained in unfixed preparations, but survive fixation. Increasingly, many diagnostically useful antibodies react with formalin-fixed paraffin-embedded materials and are available from commercial companies.

TISSUE AND SECTION PREPARATION

Paraffin sections should not be directly heated on a slide hot plate but dried overnight, at 37°C or 56°C. Tissue processing can be as harmful as fixation to antigens, and tissues which will not survive routine processing should be pre-fixed, frozen and cut in a cryostat. Protease treatment may be necessary for such preparations.

Cryostat sections should be air-dried at room temperature for several hours. Sections are fixed according to the antigens to be demonstrated and air-dried before applying the technique or placing in buffer. Cryostat sections, once wet, should not be allowed to dry during the incubating procedure, as this results in patchy staining and poor tissue architecture.

Resin sections

Epoxy resin-embedded sections can be incubated in the same way as paraffin sections but the resin is first removed by saturated alcoholic sodium hydroxide.

Glycol methacrylate sections are often used for thin sectioning at light microscopical level and give excellent morphology. Unfortunately the polymerized methacrylate cannot be dissolved, so antibodies do not reliably penetrate sections. An adaptation of the resin to yield a wider-meshed polymer has been reported that allows reliable immunocytochemistry after careful fixation and processing (van Goor et al 1988).

Section adhesion

Sections for immunocytochemistry should be picked up on slides coated with a 0.01% aqueous solution of a high molecular weight (150 000) poly-L-lysine, particularly if protease treatment is to be used, to prevent section loss.

Treatment of sections for endogenous peroxidases

It is usually necessary to treat sections before immunochemical staining to remove any endogenous peroxidases that will cause a pseudo-reaction (see above). These enzymes are present in many normal and pathological tissues. If not removed they will react with the substrate being used to localize the enzyme tracer, and produce a false positive reaction. The treatment of sections in methanol containing 0.3% hydrogen peroxide for 30 min at room temperature aims at removing this endogenous peroxidase activity without affecting the reactivity of the antigens.

Unmasking of reactivity using proteolytic enzymes

A problem of immunoperoxidase techniques can be the variable results that are obtained with formalin-fixed material, formaldehyde affecting some, but not all, of the antigens. Mepham et al (1979) published work showing that enzymatic pre-treatment reactivated the antigens as well as enhancing the staining reaction and improving the reliability of the immunoperoxidase methods. There are several factors that affect the pre-treatment time with enzymes. Mepham et al (1979) compared the effects of different enzymes at varying concentrations, temperature, and other factors. Their conclusions are shown in the trypsin method below; over-incubation will increase non-specific background staining. Trypsinization is not required when the tissues have been fixed and processed by a method that is known not to affect the reactivity of the antigen being demonstrated. Even so, it will be found that, in practice, some antisera require trypsinization routinely whilst others do not. The commercial suppliers' antisera protocols should be consulted in this context, as these usually give some guidance on the necessity for prior enzyme treatment.

The following table is drawn from our experience, for workers using a particular antiserum for the first time.

Table 12.1   Antisera and need for trypsinization

Polyclonal antisera		Monoclonal antisera	
Cytokeratin	trypsin	LCA	no trypsin
CEA	no trypsin	EMA	no trypsin
S100	no trypsin	Vimentin	no trypsin
PSA	no trypsin	Desmin	trypsin
PSAP	no trypsin	MB2	no trypsin
PGP 9.5	no trypsin	UCHLI	no trypsin
Thyroglobulin	no trypsin	L26	no trypsin
α-fetoprotein	trypsin	CAM 5.2	trypsin
Muramidase	trypsin	Factor VIII-related antigen	trypsin
α₁-anti-trypsin	trypsin	BER H2	trypsin
Immunoglobulins	trypsin	β-HCG	no trypsin

Background staining

This is seen in two forms—specific staining, e.g. fibrinogen in blood vessels, or non-specific, involving the affinity of some tissue structures, notably reticulin and collagen, for the antisera used in the staining methods. Normal swine serum is often used as a preliminary step in immunoperoxidase techniques to minimize connective tissue staining. The complex subject of background staining is discussed by Robinson et al (1990).

Dilutions

To obtain optimal staining and to prevent a non-specific precipitation of antibody on to sections, it is necessary to use each antiserum at the correct dilution as incorrect dilutions can produce false negatives. In the PAP technique the concentration of the primary specific antiserum is varied; the bridging molecule and PAP are kept constant and a dilution of 1:20 is used for the bridging molecule and 1:60 for the PAP solution. It is important to establish the optimal dilution for each new batch of antiserum. It is often helpful, initially, to consult the commercial suppliers' protocols.

Storage

Antisera which are not destroyed by freezing are frozen undiluted, or at dilutions of 1:2–1:10, and stored at $-20°C$ in aliquots suitable for subsequent dilution. Antisera that are destroyed by freezing are stored at $4°C$ in a buffer solution containing extra protein, i.e. 0.1 % bovine serum albumin, and 0.1 % sodium azide to prevent bacterial contamination. The added protein competes with the antibody for non-specific attachment sites on the walls of the storage vessel. Alternatively, it is sometimes convenient to store antisera at their working dilution in buffer (phosphate- or Tris-buffered saline, pH 7.0–7.6) containing azide and albumin.

STAINING METHODS

The practice of immunocytochemical staining is not difficult as it is a straightforward incubation and rinse sequence, with no differentiation necessary. It is important that at no stage are any of the solutions allowed to evaporate off the sections.

Washing

It is important that adequate washing occurs between each stage of the technique. If this is not done a formation of antigen-antibody complexes will precipitate onto the sections. Between each stage a Tris-buffered saline solution is used.

PREPARATION OF DAB (Graham & Karnovsky 1966)

Solutions

Add 5 mg DAB (see p. 266) to 10 ml 0.05 M Tris/HCl buffer, pH 7.6 (see Appendix 3) and stir until the solid dissolves. Add 0.1 ml of freshly prepared 1 % hydrogen peroxide.

This medium should be used immediately after preparation, and 5 min incubation at room temperature is generally sufficient. The reaction end-product, which is brown in colour, resists alcohol dehydration and clearing in xylene. Due to the possible carcinogenic nature of the salt it is advisable to work in a fume cupboard, use disposable vessels for weighing and mixing, and to wear disposable rubber gloves during preparation of the medium and subsequent incubation.

TRYPSIN DIGESTION METHOD (Mepham et al 1979)

Notes

The trypsinization medium is freshly prepared as its activity decreases with time. As the time for treatment is different for all specimens, it is necessary to treat a series of slides for varying durations; for most tissues optimum digestion occurs within 15–30 min and, therefore, digestion times of 10, 20 and 30 min are recommended.

Solutions

Add 0.1 g trypsin (pancreatic type II, Sigma) to 100 ml 0.1 % calcium chloride and mix thoroughly with a magnetic stirrer. With continuous stirring, add 0.1 M sodium hydroxide until a pH of 7.8 is reached. Place the working solution in a Coplin jar and equilibrate to 37°C in a water bath before use.

Technique

1. Equilibrate temperature of section to 37°C by placing in distilled water at 37°C for 10 min.
2. Place in the digestion solution for 10–30 min at 37°C.
3. Wash in running cold water for 15 min and proceed with the appropriate immunocytochemical technique.

INDIRECT IMMUNOFLUORESCENT TECHNIQUE FOR AUTO-ANTIBODIES

Notes

Fresh cryostat sections are obtained from a composite block of rat tissues consisting of liver, kidney and stomach and separate cryostat sections of human thyroid. Air-dry the sections for 20 min at room temperature; an electric fan will help the drying.

The sections are not allowed to dry after Step 1 of the method. Control sections must always be prepared similarly to the test sections. Parallel sections should be treated with known positive and negative sera as well as phosphate-buffered saline in Step 3. Positive sera are usually re-examined quantitatively using doubling dilutions of serum, with the final titre being the last dilution to show positive fluorescence. Antisera are pipetted into aliquots and stored at −20°C or below, and for use should be spun down hard to remove protein particles (e.g. 4500 r/min 0.5–1 h) to reduce non-specific background staining. Ring the sections with a felt tip pen:(a) to identify site of section and (b) to conserve the reagents.

Tris-buffered saline, see below, is used in the washes and for the dilution of the serum. The dilution of the test and control serum should be determined for each batch as different suppliers' antisera will show variation in optimal dilution (a dilution of sera 1:5 with buffer is a good starting point).

Solutions

Tris-buffered saline pH 7.6:

Distilled water	1 litre
Sodium chloride	8.1.g
Tris (hydroxy methylamine)	0.6 g
1 M HCl	4.2 ml

If necessary adjust pH to 7.6 with either M HCl or 0.2 M Tris solution

Fluorescein-labelled anti-human globulin

This may be mono- or polyvalent; the latter is normally used for routine serum investigation.

Technique

1. The test and control diluted sera are applied to the air-dried cryostat sections in a covered moistened container for 20 min.
2. Wash well in Tris-buffered saline (two changes) for 15 min (mechanical agitation is recommended).
3. Remove excess Tris-buffered saline.
4. Apply the diluted fluorescein-labelled anti-human globulin to the sections in the container for 20 min.
5. Wash in Tris-buffered saline for 20 min with at least one change.
6. Mount sections in buffered glycerol.
7. Examine in the fluorescence microscope.

Results

Auto-immune antibodies against tissue components will produce a bright yellow fluorescence at site.

The colour of the resulting fluorescence can be varied by the choice of filters used in the microscope.

INDIRECT TECHNIQUE TO DEMONSTRATE TISSUE ANTIGENS

Notes

Both this and the techniques following are *examples* of suitable schemes for demonstrating a wide range of tissue antigens. The various steps of the techniques remain unchanged. It is the primary antiserum that will need to be appropriate to the antigen to be demonstrated (this will appear brown) and if a secondary antiserum is involved it will need to be of the appropriate species (this does not apply to the Indirect Technique).

The following controls are recommended:

a. Treat an un-treated section with DAB to check for endogenous peroxidase activity and the effectiveness of the methanol/hydrogen peroxide treatment.
b. Omit the primary antiserum.
c. Pre-absorb the primary antiserum overnight with excess antigen.
d. Replace the primary antiserum with a rabbit antiserum directed against an unrelated antigen, e.g. rabbit anti-gastrin serum.
e. Block the binding of the conjugated antiserum by incubating for 30 min in unconjugated swine anti-rabbit IgG, diluted 1:20 with Tris/saline, after Step 7 in the following sequence. Then wash in Tris/saline and go to Step 8.
f. If available, include a known positive control.

Solutions

0.3% hydrogen peroxide in absolute methanol
Trypsin solution (see p. 271) if required
3% normal swine serum in Tris saline
Primary rabbit antiserum
Peroxidase-conjugated swine anti-rabbit IgG
DAB medium, see above
Tris/saline buffer pH 7.6 (see p. 272)

Technique

1. Sections to absolute alcohol.
2. Inhibit endogenous peroxidase activity by incubating in the hydrogen peroxide in absolute methanol for 30 min.
3. Hydrate sections through graded alcohols and wash in running water for 15 min.
4. Incubate sections in the normal swine serum diluted in Tris/saline for 15 min.
5. Drain off excess normal swine serum in Tris/saline.
6. Incubate sections in primary antiserum diluted 1:1000, 1:500, 1:250, 1:100 and 1:50 in 1% normal swine serum in Tris/saline for 30 min.
7. Jet wash off excess antiserum and wash slides in Tris/saline for three 2 min changes.
8. Incubate in peroxidase-conjugated swine anti-rabbit IgG diluted 1:20 in Tris/saline for 30 min.
9. Jet wash off excess antiserum and wash slides in Tris/saline for three 2 min changes.
10. Incubate sections in DAB medium for 5 min.
11. Wash in running water for 10 min.
12. Counterstain in an alum haematoxylin, dehydrate, clear and mount.

Results

Reaction product	brown
Nuclei	blue

PEROXIDASE-ANTI-PEROXIDASE (PAP) TECHNIQUE

Notes

The recommended controls are similar to those outlined with the indirect method. The exception is that the staining blocking control, i.e. control (e), is undertaken with rabbit IgG for 30 min at a 1:20 dilution in Tris/saline after Step 9 in the sequence below.

If either technique results in negative test and negative positive control sections, try less dilute primary antiserum. If the reaction continues to be negative, try controlled trypsin digestion (see p. 271); this is undertaken after Step 3 in both schedules. If this fails, it will be necessary to study systematically the effect of various fixative solutions on the preservation of the antigen. If fixed tissues are still negative, it will be necessary to use fresh frozen sections but remember that there is likely to be extensive diffusion of some antigens in unfixed cryostat sections. If the technique does not work on these sections, re-check the avidity of all antisera.

Solutions

0.3% hydrogen peroxide in absolute methanol
Trypsin solution (see p. 271) if required
3% normal swine serum in Tris/saline
Primary antiserum (e.g. rabbit anti-human IgM)
Swine anti-rabbit IgG
PAP complex
DAB medium (see p. 270)
Tris/saline buffer pH 7.6 (TBS) (see p. 272)

Technique

1. Sections to alcohol.
2. Block endogenous peroxidase activity by incubating in hydrogen peroxide solution for 30 min.
3. Hydrate sections by passing through graded ethanol series and wash in running water for 15 min.
4. Incubate sections in the normal swine serum diluted in Tris/saline for 15 min.
5. Drain off excess Tris-buffered normal swine serum.
6. Incubate sections with primary antiserum diluted 1:2000 1:1000, 1:250 and 1:100 in 1% normal swine serum for 30 min.
7. Jet wash off excess antiserum and then wash slides in Tris/saline for three 2 min changes.
8. Incubate sections in swine anti-rabbit IgG diluted 1:20 for 30 min.
9. Jet wash off excess antiserum and then wash slides for three 2 min changes.
10. Incubate sections in PAP complex diluted 1:60 in 1% normal swine serum in Tris/saline for 30 min.
11. Jet wash off excess complex and wash in Tris/saline for three 2 min changes.
12. Incubate sections in DAB medium for 5 min.
13. Wash sections in running water for 10 min.
14. Counterstain in alum haematoxylin, dehydrate, clear and mount.

Results

Reaction product	brown
Nuclei	blue

ALKALINE PHOSPHATASE ANTI-ALKALINE PHOSPHATASE TECHNIQUE (APAAP)

Notes

The reaction end-product may be enhanced by repeating Steps 5–8 once or twice with a reduction of the incubation times to 10 minutes. As the alkaline phosphatase tracer is not human in origin, endogenous alkaline phosphatase activity can be blocked by including levamisole in the substrate solution.

Solutions

Normal swine serum (NSS)
Tris-buffered saline (TBS) (see p. 272)
Primary antibody
Bridging antibody
Alkaline phosphatase substrates
   The methods for the visualization of alkaline phosphatase activity are based on the coupling of substituted naphthol to a suitable diazonium salt. The most commonly used diazonium salts are fast red TR and hexazotized new fuchsin.

Fast red TR:

Naphthol AS-MX phosphate, free acid	2 mg
N, N-dimethyl formamide	0.2 ml
0.1 M Tris buffer pH 8.2	9.8 ml
Levamisole	2.4 mg
Fast red TR salt	10 mg

Dissolve the naphthol AS-MX phosphate in the N, N-dimethyl formamide and then add the Tris buffer. Add and dissolve the levamisole and fast red TR salt and immediately filter on to the sections. Incubate the sections for 10–20 min and, as the bright red reaction product is soluble in alcohol, mount in an aqueous medium. A blue reaction product can be obtained by using 2.1 mg fast blue BB salt instead of fast red TR. Haematoxylin is not a suitable counterstain with this salt.

Hexazotized new fuchsin:

Naphthol AS-BI phosphate	5 mg
N,N-dimethyl formamide	60 ml
0.05 M Tris buffer pH 8.7	10 ml
1 M levamisole	10 ml
4% sodium nitrite (freshly prepared)	50 ml
5% new fuchsin in 2 M HCl	20 ml

It is advisable to make up this substrate in a fume cupboard. Add the new fuchsin to the sodium nitrite, mix for 30–60 s and then add the Tris buffer and levamisole. Immediately before staining, add the naphthol AS-BI phosphate dissolved in the N, N-dimethyl formamide and filter directly on to the sections. Incubate the sections for 10–20 min. The reaction end-product is bright red and the sections may be rapidly dehydrated, cleared and mounted in a permanent medium.

Technique

1. Incubate in normal swine serum diluted 1:5 with TBS for 20 min.
2. Drain off the normal swine serum.
3. Incubate in the primary antibody at the optimal dilution, using 1:20 normal swine serum in TBS as diluent, for 30 – 45 min.
4. Wash off the excess antiserum with TBS and then wash in TBS for three 5 min changes.
5. Incubate in unconjugated bridging antibody at the optimal dilution, using 1:20 NSS in TBS as diluent, for 30 – 45 min.
6. Jet wash off excess antiserum with TBS and then wash in TBS for three 5 min changes.
7. Incubate in alkaline phosphatase anti-alkaline phosphatase complex at the optimal dilution, using 1:20 NSS in TBS as diluent, for 30 – 60 min.
8. Wash off the excess antiserum with TBS and then wash in TBS for three 5 min changes.
9. Incubate in the substrate medium of choice (see Notes).
10. Wash in running tap water.
11. Counterstain and mount as appropriate.

Results

Reaction product with fast red TR and new fuchsin	red
Reaction product with fast blue BB	blue
Nuclei	according to counterstain

AVIDIN-BIOTIN TECHNIQUE

Solutions

0.3% hydrogen peroxide in methanol
Trypsin solution
3% normal swine serum in pH 7.6 Tris/saline buffer
Primary antiserum: either rabbit polyclonal or mouse monoclonal diluted as appropriate in pH 7.6 Tris/saline buffer
Biotinylated secondary antiserum
  Usual dilution is either 1 in 500 or 1 in 200 with antibody diluent I. Swine anti-rabbit is used for polyclonal antisera, and rabbit anti-mouse for the monoclonal.
Phosphate saline buffer pH 7.4
Antibody diluent I
  Dissolve 0.75 g bovine serum albumin in 75 ml Tris/saline buffer pH 7.6; add 50 ml of 10% aqueous sodium azide.
Antibody diluent II

Dissolve 0.75 g bovine serum albumin in 75 ml Tris buffer pH 7.2; add 50 ml of 10% aqueous sodium azide and 7.5 ml of normal swine serum.

Avidin-biotin complex (ABC reagent)

Supplied as a kit: prepare according to instructions at least 30 min before use.

DAB medium (see p. 270)

Mayer's haematoxylin (see p. 25)

Technique

1. Test and control sections to water.
2. Treat with the hydrogen peroxide solution for 20 min.
3. Wash in tap water for 5 min.
4. If trypsinization is necessary (see Table 12.1, p. 261), treat with the pre-heated solution for 12 min (see Notes, p. 261) at 40°C.
5. Wash in tap water for 5 min.
6. Wash in phosphate-buffered saline pH 7.4 for 5 min.
7. If using the rabbit polyclonal primary antiserum, treat with normal swine serum diluted to 1 in 5 with antibody diluent II for 15 min (this blocks non-specific reactivity). Drain slides.
8. Treat all sections with the required primary antiserum for 30 min. Negative control slides will be treated with antibody diluent I only.
9. Wash in pH 7.4 phosphate-buffered saline for two periods of 5 min each.
10. Treat with the appropriate secondary antiserum for 30 min.
11. Rinse sections in phosphate-buffered saline pH 7.4.
12. Treat with the prepared ABC reagent for 30 min.
13. Rinse sections in phosphate-buffered saline pH 7.4.
14. Treat sections with DAB medium for 10 min.
15. Wash well in tap water and stain nuclei with Mayer's haematoxylin for 10–30 s then blue (do not differentiate in acid-alcohol).
16. Dehydrate, clear and mount as desired.

Results

Reaction product	brown
Nuclei	blue

IMMUNOGOLD TECHNIQUES

DIRECT TECHNIQUE

Note

Step 7 is not necessary if pre-treatment with iodine and thiosulphate has been performed.

Solutions

Lugol's iodine (see p. 59)

2.5% aqueous sodium thiosulphate

Normal goat serum (NGS)

Diluted 1:20 in 0.1% bovine serum in Tris-buffered saline pH 8.2.

Gold-conjugated primary antibody (BSA in TBS)
 At optimal dilution in 0.1% bovine serum in Tris-buffered saline pH 8.2.
Tris-buffered saline pH 8.2 (TBS)
0.1 M phosphate-buffered saline (PBS)
2% glutaraldehyde in 0.1 M phosphate-buffered saline

Technique

1. Sections to water. If required, treat sections with Lugol's iodine for 5 min, clear with the sodium thiosulphate solution and then wash well in running tap water.
2. Incubate in 1:20 normal goat serum in 0.1% bovine serum albumin in Tris-buffered saline pH 8.2, for 10 min.
3. Drain off excess bovine serum in Tris-buffered saline.
4. Incubate in gold-conjugated primary antibody at optimal dilution in 0.1% bovine serum albumin in 0.1 M phosphate-buffered saline for 60 min.
5. Wash off the excess antiserum with BSA in TBS and then wash in BSA in TBS for three 5 min changes.
6. Wash in 0.1 M phosphate-buffered saline for three 2 min changes.
7. Post-fix with 2% glutaraldehyde in PBS for 10–15 min.
8. Wash well in distilled water and, if required, enhance with silver (see silver enhancement below).
9. Counterstain, dehydrate, clear and mount as desired.

Results

Reaction product	purple
Nuclei	according to counterstain

INDIRECT TECHNIQUE

Note

Step 7 is not necessary if pre-treatment with iodine and thiosulphate has been performed.

Solutions

Lugol's iodine (see p. 59)
2.5% aqueous sodium thiosulphate
Bovine serum albumin (BSA)
Normal goat serum (NGS)
 Diluted 1:20 in 0.1% bovine serum in Tris-buffered saline pH 8.2.
Gold-conjugated primary antibody (BSA in TBS)
 At optimal dilution in 0.1% bovine serum in Tris-buffered saline pH 8.2.
0.1 M phosphate-buffered saline (PBS) pH 7.6
Tris-buffered saline pH 8.2 (TBS)
2% glutaraldehyde in 0.1 M phosphate-buffered saline
Primary antibody
 At optimal dilution in 0.1% bovine serum albumin in Tris-buffered saline pH 8.2 (BSA in TBS).

Technique

1. Sections to water. If required, treat sections with Lugol's iodine for 5 min, clear with the sodium thiosulphate solution and then wash well in running tap water.
2. Incubate 1:20 normal goat serum (NGS) in 0.1% bovine serum albumin in TBS, pH 8.2, for 10 min.
3. Drain off excess bovine serum in Tris-buffered saline.
4. Incubate in primary antibody at optimal dilution in BSA in TBS for 60 min.
5. Wash off the excess antiserum with BSA in TBS and then wash in BSA in TBS for three 5 min changes.
6. Incubate in gold-conjugated secondary antibody at optimum dilution in BSA in TBS for 60 min.
7. Wash off the excess antiserum with BSA in TBS and then wash in BSA in TBS for three 2 min changes.
8. Wash in 0.1 M phosphate-buffered saline (PBS), pH 7.6, for three 2 min changes.
9. Post-fix with 2% glutaraldehyde in PBS for 10–15 min.
10. Wash well in distilled water and, if required, enhance with silver (see silver enhancement below).
11. Counterstain, dehydrate, clear and mount.

Results

Reaction product	purple
Nuclei	according to counterstain

SILVER ENHANCEMENT TECHNIQUE

Note

The intensity of the gold label in immunogold techniques can be enhanced by using the following silver method.

Solutions

2 M citrate buffer:

Trisodium citrate	2.35 g
Citric acid	2.55 g
Distilled water	10 ml

Silver solution:

Silver lactate	0.11 g
Distilled water	15 ml

Hydroquinone solution:

Hydroquinone	0.95 g
Distilled water	15 ml

Gum acacia:

50% solution of gum acacia	7 ml

Working silver enhancement solution:

Silver lactate solution	15 ml
Hydroquinone solution	15 ml
2 M citrate buffer	10 ml
Distilled water	60 ml
50% aqueous solution of gum acacia	7 ml

Technique

1. Rinse the sections in 2 M citrate buffer for 2 min.
2. Incubate the sections in freshly prepared silver enhancement solution at room temperature and protected from the light for approximately 3 min.
3. Fix in a 1:10 dilution of fixing solution (Janssens Pharmaceuticals Ltd.) for 2 min.
4. Wash well in running tap water.

Results

Reaction product	black
Nuclei	according to counterstain

EPOS TECHNIQUE

A recent development by the Dako Company is the EPOS (Enhanced Polymer One Step) immunocytochemical system. It is a streamlined method which holds great promise for the future in terms of simplicity and speed of reaction.

In essence, it consists of a direct, single application staining technique which is sold in a kit form and contains the EPOS reagent, which is a peroxidase-linked primary antibody plus optimized blocking agents. These latter obviate the need for subsequent second and third antibody layers. Normal DAB visualization of bound antibody follows in the usual way. The EPOS application is preceded by the standard hydrogen peroxide blockage of endogenous peroxidase, also trypsinization, if this is needed.

The range of available EPOS antibodies will undoubtedly grow with time, and initial results in our hands are encouraging.

Table 12.2   Uses of immunocytochemistry

Demonstration of immunoglobulins of lymphoreticular origin	Multiple myeloma, Hodgkin's disease, lymphomas, etc.
Skin diseases (bullous disorders), e.g. pemphigus vulgaris and bullous pemphigoid	IgG on prickle cell junctions, IgG on basement membranes
Identification of hormone-containing cells and tumours	Gastrin, calcitonin, testosterone, etc.
Tumour and cell markers	α_1-antitrypsin, α-fetoprotein, carcino-embryonic antigen, Factor VIII-related antigen
Identification of organisms	Hepatitis B[2] antigen, *Herpes simplex*, *L. pneumophila*[1]

[1] Currently the most satisfactory means of demonstrating *L. pneumophila* seems to be the use of direct immunofluorescence on imprint smears or paraffin sections, employing a rabbit anti-*L. pneumophila* group 1. IgG conjugated with FITC.
[2] Immunoperoxidase technique for hepatitis B surface antigen. (We have had good results with the Dako PAP Kit.)

Table 12.3   Autoimmune disease

Examples of disease	Predominant antigen
Hashimoto's	Thyroglobulin
Chronic active hepatitis	Smooth muscle
Rheumatoid arthritis	IgG and nuclear antigens
Goodpasture's syndrome	Basement membranes
Primary biliary cirrhosis	Thyroid and kidney mitochondria
Systemic lupus erythematosus	DNA: nuclear proteins
Pernicious anaemia	Gastric parietal cells, intrinsic factor

DIAGNOSTIC IMMUNOCYTOCHEMISTRY (*Dr. R. W. Stirling*)

No single development has had such a revolutionary effect on histopathology as immunocytochemistry. The initial work with polyclonal antibodies fuelled, and has been largely superseded by, the work of Sternberger (1969). The explosion of monoclonal antibodies that has followed, combined with enhancement techniques like the avidin-biotin complex method (Hsu et al 1981), has led to a confusing embarrassment of riches being made available to histopathologists. Acquiring sufficient knowledge about the specificity of the antibodies and their potential for diagnostic applications keeps all diagnostic histopathologists occupied. The other side of the equation is the high cost of many of the antibodies, which precludes all laboratories stocking a vast array of the antisera. Antibody sharing schemes operate in some areas, allowing a wider spectrum of antisera to be stocked by more laboratories. Specialized centres also justify a more comprehensive and full antibody panel, e.g. for lymphoma and soft tissue tumour work.

USES

1. Research applications.
2. Lymphoma.
3. Poorly differentiated tumours.
4. Soft tissue tumours.
5. Mesothelial proliferation versus disseminated carcinoma.
6. Germ cell tumours.

Certain fundamental principles apply to diagnostic uses of immunocytochemistry:

- The results must be interpreted in conjunction with the morphology and differential diagnosis generated from routine and special stains.
- Positive results are in general terms more helpful than negative results.
- Adequate relative control sections should be performed with every diagnostic run as there are many steps where errors can occur and cause erroneous results.
- Expected results in test sections should be checked, e.g. that nerves are S100-positive and epithelial elements are positive with epithelial markers.
- Edge effects are seen around the edges of sections where there is often an apparent area of positivity produced by artefactual trapping of the label. This is particularly important in small biopsies where a larger proportion of the material is at the edge of the section.

Research applications

There are many antibodies available which mark basement membrane and subcellular structures; immunogold silver staining (Faulk & Taylor 1971) may be required to demonstrate these reactions. Their applications in research are legion.

Lymphomas

There is a vast confusing array of antibodies for immunotyping non-Hodgkin's malignant lymphomas. The spectrum was well-reviewed by Chan et al (1988). The introduction of cluster of differentiation (CD) numbers has facilitated easier comparison of antibodies offered by the various companies.

The commonly used antibodies (Table 12.4) are applicable for use on paraffin sections. Immunotyping of lymphomas is currently more advanced than required for treatment modalities, with most haematologists being content with a diagnosis of high or low grade lymphoma plus the cell lineage (B or T). A full comprehensive panel of antibodies is only justifiable, both on cost and usefulness, at specialist centres. Referral of problem cases to these centres maintains their expertise, justifies their resources with a steady throughput of cases, and produces an expanding pool of research material.

Table 12.4   Antibodies in common usage at non-specialized centres

Antibody	Type	Specificity
LCA (CD45)	monoclonal	Pan lymphocyte marker
L26	monoclonal	Pan B cell marker
UCHL1	monoclonal	Pan T cells with granulocytes and macrophages
CD3	polyclonal	T lymphocytes
BerH2 (CD30)	monoclonal	Reed–Sternberg cells, Ki1 lymphoma, myeloid and erythroid precursors

At a District General Hospital, the important questions to be answered are:

- Is it a lymphoma?
- Is classification adequate to allow treatment and future comparison of response between similar groups of lymphomas?

Routine light microscopy combined with reticulin stains remains the initial mainstay for diagnosis. Loss of the normal architectural arrangement of the cortical germinal centres (B cell areas) and the paracortex (T cell areas) is a feature of lymphomas but is also present in some reactive conditions, e.g. glandular fever. It is in separating the reactive conditions that immunocytochemistry plays its most important role.

Demonstration of monoclonality in B cell lymphomas, by restriction of light chain production, is dramatic evidence. This has been one of the more fickle and subtle reactions for departments to perfect, however the EPOS technique (Dako Ltd.) has given enhanced results. Separation into high and low grade lymphomas is largely made on the morphology of the proliferating cell types, although proliferation markers are available, but not in routine use outside the specialized centres.

In conjunction with the morphology UCHLI (CD45RO), CD3 and L26, used as a panel of antibodies, will usually allow correct assignment of the cell lineage of most lymphomas.

Poorly differentiated tumours

Differentiation of such tumours forms a most valuable use of immunocytochemistry. Recognition of anaplastic carcinomas from lymphomas can have life-saving consequences in critically ill patients with disseminated tumours, as lymphomas respond rapidly to chemotherapy whereas carcinomas usually have a limited response. Biopsies in these circumstances are often small and distorted, making morphological assessment problematic. Application of a panel of antibodies will help to clarify the origin of the tumour and then permit further appropriate investigations. An initial panel of antibodies suitable for paraffin-fixed tissue is suggested in Table 12.5. Intermediate filaments are a part of the major cytoskeletal system of cells. There are five subgroups: vimentin, desmin, cytokeratin, neurofilament protein and glial fibrillary protein. The production of these intermediate filaments gives an indication of the line of differentiation of the cell:

Table 12.5   Initial panel for anaplastic tumours

Antibody	Tumour type
Leukocyte common antigen (CD45)	Lymphoid cells
CAM 5.2 (cytokeratin)	Epithelial cells
EMA (epithelial membrane antigen)	Epithelial cells
S100 protein	Neural / melanocytic cells
Vimentin	Mesenchymal / melanocytic cells

- Vimentin is the intermediate filament associated with mesenchymal cells, being found in virtually all sarcomas but also some epithelial and mesothelial tumours.
- Desmin is found in cardiac, skeletal and smooth muscle.
- Cytokeratin is a group of 19 separate polypeptides with variable molecular weight. They are found in epithelia, mesothelioma and some soft tissue tumours. The most common antibody used is CAM 5.2, which detects the mid-range of cytokeratins.
- Neurofilament protein is found in most but not all neuronal cells. It has been identified in neuroblastoma, ganglioneuroma and paragangliomas.
- Glial fibrillary acidic protein is the intermediate filament found in glial cells and is mainly confined to the central nervous system.

These antibodies will usually allocate tumours into broad groups, namely epithelial, mesenchymal and lymphoid. A few tumours will give weak reactions in one group plus reaction in another, e.g. malignant melanoma (vimentin-positive, S100-positive, CAM 5.2 weak positive). Anaplastic lymphoma and plasma cell tumours (previously mentioned) are negative with LCA but weakly positive with epithelial membrane antigen, suggesting an epithelial tumour. The degree of positivity is not as strong as usually expected, they are also CAM 5.2-negative. After interpretation of the first panel of antibodies the results should be evaluated in conjunction with the morphology and the differential diagnosis constructed from the original H & E sections.

Table 12.6 suggests antibodies to evaluate further the subgroups produced from the first panel. Included in this panel are two relatively organ-specific antibodies, prostatic acid phosphatase (PSAP) and thyroglobulin. PSAP is sensitive and will stain even poorly differentiated carcinomas. Prostate-Specific Antigen (PSA) shares similar specificity. Thyroglobulin is also specific but tends to be lost in poorly differentiated tumours. Discussion of the antibodies for soft tissue tumours will follow in the next section.

Table 12.6 Further panel of antibodies

Initial group	Further antibodies
Lymphoid	CD3, UCHL1, L26, Ber H2
Epithelial	PSAP, thyroglobulin, CEA, PGP 9.5
Mesenchyme	Myoglobin, desmin, Factor VIII-related antigen, α_1-antitrypsin

Carcino-embryonic antigen (CEA), a glycoprotein, is widely distributed in inflamed and dysplastic endoderm. Positive reactions are relatively unhelpful in specifying a site of a tumour, however, if negative, a carcinoma is unlikely to be of large bowel origin. Protein gene product (PGP 9.5) is a cytoplasmic neurone-specific protein and is a reliable marker of neuroendocrine activity as seen in gastrointestinal carcinoid tumours, small cell carcinomas of lung or neuroendocrine differentiation in tumours of other sites. Epithelial membrane antigen (EMA) is a glycoprotein present in the human milk fat globule membrane. It is a good marker of epithelia, especially adenocarcinomas, but as previously mentioned is present in some lymphomas.

S100 protein is an acidic protein of unknown function found in the central and peripheral nervous system. Its main use is in the soft tissue tumours, but it is also expressed in melanomas and Langerhans cells.

Soft tissue tumours

These tumours are uncommon in routine practice at District General Hospitals and like lymphomas are applicable for referral to specialist centres where a more comprehensive panel of specialist antibodies can be utilized. These are beyond the scope of this chapter. However a restricted panel of antibodies combined with standard special stains and careful evaluation of multiple H & E sections will allow characterization of most tumours encountered.

Vimentin is the generic intermediate filament of mesenchymal cells and does not help in further characterization. Desmin—the intermediate filament of smooth and skeletal muscle—is not usually positive in leiomyosarcomas but is found in a substantial proportion of rhabdomyosarcomas even when rhabdomyoblasts can not be identified (Altmannsberger et al 1985). Cytokeratins (CAM 5.2) are present in the epithelial areas and in the spindle cell areas of synovial sarcoma. The latter feature is useful in the identification of monophasic synovial sarcoma. Epithelioid sarcoma and chordoma also display cytokeratin positivity. Epithelial membrane antigen (EMA) is found in the glandular and spindle areas of synovial sarcoma (vimentin positivity is lost in the glandular areas). Epithelioid sarcoma is also EMA-positive.

Factor VIII-related antigen, a glycoprotein synthesized by endothelial cells, is demonstrable in vascular tumours and lymphangiomas. Kaposi's sarcoma gives a variable reaction, as do more poorly differentiated angiosarcomas.

S100 protein is a useful neural marker but it is more consistently positive in benign neural tumours than poorly differentiated malignant nerve sheath tumours (Wick et al 1987). Positive reactions are seen with chordomas which, combined with cytokeratin positivity, produce a phenotype distinctive from chondrosarcoma.

Mesothelial proliferations versus disseminated adenocarcinoma

The wide spectrum of appearances produced by benign and malignant mesothelial proliferations, combined with the small size of pleural biopsies, makes this an ideal situation for immunocytochemistry. It is however unfortunate that proliferating mesothelial cells and adenocarcinomas can often share a similar immunophenotype. CAM 5.2, EMA and CEA in combination have been suggested as a possible means of separating these entities but are not without significant overlap. A relatively new antibody AuA1, well described by Soosay et al (1991), is found in most adenocarcinomas but not in benign or malignant mesothelial proliferations.

Germ cell tumours

The morphology of most germ cell tumours is diagnostic and with modern chemotherapeutic regimes the prognosis of all subgroups of teratomas is now good. Due to the diverse lines of cell differentiation seen with teratomas many antigens may be expressed. Some of these can be utilized to aid diagnosis of the more problematic cases. Placental alkaline phosphatase (PLAP), unlike other alkaline phosphatases, is heat-stable. It is membrane-bound and expressed in the placenta, embryonic germ cells, germ cell tumours and some non-germ cell tumours. Strong membrane staining is seen in classic seminomas and a high percentage of non-seminomatous germ cell tumours (Mostofi et al 1987). PLAP is not seen in spermatocytic seminomas. Carcinoma-in-situ of the testis can be highlighted by demonstration of PLAP positivity of the intratubular cells. α-Fetoprotein (AFP), a glycoprotein produced by fetal liver and yolk sac, is a useful serum marker for patients with non-seminomatous germ cell tumours as up to 75% can show elevated levels. Immunocytochemistry can be used to demonstrate areas of production; most often these are where yolk sac differentiation can be seen. Human chorionic gonadotrophin (HCG) similarly is a glycoprotein which can be measured in serum. The β subunit is specific, and elevated serum levels (except in pregnancy) correlate well with trophoblastic tumours or trophoblastic elements within germ cell tumours. Immunocytochemistry with β-HCG antibodies will highlight areas of choriocarcinoma and also scattered syncytiotrophoblast cells within seminomas (Heyderman 1986).

Immunocytochemistry as described in the previous sections has an important role to play in aiding diagnosis in problem areas. It has a complementary role alongside conventional special stains which are by no means circumvented and are still most useful. The diagnostic return from any investigation must, however, be considered in conjunction with the expense of the technique when all hospital budgets are stretched and all histopathology laboratories are competing for work in the NHS marketplace. Cost must unfortunately be considered and immunocytochemistry is expensive in both technical time and reagents.

REFERENCES

Altmannsberger M, Weber K, Droste R, Osborn M 1985 Desmin as a specific marker for rhabdomyosarcomas of human and rat origin. American Journal of Pathology 118: 85–95

Chan J K C, Ng C S, Hui P K 1988 A simple guide to the terminology and application of leucocyte monoclonal antibodies. Histopathology 12: 461–480

Cordell J L, Falini B, Erber W Wn et al 1984 Immunoenzymatic labelling of monoclonal antibodies using immune complexes of alkaline phosphatase and monoclonal anti-alkaline phosphatase (APAAP complexes). Journal of Histochemistry and Cytochemistry 32: 219–229

De Mey J, Moeremans M 1986 Raising and testing polyclonal antibodies for immunocytochemistry. In: Polack J M, Van Noorden S (eds) Immunocytochemistry, modern methods and applications. Wright, Bristol, pp 71–89

Faulk W, Taylor G 1971 An immunocolloid method for the electron microscope. Immunochemistry 8: 1081–1083

Graham R C, Karnovsky M J 1966 The early stages of absorption of injected horseradish peroxidase in the proximal tubules of mouse kidney. Ultrastructural cytochemistry by a new technique. Journal of Histochemistry and Cytochemistry 14: 291

Guesdon J L, Terynck T, Avrameas S 1979 The use of avidin-biotin interaction in immunoenzymatic techniques. Journal of Histochemistry and Cytochemistry 27: 1131–1139

Heyderman E 1986 Tumour markers. In: Polak J M, Van Noorden S (eds) Immunocytochemistry, modern methods and applications, 2nd edn. Wright, Bristol, pp 502–532

Heyderman E, Monaghan P 1979 Immunoperoxidase reactions in resin embedded sections. Investigative Cell Pathology 2: 312–332

Holgate C, Jackson P, Cowen P, Bird C 1983a Immunogold-silver staining: a new method of immunostaining with enhanced sensitivity. Journal of Histochemistry and Cytochemistry 31: 938–944

Holgate C, Jackson P, Lauder I, Cowen P, Bird C 1983b Surface membrane staining of immunoglobulins in paraffin sections of non-Hodgkin's lymphomas using immunogold-silver staining techniques. Journal of Clinical Pathology 36: 742–746

Holgate C S, Jackson P, Pollard K, Lunny D, Bird C C 1986 Effect of fixation on T and B lymphocyte surface membrane demonstration in paraffin processed tissue. Journal of Pathology 149: 293–300

Hsu S M, Raine L, Fanger H 1981 Use of avidin-biotin-peroxidase complex (ABC) in immunoperoxidase techniques: a comparison between ABC and unlabelled antibody (PAP) procedures. Journal of Histochemistry and Cytochemistry 29: 577–580

Mason T E, Pfifer R F, Spicer S S, Swallow R A, Dreskin R B 1969 An immunoglobulin enzyme bridge method for localising tissue antigens. Journal of Histochemistry and Cytochemistry 17: 563

Mepham B L, Frater W, Mitchell B S 1979 The use of proteolytic enzymes to improve immunoglobulin staining by the P.A.P. technique. Histochemical Journal 11: 345

Mostofi F K, Sesterhenn I A, Davis C J 1987 Immunopathology of germ cell tumours of the testis. Seminars in Diagnostic Pathology 4: 320

Pollard K, Lunny D, Holgate C S, Jackson P, Bird C C 1987 Fixation, processing and immunohistochemical reagent effects on preservation of T-lymphocyte surface membrane antigens in paraffin-embedded tissue. Journal of Histochemistry and Cytochemistry 35: 1329–1338

Robinson G, Ellis I O, MacLennan K A 1990 Immunocytochemistry. In: Bancroft J D, Steven A (eds) Theory and practice of histological techniques, 2nd edn. Churchill Livingstone, Edinburgh

Soosay G N, Griffiths M, Papadaki L, Happerfield L, Bobrow L 1991 The differential diagnosis of epithelial-type mesothelioma from adenocarcinoma and reactive mesothelial proliferation. Journal of Pathology 163: 299–305

Sternberger L A 1969 Some new developments in immunocytochemistry. Mikroskopie 25: 346–361

Sternberger L A, Hardy P H, Cuculis J J, Meyer H G 1970 The unlabelled antibody enzyme method of immunohistochemistry: preparation and properties of a soluble antigen-antibody complex (horseradish peroxidase-antiperoxidase) and its use in identification of spirochaetes. Journal of Histochemistry and Cytochemistry 18: 315

Sternberger L A, Sternberger N H 1986 The unlabelled antibody method: comparison of peroxidase-antiperoxidase with avidin-biotin complex by a new method of quantification. Journal of Histochemistry and Cytochemistry 34: 599–605

Suffin S C, Muck K B, Yong J C, Lewin K, Porter D D 1979 Improvement of the glucose oxidase immunoenzyme technic. American Journal of Clinical Pathology 71: 492–496

van Goor H, Harms G, Gerrits P O, Kroese F G M, Poppema S, Grond J 1988 Immunohistochemical antigen demonstration in plastic-embedded lymphoid tissue. Journal of Histochemistry and Cytochemistry 36: 115–120

van Noorden S 1990 Principles of immunostaining. In: Filipe M I, Lake B D (eds) Histochemistry in pathology, 2nd edn. Churchill Livingstone, Edinburgh, pp 31–47

Weir D M 1973 Immunology for undergraduates, 3rd edn. Churchill Livingstone, Edinburgh

Wick M R, Swanson P E, Scheithauer B W, Manivel J C 1987 Malignant peripheral nerve sheath tumour: An immunohistochemical study of 62 cases. American Journal of Clinical Pathology 87: 425–433

13. Enzyme histochemistry

INTRODUCTION

For enzyme histochemistry to be applied to tissue sections suitable preparation of the tissue is necessary. The way the tissue is handled and the subsequent sections produced, depends upon the information required from the preparation. Surgical specimens require specialized fixation, handling and processing. Muscle biopsies require enzyme methods to produce a definite diagnosis, most of the methods being applied to unfixed sections.

It is important to be aware of the different techniques available. As a rule there is little point in applying enzyme methods to paraffin-embedded tissue but there are a few exceptions to this statement (see below). The range of methods of preservation of the tissue and enzyme at our disposal is considerable—the first decision to be made being, is the tissue to be fixed or frozen? Tissues frozen to $-70°C$ or below are well-preserved and there is little loss of enzyme activity; the tissue can be stored for some time. Alternatively a fixative is used, with the choice governed by the subsequent method. Freezing for preservation is employed where fixation or subsequent processing will affect the results of the demonstrating method, as with the ATPase methods in muscle biopsy specimens. Most specimens are fixed on arrival in the laboratory: formaldehyde-based fixatives are suitable for most techniques. The drawbacks of routine processing on tissue constituents are shown in Table 13.1, modified from Bancroft (1975).

Table 13.1   Effects of tissue processing

Fixation at 20°C	Loss of enzyme activity, some carbohydrates. Denaturation of proteins (depending upon fixative and length of fixation). Diffusion of enzymes, carbohydrates.
Dehydration in alcohol	Loss of enzyme activity (room temp). Shrinkage, hardening. General diffusion of enzymes. Loss of lipids.
Clearing in xylene, chloroform, toluene, etc.	Loss of enzyme activity, lipids. Shrinkage, hardening of tissue blocks.
Wax embedding 56–60°C	Loss of enzyme activity, loss of lipids. Shrinkage and hardening.

FROZEN SECTIONS

The rapid development of the cryostat over the last 30 years or so has been due to the expansion of histochemistry and the need to increase the quality of sections produced as 'urgent frozen sections'. The principle involved is simple in comparison with paraffin wax embedding. The water in the tissue is frozen and as ice

289

produces a firm block of tissue, the ice acts as the embedding medium. The consistency of frozen blocks is affected by two factors: firstly as in paraffin sections by the nature of the tissue, and secondly by the amount of water in the tissue. Tissues that have a low water content section better at colder temperatures; those with a higher content, being harder due to more ice crystals, section better at higher temperatures. It is possible to improve sectioning of frozen blocks in the cryostat by adjusting the temperature of the block tissue (see Table 13.2). Fixed tissue, of any nature, is sectioned at –5 to –10°C.

FREEZING UNFIXED TISSUE

The more rapidly the tissue is frozen the better its appearance under the microscope. In the freezing of muscle biopsies it is imperative that a solution such as isopentane, super-cooled by liquid nitrogen is used, to avoid an ice crystal artefact being produced. Other tissues can be frozen by carbon dioxide gas.

Table 13.2 Cutting temperatures of unfixed frozen tissue in the cryostat

Tissue	Optimal sectioning temperatures
Brain	–12°C
Lymph node, liver, kidney, spleen	–15 to –18°C
Muscle, thyroid	–20 to –22°C
Breast, skin	–25 to –28°C
Breast with fat, adipose tissue	–30°C or below

FREEZING FIXED TISSUE

Due to the water in the tissue it is advisable to freeze the tissue slowly to avoid tissue disruption. In most instances it will be wise to place the tissue in the cryostat and allow it to freeze.

FIXATION BEFORE FREEZING

For the demonstration of hydrolytic enzymes it is advisable to use controlled fixation before freezing and sectioning; without this, diffusion of the reaction product occurs.

FIXATION OF TISSUE FOR ENZYME DEMONSTRATION

Solutions

4% formal calcium:

Conc. formalin	4 ml
Distilled water	96 ml
Calcium chloride	1 g

Further calcium chloride is added if necessary until the pH reaches 7.0.

Gum sucrose:

Gum acacia	2 g
Sucrose	60 g
Distilled water	200 ml

Allow to dissolve and store at 4°C.

Formaldehyde-gelatin mixture:

1% aqueous gelatin	25 ml
2% formalin	25 ml

Technique

1. Cut a small block of fresh tissue.
2. Place in formal calcium solution overnight.
3. Blot dry, wash in tap water for 2 min, blot dry.
4. Place in gum sucrose solution at 4°C for 24 h.
5. Blot dry.
6. Attach blocks to cryostat holder and freeze by standing in the cryostat.
7. Section at 8–10 mm at –10°C.
8. Pick up sections on slides or coverslips pre-coated with formaldehyde-gelatin mixture; allow to dry before incubating.

PRINCIPLES OF ENZYME HISTOCHEMISTRY

Enzyme histochemistry has developed into a significant part of histopathology, with roots in both histology and biochemistry. The expansion of the subject at one time was most marked in the demonstration of enzymes, see Table 13.3. Enzymes are protein catalysts for the chemical reactions that occur in biological systems and are necessary for the normal metabolic processes within tissues. Enzymes have long been assayed biochemically; in the first edition of Pearse (1953) methods existed for 18 enzymes, this number has now increased to well over 100. Many early methods demonstrated hydrolytic enzymes; the largest expansion in recent years has been in the demonstration of the oxidative enzymes.

Table 13.3   Commonly demonstrated enzymes

Oxidoreductases	Hydrolases
Oxidative (transfer of electrons)	**Hydrolytic** (addition or removal of water)
Examples:	*Examples:*
Dehydrogenases: succinate, malate, isocitrate.	Specific phosphatases: ATPase, glucose-6-phosphatase. Alkaline and acid phosphatases, esterases.

APPLICATIONS

Enzyme methods are not often applied to routine surgical material due to the partial or total loss of activity after paraffin processing. A few enzymes are identifiable, such as chloroacetate esterase which is used to demonstrate mast cells and certain white blood cells. Cryostat sections of frozen material are required for most enzyme methods and retrospective investigations are not usually feasible. If good communications exist between clinician and pathologist then most enzyme techniques can be applied to freshly received tissue. The current uses of enzyme histochemistry in surgical laboratories are:

1. Muscle biopsies using mainly oxidative enzymes to demonstrate muscle fibre sizes
2. Demonstration of white blood cells of the myeloid series, using chloroacetate esterase
3. Detection of ganglia in Hirschsprung's disease using non-specific esterase
4. Jejunal biopsy in cases of gluten enteropathy
5. As immunocytochemical markers.

PRESERVATION

Due to the labile nature of enzymes their preservation is a problem. Enzymes react in various ways to outside influences; mitochondria, which contain many oxidative enzymes, are damaged rapidly when denied a blood supply. The membranes become damaged and a loss of enzyme activity occurs, so as little time as possible is wasted in preparing tissue for this type of histochemical technique. Lysosomes, containing many hydrolytic enzymes, are damaged by freezing and thawing of tissue, and enzymes diffuse from the damaged organelles. This is the main cause of the gross diffusion artefact seen in post-fixed sections of acid phosphatase demonstration. Careful fixation of tissue at 4°C and treatment in gum sucrose before incubation help to retard diffusion. The fixative localizes the enzyme and protects it from the effects of freezing and thawing.

Most mitochondrial enzymes are destroyed by normal histological fixation, but are much less sensitive to the effects of freezing and thawing, as this appears not to rupture the mitochondrial membrane. A loss of enzyme activity occurs when tissue is left at room temperature, so rapid handling of tissue is important. The damage caused to some of the mitochondrial enzymes can be avoided by the use of hypertonic protection media such as polyvinyl pyrrolidone (PVP), first described by Novikoff (1956) and now used with sucrose. Different enzymes react in varying degrees to the damaging agents discussed as some of them are more resistant; alkaline phosphatase is better able to withstand the effects of fixation than acid phosphatase. Often a choice has to be made for hydrolytic enzymes when fixation, leading to some enzyme loss but better localization, is to be preferred to post-fixation or no fixation, with little or no loss of enzyme activity but considerable enzyme diffusion. In general, rapid cross-linkage aldehydic fixatives such as glutaraldehyde should be avoided. Dehydrogenases are demonstrated on unfixed sections.

FACTORS AFFECTING ENZYME ACTIVITY

Temperature

The optimal temperature for most enzyme reactions is 37°C. At higher temperatures enzymes are rapidly denatured. Lower temperatures, between 4 and 30°C, can be usefully employed in histochemistry for the rate of the enzymic reaction is slowed and, for active enzymes, a better localization obtained.

pH

Enzymes have a pH at which the rate of the reaction is optimal. For most enzymes this is in the range 7.0–7.2. Alkaline phosphatases at 9.2 and acid phosphatases at 5.0 are exceptions.

Inhibitors

Enzyme activity in sections can be destroyed by using chemical substances known as inhibitors. There are three main types of inhibitor:

1. Specific inhibitors, e.g. eserine for cholinesterases.
2. Non-specific inhibitors, e.g. heat for all enzymes.
3. Competitive inhibitors, e.g. chemicals competing with the substrate for active enzyme sites.

Specific inhibitors affect reactive sites of enzyme molecules. Non-specific inhibitors destroy the enzyme reaction by denaturing the protein enzyme.

Activators

These are chemicals that are used to promote enzyme activity. An example is magnesium ions, used in the Gomori metal precipitation technique for alkaline phosphatase.

TECHNIQUES FOR DEMONSTRATION

The basic principle in most enzyme histochemical techniques is that the enzyme in the tissue is presented with its own specific substrate in the incubating medium and a reaction takes place. Unfortunately, the immediate product of this reaction, the primary reaction product (PRP), is frequently invisible. It is then coupled with another substance so that an insoluble and visible final reaction product (FRP) is produced at the site of the enzyme activity. The coupling substance can vary; for example, diazonium salts in the demonstration of the phosphatases ('azo dye methods'), tetrazolium salts in the demonstration of dehydrogenases, and inorganic chemicals such as ammonium sulphide in the metal precipitation techniques.

Three basic techniques are available for the demonstration of enzymes:

1. Metal precipitation techniques.
2. Simultaneous coupling using diazonium salts.
3. Post-incubation coupling using diazonium salts.

Metal precipitation

This technique is commonly applied to the demonstration of phosphatases (see later). The phosphate ions released as a result of the enzyme reaction with the substrate combine with a suitable metallic cation to produce an insoluble precipitate of metal phosphate. Phosphates produced are usually invisible but are rendered visible by converting them to black sulphides by treatment with ammonium sulphide. Metallic cations frequently used for combining with the released phosphate are calcium and lead. This technique is a type of simultaneous coupling, but using metallic ions instead of diazonium salts.

Simultaneous coupling using diazonium salts

This occurs when an incubation mixture containing a substrate and a diazonium salt is applied to suitable sections in a buffered solution. The enzyme present in the section hydrolyzes the substrate and this immediately couples with a diazonium salt to produce the final reaction product, which is seen as a visible, coloured deposit under the microscope. This type of method (see Fig. 13.1) is exemplified by azo dye methods for phosphatases.

The PRP is colourless and the FRP is coloured. The substrate is soluble in water or in the buffer medium to an extent that there is sufficient substrate available in solution for the enzyme to hydrolyze. The histochemical method is performed at a pH at which the enzyme shows maximal activity and at which the substrate has adequate solubility. The diazonium salt also has an optimal pH for its most efficient rate of coupling, and this is considered when the pH at which the method is to be performed is chosen. The PRP must be fairly insoluble; if it is too soluble it will not all couple with the diazonium salt. The quantity of the substrate and diazonium salt in the incubating medium is also important. Too much of either will cause inhibition of the rate of hydrolysis of the substrate on one hand, and inhibition of the formation of the FRP on the other.

Post-incubation coupling using diazonium salts

In this type of procedure the enzyme hydrolyzes the substrate and produces an insoluble PRP. The subsequent coupling is carried out in a separate solution. This type of method relies upon the PRP remaining at the initial site of the hydrolysis and it is important that diffusion of the PRP does not occur during the coupling process. Post-incubation coupling has theoretical advantages. The optimal pH for the initial substrate enzyme reaction can be attained in the first incubation, say pH 7.0, and a possibly different optimal pH for the coupling can be produced in the second (coupling) stage, e.g. pH 9.1. The method avoids the deleterious effects that diazonium salts may have upon the initial reaction, and avoids the effects of these diazonium salts when the incubation time is long, for many workers consider that these salts tend to inactivate enzymes or interfere with hydrolysis. Long exposure of tissue to diazonium salts in acid or alkaline solutions produces non-specific staining. The serious drawback to this type of method results from the solubility of the PRP leading to excessive diffusion between the two stages. Localization may be poor unless the PRP is reasonably insoluble.

Self-coloured substrate

There are few methods using this type of procedure. The substrate is a coloured but soluble substance, and the effect of the enzyme to be demonstrated is to remove the solubilizing group without interfering with the colour. The PRP is therefore coloured and insoluble, and no coupling stage is necessary. The insoluble coloured reaction product is precipitated at the site of enzyme activity.

DIAZONIUM SALTS

Diazonium salts are prepared by treating primary aromatic amines with an acid solution of sodium nitrite. The resulting salt, generally a chloride, reacts readily with phenols or with aryl amines to produce a corresponding intensely coloured insoluble azo dye. Diazonium salts are stored in a cool dark place and renewed at 6-monthly intervals. During incubation it is important to choose conditions carefully so that combination of the reactants takes place as rapidly as possible, and that the product formed remains insoluble through subsequent processing. Failure in either of these respects reduces the accuracy of localization of the enzyme activity.

The rate of coupling of diazonium salts depends not only on the chemical nature of the diazonium salt used, but also on the pH of the incubating medium, as well as the optimal pH for enzyme activity; this determines to a large extent the choice of diazonium salt. Precision in locating the sites of enzyme activity also depends upon the concentration of diazonium salt used. There is an average optimal concentration for diazonium salts in the incubating solution. If the concentration is less than optimal, diffusion of the PRP may be a problem. If the concentration is much greater than optimal then inhibition of enzyme activity may occur and the risk of non-specific background staining becomes increased.

THE USE OF CONTROLS

Controls are a necessary part of enzyme histochemistry. Substrates, diazonium salts and chemical solutions deteriorate with time so a positive control should be carried through when incubating test sections, to show that all the chemical solutions are working. Occasionally, also, false positives may be produced. Omission of the substrate from the incubating medium and the inclusion of specific enzyme inhibitors are adequate negative control measures. If further controls are deemed necessary, competitive inhibitors may be added to the incubating solution. Sections may also be pre-treated by immersing them in boiling water for a few minutes, and then processing through the rest of the method, or by 'incubating' in distilled water. In each case, the absence of reaction product indicates that the positive results obtained with the authentic techniques are yielding useful information about the distribution of the enzyme. Non-specific background staining is also excluded as a possible source of error if control sections give negative results. Any activity in negative control sections is regarded as a false result.

PHOSPHATASES

Phosphatases are present in a variety of animal and plant tissues and are responsible for the hydrolysis of organic phosphate esters. Some phosphatases act specifically on a single substrate (specific phosphatases). Of these, a number can be demonstrated by reliable histochemical techniques. An example of a specific phosphatase is adenosine triphosphatase, which specifically hydrolyzes adenosine triphosphate.

The remainder, whose substrate specificity is less limited, are divided into two groups: those exhibiting optimal activity at high pH values (alkaline phosphatases) and those exhibiting optimal activity at low pH values (acid phosphatases).

The hydrolysis of organic phosphate esters during incubation is the basis for enzyme histochemical reactions. The released phosphate ions or the remaining organic residue is made visible by a variety of means. Phosphate ions are precipitated as insoluble salts, i.e. lead or calcium phosphate, and then converted to coloured sulphides that are visible under the microscope. This is the basis of the many Gomori-type metal precipitation techniques. Alternatively, the alcoholic residue of the substrate, after enzymatic hydrolysis, reacts with a diazonium salt to produce a highly coloured insoluble azo dye. Phosphate esters of α-naphthol or its derivatives are the most commonly used substrates in the azo dye techniques.

Coupling may take place during incubation (simultaneous coupling) or after incubation (post-coupling). The relative merits have been discussed earlier. In the demonstration of phosphatases Pearse (1960) states that the average optimal concentration of the diazonium salt is 1 mg per 1 ml of incubating solution. If the concentration is less, diffusion of the primary reaction product α-naphthol may occur; if the concentration is greater, inhibition of PRP formation occurs, and non-specific background staining is seen.

The pH of the final incubating solution is critical; for example acid phosphatases and alkaline phosphatases exhibit optimal activity at pH 5.0 and pH 9.2 respectively. The optimal pH values for glucose-6-phosphatase and 5'-nucleotidase are at pH 6.5 and pH 7.5–8.5 respectively whilst adenosine triphosphatase has an optimal pH of 7.2.

Adequate controls are used to eliminate the possibility of failure of the method, and of producing false positives. In phosphatase histochemistry the general points made on page 292 should be considered. In addition, false positive reactions can be obtained if calcium or iron is present in the tissues.

ALKALINE PHOSPHATASES

These enzymes, exhibiting optimum activity at an alkaline pH of 9.0–9.6, are widely distributed throughout the tissues, kidney making an ideal control. They are activated by magnesium, manganese and cobalt ions. Cyanide and cysteine inhibit alkaline phosphatase activity and may be incorporated in the incubating medium to provide a negative control.

METAL PRECIPITATION TECHNIQUES: GOMORI CALCIUM PHOSPHATE METHOD (Gomori 1951)

Notes

The first methods for the demonstration of alkaline phosphatases were described by two people independently in 1939. Gomori and Takamatsu provided the incentive for further study with the publication of these methods, and a variant of the Gomori technique published in 1952 is still in use today. The incubating medium includes sodium β-glycerophosphate, calcium nitrate and magnesium chloride.

If a section is placed in an incubating solution containing a substrate (sodium β-glycerophosphate) and calcium ions (calcium nitrate), plus an activator for the phosphatase (magnesium chloride), a precipitate of calcium phosphate is formed at the sites of enzyme activity. Alkaline phosphatase liberates phosphate from the sodium β-glycerophosphate and combines with calcium ions to form calcium phosphate. This precipitate is treated with cobalt nitrate to produce cobalt phosphate, which is then treated with dilute ammonium sulphide to form cobalt sulphide. This is visible as a black deposit. The reactions can be summarized in the following flow diagram (Fig. 13.1).

Alkaline phosphatase

Sodium β-glycerophosphate	------➤	Phosphate ions
Phosphate ions + calcium ions	------➤	Calcium phosphate
Calcium phosphate + cobalt ions	------➤	Cobalt phosphate
Cobalt phosphate + sulphide ions	------➤	Cobalt sulphide (black fine precipitate)

Fig. 13.1   The Gomori calcium phosphate method for demonstrating alkaline phosphatases.

It is advisable to make up solutions immediately before use. The final pH of the solution is critical; if pH values less than 9.0 are employed the intensity of the final reaction product is reduced. Localization is also adversely affected owing to the solubility of calcium phosphate at the lower pH. Incubation is carried out at 37°C. Duration is determined by experiment, and varies with the type of tissue. Unnecessarily long incubation times should be avoided as this favours diffusion, especially in unfixed sections. Shorter times are required for cryostat sections, longer for fixed and paraffin-processed material.

Solutions

Incubating medium:

2% sodium β-glycerophosphate	2.5 ml
2% sodium veronal	2.5 ml
2% calcium nitrate	5.0 ml
1% magnesium chloride	0.25 ml
Distilled water	1.25 ml

The final pH of the incubating medium should be between 9.0 and 9.4.
2% aqueous cobalt nitrate
1% ammonium sulphide
2% aqueous methyl green (chloroform extracted)

Technique

1. After suitable fixation, bring sections to water and incubate at 37°C for 45 min to 6 h.
2. Wash well in distilled water.
3. Repeat wash.

4. Treat section with the cobalt nitrate solution for 3 min.
5. Wash well in distilled water.
6. Repeat wash.
7. Immerse sections in the ammonium sulphide solution for 2 min.
8. Wash well in distilled water.
9. Counterstain in the methyl green solution for 5 min.
10. Wash well in running tap water.
11. Mount in an aqueous mountant.

Results

Alkaline phosphatase activity	brownish black
Nuclei	green

AZO-DYE METHODS

Simultaneous coupling method

This method, described by Menton et al (1944), has been modified and improved upon by most people, notably Gomori (1951). It employs sodium α-naphthyl phosphate as the substrate and a suitable diazonium salt; the solution is buffered to pH 9.2. The enzyme liberates α-naphthol from the substrate that is coupled to a diazonium salt producing an insoluble azo dye at the sites of enzyme activity (Fig. 13.2).

Alkaline phosphatase

Sodium α-naphthyl phosphate   ---▶ Primary reaction product (α-naphthol)
(PRP) α-naphthol + diazonium salt   ---▶ Final reaction product (coloured precipitate)

Fig. 13.2   The simultaneous coupling method for demonstrating alkaline phosphatases.

ALKALINE PHOSPHATASE: AZO-DYE COUPLING METHOD (SIMULTANEOUS COUPLING)

Solutions

Incubating solution:

Sodium α-naphthyl phosphate	10 mg
0.1 M Tris buffer (stock solution), pH 10.0	10 ml
Diazonium salt (fast red TR)	10 mg

The final pH of the incubating medium should be between 9.0 and 9.4. Sodium α-naphthyl phosphate is dissolved in buffer, the diazonium salt is added and the solution well mixed, filtered and used immediately.

2% aqueous methyl green, (chloroform extracted)

Technique

1. After fixation, bring sections to water, incubate at room temperature for 10–60 min.
2. Wash in distilled water.

3. Counterstain in the methyl green solution for 5 min.
4. Wash in running tap water.
5. Mount in an aqueous mountant.

Results

Alkaline phosphatase activity	reddish brown
Nuclei	green

SIMULTANEOUS COUPLING METHOD USING SUBSTITUTED NAPHTHOLS

Gomori introduced substituted naphthols for the demonstration of alkaline phosphatases; further developmental work was by Burstone (1958, 1961). Gomori studied three substituted naphthol esters: AS-BI, AS-CL and AS-TR phosphate. The esters are hydrolyzed rapidly by alkaline phosphatases, yielding extremely insoluble naphthol derivatives. They react with a diazonium salt to produce an insoluble azo dye at the site of activity.

The localization with substituted naphthols is superior to alternative methods, and they couple with diazonium salts over a wide pH range. Stock solutions of substituted naphthol phosphates are produced by dissolving the compound in dimethylformamide (DMF) and adding distilled water and buffer to pH 8.3. The solutions keep at 4°C or for several months. To apply the reaction, add a suitable diazonium salt (e.g. fast red TR, fast blue RR) to the required amount of incubating solution in the ratio of 1mg/1ml. The incubating solution is prepared immediately before use. Incubation time is variable, in a range of 5–30 min.

ALKALINE PHOSPHATASE: NAPHTHOL AS-BI METHOD (SIMULTANEOUS COUPLING WITH SUBSTITUTED NAPHTHOLS)

Solutions

Stock solution:

Naphthol AS-BI phosphate	25 mg
N:N'-dimethylformamide	10 ml
Distilled water	10 ml
1 M sodium carbonate	2–6 drops

The reagents are added in the above order, sufficient molar sodium carbonate being added until the pH is 8.0; then add:

Distilled water	300 ml
0.2 M Tris buffer, pH 8.3	180 ml

The solution, which is faintly opalescent, is stable for many months.

Incubating solution:

Stock naphthol AS-BI	10 ml
Fast red TR	10 mg

Shake well, filter and use immediately.
2% aqueous methyl green (chloroform extracted)

Technique

1. After fixation, bring sections to water and incubate in the incubating solution at room temperature for 5–15 min.
2. Wash in water.
3. Counterstain in the methyl green solution for 5 min.
4. Wash well in running tap water.
5. Mount in an aqueous mountant.

Results

Alkaline phosphatase activity	red
Nuclei	green

ALKALINE PHOSPHATASE BCIP-NBT METHOD (from Filipe & Lake 1990)

Notes

The intestinal enzyme is resistant to formalin fixation and this method demonstrates the brush border in paraffin sections of small bowel. Avoid heat as much as possible when preparing paraffin sections.

Incubation solution:

5-Bromo-4-chloro-3-indolyl phosphate in 0.5 ml dimethylformamide	2.5 mg
0.2 M veronal acetate buffer pH 9.5	10 ml
Nitro BT	5 mg
1 M magnesium chloride	0.08 ml

Method

1. Paraffin sections to water, wash cryostat sections.
2. Incubate at 37°C for 10–30 min.
3. Wash.
4. Counterstain lightly with Mayer's haematoxylin (see p. 25) 2 min.
5. Wash, dehydrate, clear and mount as desired.

Results

Alkaline phosphatase activity	dark blue to black
Nuclei	blue

ACID PHOSPHATASES

These enzymes received less attention originally than alkaline phosphatases and only in recent years have the methods for their demonstration become reliable. The problem is the high solubility of acid phosphatases and difficulty in obtaining accurate localization of the final reaction product. Simultaneous coupling azo-dye methods are also beset by the difficulty of finding diazonium salts that couple efficiently under the acidic conditions necessary for optimal enzyme activity.

The enzymes are distributed widely throughout the body; proximal convoluted tubule lining cells of the kidney and liver hepatocytes being particularly rich.

Histiocytes also contain significant amounts of acid phosphatase, as do osteoclasts of bone. The latter cells contain a form of the enzyme that is resistant to extraction by solutions used in fixation, decalcification and tissue processing. Fluoride ions inhibit these enzymes, and the inclusion of sodium fluoride in the incubating medium affords a reliable control measure. As with alkaline phosphatase, there are two reliable types of technique for the demonstration of these enzymes, the Gomori lead phosphate methods, and the azo-dye coupling methods using simultaneous coupling.

GOMORI LEAD PHOSPHATE METHOD (Gomori 1941)

Notes

This method was first introduced by Gomori (1941). Calcium phosphate, which is formed at the site of activity in the alkaline phosphatase technique (see p. 296), cannot be used in this instance due to its solubility at acid pH levels. Lead nitrate is therefore used to precipitate the phosphate ions (Fig. 13.3).

The section is incubated in a medium containing sodium-β-glycerophosphate as substrate and lead nitrate; no activator is required. The enzyme splits phosphate ions from the substrate and these form an insoluble precipitate of lead phosphate at the site of enzyme activity. The sections are treated with a dilute solution of ammonium sulphide and the precipitate converted to lead sulphide, which is visible under the microscope as a dense brown-black deposit. The deposit is granular, and if the optimal conditions for the method have been fulfilled, the granules should be small.

Acid phosphatase

Sodium-β-glycerophosphate ------▶ Phosphate ions
Phosphate ions + lead ions ------▶ Lead phosphate
Lead phosphate + sulphide ions ------▶ Lead sulphide (fine brown-black deposit)

Fig. 13.3   The Gomori lead phosphate method for demonstrating acid phosphatases.

The incubating medium is made up fresh for each batch of sections to be incubated. It is convenient to keep the individual reagents in stock solutions and stored at 4°C. The preparation of the incubating solution is important and it is necessary to use reagents of a high grade to obtain satisfactory results. The method works best at a pH of 4.8–5.0. If the pH is increased much above 5.5, it is possible to demonstrate phosphatases other than acid phosphatases. Incubation is carried out at 37°C for 30 min to 6 h, depending on the method of preparation of the material and the tissue used.

Solutions

Incubating solution:

0.5 M veronal acetate buffer, pH 5.0	10 ml
Sodium-β-glycerophosphate	32 mg
Lead nitrate	20 mg

The lead nitrate must be dissolved in the buffer before the β-glycerophosphate is added. The pH of the incubating medium should be approximately 5.0.
1% ammonium sulphide (fresh)

Technique

1. Place sections in the incubating medium at 37°C for $\frac{1}{2}$ – 2 h.
2. Wash in distilled water.
3. Immerse in the ammonium sulphide solution for 2 min.
4. Wash well in distilled water.
5. Counterstain in either 2% methyl green, or Mayer's carmalum (see p. 28) for 5 min.
6. Wash in tap water.
7. Mount in an aqueous mountant.

Results

Acid phosphatase activity	black
Nuclei	green or red

AZO-DYE SIMULTANEOUS COUPLING METHOD

The principle employed in the corresponding technique for alkaline phosphatase is used for the demonstration of acid phosphatase. The substrate is sodium α-naphthyl phosphate (1-naphthyl phosphoric acid) dissolved in 0.1 M veronal acetate buffer at pH 5.0. α-Naphthol is released at the site of enzyme activity and coupled with a suitable diazonium salt.

The difficulty with azo-dye methods for demonstrating acid phosphatases is to find a diazonium salt to couple satisfactorily at a low pH. Grogg & Pearse (1952) carried out a comprehensive study of different diazonium salts and their performance in the acid phosphatase technique. They concluded that fast garnet GBC gave the best results, and recommended its use with this method. The localization is inferior to using substituted naphthol as a substrate and hexazonium pararosanilin as coupler.

ACID PHOSPHATASE: AZO-DYE COUPLING METHOD (SIMULTANEOUS COUPLING)

Solutions

Incubating solution:

Sodium α-naphthyl phosphate	10 mg
0.1 M acetate buffer, pH 5.0	10 ml
Fast garnet GBC	10 mg

Sodium α-naphthyl phosphate is dissolved in the buffer and the diazonium salt added. The solution is filtered and used immediately.

2% aqueous methyl green (chloroform extracted)

Technique

1. Incubate sections at 37°C for 15–60 min.
2. Wash in distilled water.
3. Counterstain in the methyl green solution for 5 min.

4. Wash in running tap water.
5. Mount in an aqueous mountant.

Results

Acid phosphatase activity	red
Nuclei	green

SIMULTANEOUS AZO-DYE COUPLING METHOD USING SUBSTITUTED NAPHTHOLS

This method, also applicable to the demonstration of acid phosphatases, was explored by Burstone (1958). The substituted naphthols he studied coupled efficiently at an acid pH, and he recommended naphthol AS-BI phosphate as the substrate of choice. Barka (1960) recommended the use of hexazonium pararosanilin as a diazonium salt in the simultaneous coupling method for acid phosphatase. This salt was first used by Davis & Ornstein (1959) for the demonstration of alkaline phosphatases and esterases. According to Barka, hexazonium pararosanilin does not inhibit the enzyme at an acid pH, and he attributed the improved localization obtained using this salt to the extreme insolubility and substantivity of the azo dye produced. The diazonium salt is prepared in two stages. First, pararosanilin hydrochloride is dissolved in distilled water and acidified with concentrated hydrochloric acid; the solution is filtered and stored at room temperature where it is stable for several months. Diazotization is then achieved by the addition of 4% aqueous sodium nitrite; it is important that the solution is freshly prepared.

Incubation is carried out at room temperature for periods of 30 min to 2 h, or at 37°C for 10–30 min, a bright red colour indicates the site of enzyme activity. Methyl green (chloroform extracted) is an ideal counterstain providing selective staining of the nuclei without affecting the colour of the final reaction product. The sections may be dehydrated rapidly through graded alcohols to xylene, and mounted in DPX. This causes little loss in staining reaction and allows permanent preparations to be made.

PREPARATION OF HEXAZOTIZED PARAROSANILIN (Davis & Ornstein 1959)

Pararosanilin solution:

Pararosanilin hydrochloride	1 g
Distilled water	20 ml
Hydrochloric acid (conc)	5 ml

The pararosanilin is dissolved in distilled water and hydrochloric acid added. The solution is heated gently, cooled, filtered and stored at 4°C.

Nitrite solution:

Sodium nitrite	2 g
Distilled water	50 ml

This solution will keep overnight at 4°C.

Incubating solution for use
Pararosanilin and nitrite solutions in equal parts; allow to stand for 30 s until the solution becomes an amber colour.

ACID PHOSPHATASE: THE NAPHTHOL AS-BI PHOSPHATE METHOD
(Burstone 1958, modified by Barka 1960) (SIMULTANEOUS COUPLING WITH SUBSTITUTED NAPHTHOLS)

Solutions

1. *Substrate solution:*

Naphthol AS-BI phosphate	50 mg
Dimethyl formamide	5 ml

2. *Buffer solution*
   Veronal acetate buffer stock A (see p. 435).

3. *Sodium nitrite solution:*

Sodium nitrite	400 mg
Distilled water	10 ml

4. *Pararosanilin stock, see p. 303*

Preparation of incubating solution

Substrate solution	0.5 ml
Buffer solution	2.5 ml
Nitrite solution	
0.4 ml of nitrite solution	
Pararosanilin stock solution total of	0.8 ml, mix before adding to rest of the incubating solution
0.4 ml stock solution	

Add 6.5 ml distilled water.
It is necessary for the success of the technique that equal parts of solutions 3 and 4 are mixed together and allowed to stand for 2 min before being added to the rest of the incubating solution.
The final pH should be between 4.7 and 5.0; it is adjusted if necessary with 0.1 M sodium hydroxide.

Technique

1. Incubate sections at 37°C for 10–30 min.
2. Wash in distilled water.
3. Counterstain in 2% methyl green (chloroform extracted) for 5 min.
4. Wash in running water.
5. Either (a) mount in an aqueous mountant, or (b) dehydrate rapidly through fresh alcohols. Clear and mount in DPX.

Results

Acid phosphatase activity	red
Nuclei	green

ADENOSINE TRIPHOSPHATASE (ATPase)

This specific phosphatase has a major application in the diagnosis of skeletal muscle biopsies. By applying the technique at different pH levels it is possible to differentiate muscle fibre types and thereby show changes in the number, size and relative proportions of the fibres. The method is applied to fresh unfixed cryostat sections as pre-fixation destroys the enzyme activity. ATPase acts on the substrate adenosine triphosphate to produce phosphate that combines with calcium ions. Ammonium sulphide converts these ions into a brown precipitate of calcium sulphide at the site of enzyme activity.

Note

The method employs lead or calcium to combine with the released phosphate; calcium is preferred when the method is used on muscle biopsies. Some workers prefer to use a 10 μm thick section, as this increases the contrast between the fibres in the final preparation.

Solutions

pH 9.4 buffer (veronal acetate):

0.1 M sodium barbitone solution	2 ml
0.18 M calcium chloride solution	2 ml
Distilled water	6 ml

Adjust pH to 9.4 with 0.1 M NaOH.
pH 4.6 buffer (veronal acetate)—as above but adjust pH to 4.6 with 0.1 M HCl.
pH 4.2 buffer (veronal acetate)—as above but adjust pH to 4.2 with 0.1 M HCl.
Incubating solution:

0.1 M sodium barbitone	2 ml
0.18 M calcium chloride	1 ml
Distilled water	7 ml
ATP (disodium salt)	25 mg

Adjust pH to 9.4 with 0.1 M NaOH.
1% aqueous calcium chloride
2% aqueous cobalt chloride
1% yellow ammonium sulphide

Technique at pH 9.4

1. Incubate section in buffer solution pH 9.4 for 15 min at room temperature.
2. Incubate in the incubating solution for 45 min at room temperature.
3. Wash in three changes of the calcium chloride solution for a total of 10 min.
4. Transfer to the cobalt chloride solution for 3 min.
5. Wash well in six changes of 0.1 M sodium barbitone.
6. Wash in tap water for 30 s.
7. Place in the yellow ammonium sulphide solution for 20–30 s.
8. Rinse well in tap water.
9. Dehydrate, clear and mount as desired.

Method (with pre-incubation at pH 4.6 and pH 4.2)

As above but replace Step 1 by incubation in buffer solution pH 4.6 or buffer solution pH 4.2. Both incubations are for 5 min at room temperature and should be followed by a rinse in buffer solution pH 9.4 for 30 s. Then resume the above method at Step 2.

Result

ATPase activity in muscle fibres—brown-black as follows:

At pH 4.2		At pH 4.6		At pH 9.4	
Type 1	+++	Type 1	+++	Type 1	+
Type 2AB	–	Type 2A	–	Type 2ABC	+++
Type 2C	++	Type 2BC	+++		

ESTERASES

Esterases are enzymes capable of hydrolyzing esters. By definition the phosphatases dealt with earlier are strictly esterases, since they hydrolyze phosphate esters. This section is devoted to those esterases that hydrolyze esters of carboxylic acids. Within this group there are many types of esterases, acting upon most substrates. There is considerable overlap between different types of esterases as many of them are capable of hydrolyzing the same substrate. This makes a classification of esterases dependent upon the application of inhibitors to the various enzyme methods.

NON-SPECIFIC ESTERASES

If the substrate is a simple ester (α-naphthyl acetate) the hydrolyzing enzyme is a non-specific esterase, but due to an overlap in activity the specific esterases such as cholinesterase are also capable of hydrolyzing these simple esters. Non-specific esterases can be further subdivided into several different groups, according to the type of ester they hydrolyze most efficiently, and according to the effect of organophosphate inhibitors.

SPECIFIC ESTERASES

The important specific esterases histochemically are cholinesterases; there are two types, acetyl cholinesterase ('true') and cholinesterase ('pseudo'). The former are capable of hydrolyzing acetyl thiocholine, whereas cholinesterases will hydrolyze esters of choline other than acetyl thiocholine more rapidly. Both enzymes are capable of hydrolyzing simple esters. Cholinesterases are differentiated from the non-specific esterases by their capacity to hydrolyze choline esters and the fact that this capacity is destroyed by the action of a specific inhibitor, eserine (10^{-5} M). Non-specific esterases are not inhibited by eserine.

LIPASES

These are esterases having the facility to hydrolyze long chain esters (esters containing fatty acids with more than seven carbon atoms in the chain). There is overlap between the lipases and non-specific esterases as both are capable of hydrolyzing simple esters.

INHIBITORS

The application of esterase inhibitors to histochemical reactions has permitted a more accurate identification of the various enzymes. The use of the specific inhibitor eserine in the identification of cholinesterases and acetyl cholinesterases has already been mentioned. The most useful esterase inhibitors are the organophosphorus compounds such as di-isopropyl fluorophosphate (DFP) and diethyl p-nitrophenyl phosphate (E600). The esterases have been subdivided into so-called A, B and C esterases, as described by Pearse (1972). The A esterases are resistant to a concentration of 1 mM of E600 but sensitive to other inhibitors. B esterases are sensitive to E600 in a concentration as low as 10 mM. The C esterases are resistant to most esterase inhibitors. The A, B and C esterases are resistant to the effects of eserine, but since the specific cholinesterases are also sensitive to low concentrations of E600 some authorities arbitrarily group them with the B esterases. The carboxyl esterases are B-type esterases, the aryl esterases are A-type esterases and the acetyl esterases are C-type esterases.

DEMONSTRATION OF ESTERASES

There is a wide range of activity of the various types of esterases. Substrates such as α-naphthyl acetate, indoxyl acetate and substituted naphthol acetate can be used in the demonstration of A, B and C esterases as well as cholinesterases.

α-NAPHTHYL ACETATE METHOD FOR NON-SPECIFIC ESTERASE

This is an azo-dye simultaneous coupling method described by Nachlas & Seligman (1949). Gomori (1950) substituted α-naphthyl acetate for β-naphthyl acetate, pointing out that the azo dye produced with the latter was soluble in water whilst that produced with α-naphthyl acetate was not. Localization of the enzyme is more precise. The method employs the diazonium salt fast blue B as the coupling agent, or hexazonium pararosanilin as suggested by Davis & Ornstein (1959). Histiocytes are rich in these enzymes.

METHOD USING FAST BLUE B

Notes

The incubating medium contains α-naphthyl acetate dissolved in acetone and is buffered to pH 7.4 with phosphate buffer. The diazonium salt, fast blue B, is included in the incubating medium in the concentration of 3 mg/1 ml. Esterase activity in the section splits the α-naphthyl acetate, releasing α-naphthol. This combines rapidly with the fast blue B salt to produce an insoluble azo dye at the site of enzyme activity. The reaction product marks the site of esterase activity, including cholinesterases; the latter can be inhibited by eserine (10^{-5} M) and a comparison made between the two sections.

Incubating solution

α-Naphthyl acetate	5mg
Acetone	0.1 ml
0.2 M phosphate buffer, pH 7.4	10 ml
Fast blue B	30 mg

The α-naphthyl acetate is dissolved in acetone, and phosphate buffer added and throughly mixed. Fast blue B is added and the solution filtered and used immediately.

Technique

1. After suitable fixation, wash in water.
2. Place in the incubating medium for 30 s to 15 min at room temperature.
3. Wash in running tap water for 3 min.
4. Counterstain in Mayer's carmalum (see p. 28) for 5 min.
5. Wash in running tap water for 3 min.
6. Mount in an aqueous mountant.

Results

Esterase activity	blue
Nuclei	red

METHOD USING PARAROSANILIN HYDROCHLORIDE

Notes

The reaction is as previously described except that the coupling agent is hexazonium pararosanilin instead of fast blue B, first used for the demonstration of esterases by Davis & Ornstein (1959). The results obtained are similar to the above technique with better localization of the final reaction product. An advantage is that sections may be dehydrated through alcohol to xylene and mounted in a synthetic mounting medium (DPX).

Solutions

Substrate solution:

α-Naphthyl acetate	50 g
Acetone	5 ml

Buffer solution

0.2 M phosphate buffer, stock solution A (see Appendix 3)

Nitrite solution:

Sodium nitrite	400 mg
Distilled water	10 ml

Pararosanilin-HCl stock solution:

Pararosanilin hydrochloride	2 g
2 M hydrochloric acid	50 ml

Heat gently, cool to room temperature and filter.

Preparation of incubating medium:

Substrate solution	0.25 ml
Buffer solution	7.25 ml
0.4 ml each of the nitrite solution and pararosanilin-HCl	
stock solutions are mixed before adding:	0.8 ml
Distilled water	2.5 ml

It is important that equal parts of nitrite and pararosanilin solutions are mixed before adding to the incubating medium. Adjust pH to 7.4, if required, with buffer solution.

Technique

1. After suitable fixation wash sections in water.
2. Incubate at 37°C for 2–20 min.
3. Wash in running water.
4. Counterstain in 2% methyl green (chloroform extracted) for 5 min.
5. Wash well in tap water.
6. Dehydrate rapidly, clear and mount in a DPX-type mountant.

Results

Esterase	reddish brown
Nuclei	green

INDOXYL ACETATE METHOD (Holt 1954)

Notes

This method demonstrates non-specific esterases and is a simultaneous coupling method with potassium ferricyanide as the coupler. The technique was introduced by Barnett & Seligman (1951) and Holt & Withers (1952). The substrate suggested in these two papers was indoxyl acetate but Holt (1954) introduced 5-bromo-4-chloro-indoxyl acetate as a substrate, and this is superior. The incubating medium consists of 5-bromo-4-chloro-indoxyl acetate, postassium ferrocyanide, potassium ferricyanide, calcium chloride and Tris buffer, pH 7.2. Esterase in the section hydrolyzes 5-bromo-indoxyl acetate to produce 5-bromo-indoxyl. This is a soluble product which is then oxidized by the potassium ferricyanide to an insoluble indigo dye. The potassium ferrocyanide that is in equimolar solution with the ferricyanide prevents over-oxidation of the indigo whilst the calcium chloride acts as an enzyme activator.

Incubating solution

5-bromo-4-chloro-indoxyl acetate	1 mg
Ethanol	0.1 ml

Tris buffer (0.2 M), pH 7.2 (see p. 434)	2 ml
Potassium ferricyanide (0.05 M) (1.6%)	17 mg
Potassium ferrocyanide (0.05 M) (2.1%)	21 mg
Calcium chloride (0.1 M) (2.1%)	11 mg
Distilled water	7.9 ml

The 5-bromo-4-chloro-indoxyl acetate is dissolved in the ethanol and the buffer is then added. The remaining chemicals are dissolved in the distilled water and the solution is mixed. It is important that the solution is freshly prepared.

Technique

1. After suitable fixation, wash section in water.
2. Incubate at 37°C for 15–60 min.
3. Rinse in tap water.
4. Counterstain in Mayer's carmalum (see p. 28) for 5 min.
5. Rinse in tap water.
6. Mount in an aqueous mountant or dehydrate, clear and mount in DPX.

Results

Esterase activity	blue
Nuclei	red

CHOLINESTERASES

These are specific esterases, two types of which can be demonstrated: acetyl cholinesterase (true cholinesterase) and cholinesterase (pseudocholinesterase). Acetyl cholinesterase is found in the nervous system and muscle and hydrolyzes the substrate acetyl thiocholine. Pseudocholinesterase will hydrolyze other esters of choline more rapidly than true cholinesterase and is found in parafollicular cells of the thyroid and other endocrine glands. The enzyme hydrolyzes acetyl thiocholine to produce thiocholine, which combines with copper ions to form copper thiocholine. This is treated with dilute ammonium sulphide to form a brown precipitate at the site of enzyme activity.

THIOCHOLINE TECHNIQUE (Gerebtzoff 1959)

Note

Both enzymes will be demonstrated by this technique. If differentiation between the two enzymes is required, then duplicate sections and two substrates are required, e.g. acetyl and butyryl thiocholine iodide to demonstrate true and pseudo-cholinesterase respectively.

Solutions

Solution (a):

0.1 M acetate buffer, pH 5.0 or 6.2 (see Appendix 3)

Solution (b):

Acetyl thiocholine iodide or butyryl thiocholine iodide	15 mg
Cupric sulphate	7 mg
Distilled water	1.4 ml

This solution is centrifuged at 4000 rpm for 15 min and the supernatant used.

Solution (c):

Glycine	375 mg
Distilled water	10 ml

Solution (d):

Cupric sulphate	250 mg
Distilled water	10 ml

Preparation of incubating medium:

Solution (a)	5 ml
Solution (b)	0.8 ml
Solution (c)	0.2 ml
Solution (d)	0.2 ml
Add distilled water	3.8 ml

The pH of the incubating medium is varied according to the tissue and the amount of activity expected in the tissue. Gerebtzoff (1959) states that tissues with high cholinesterase activity are incubated at pH 5.0 and other tissues at 6.2. *2% ammonium sulphide*

Technique

1. Incubate sections at 37°C for 10–90 min.
2. Rinse in two changes of distilled water.
3. Treat sections with the ammonium sulphide solution for 2 min.
4. Wash well in distilled water.
5. Counterstain if required in either methyl green for 5 min or Mayer's haematoxylin for 2 min or Mayer's carmalum for 5–30 min.
6. Wash in tap water.
7. Mount in an aqueous mountant.

Results

Cholinesterase activity	brown
Nuclei	green, blue or red according to nuclear dye used

LIPASE

Lipases are a group of enzymes having the ability to hydrolyze long chain esters, particularly those containing saturated fatty acids. The enzymes are located in the exocrine pancreas and in smaller amounts in the liver hepatocytes and adrenal cortex. There is an overlap in the demonstration of lipases and non-specific esterases as both hydrolyze the same substrate. This method depends upon the enzyme hydrolyzing Tween 60 to produce fatty acids; these are combined with calcium ions to form insoluble calcium soaps which are treated with lead ions and converted by ammonium sulphide to form a dark brown deposit of lead sulphide at the site of enzyme activity.

TWEEN METHOD

Notes

It is necessary to employ a control section which is passed through the technique, but the incubating medium will lack the Tween substrate. Comparisons are made between test and control sections and no staining should be seen in the control. Formalin-fixed frozen sections work well and acetone-fixed paraffin sections give acceptable results. Exocrine pancreas is the most suitable control tissue.

Solutions

Solution (a):
  Tris buffer, pH 7.2

Solution (b):

Tween 60	5 g
Tris buffer, pH 7.2	100 ml
Thymol	1 crystal

Solution (c):

Calcium chloride	200 mg
Distilled water	10 ml

Incubating medium:

Solution (a)	9 ml
Solution (b)	0.6 ml
Solution (c)	0.3 ml

1% aqueous lead nitrate
1% ammonium sulphide
Mayer's carmalum (see p. 28)

Technique

1. After suitable fixation, bring sections to water.
2. Incubate at 37°C for 2–8 h. If paraffin sections are used, leave for 24 h at 37°C.
3. Rinse sections in three changes of distilled water.
4. Place sections in pre-heated lead nitrate solution at 55°C for 10 min.
5. Rinse sections in distilled water for 2 min.
6. Wash in tap water for 10 min.
7. Place sections in the ammonium sulphide solution for 3 min.
8. Rinse in distilled water.
9. Wash in tap water.

10. Counterstain in Mayer's carmalum for 5–30 min.
11. Wash in tap water for 1 min.
12. Mount in an aqueous mountant.

Results

Lipase activity	yellow to brown-black
Nuclei	red

CHLOROACETATE ESTERASE

This esterase can resist the effects of paraffin processing. The technique demonstrates mast cells and white cells of the myeloid series, but early cells of the myeloid series may not react. Immunocytochemistry may prove more effective.

Notes

The pH of the incubating medium must be below 7.1. The incubation time varies according to the type of sections used; frozen sections show strong activity after 5 min while paraffin sections will require longer. Mast cells stain rapidly while myeloid cells, if in paraffin sections, may take several hours. If the method given below fails to work on paraffin sections the alternative method that follows can be tried. Stevens (1983) showed that a positive result can be obtained on bony fragments after a short decalcification in EDTA. In our hands acidic decalcification will markedly weaken the reaction.

Incubating solution

Naphthol AS-D acetate (dissolved in 0.5 ml dimethylformamide)	5mg
Distilled water	25 ml
0.2 M Tris buffer (pH 7.1)	25 ml
Fast blue RR salt	30 mg

Mix reagents in the order given, shake well and filter. Check that the pH is below 7.1.

Technique

1. Paraffin sections to water.
2. Incubate sections in freshly filtered incubating solution at room temperature 5 min to several hours.
3. Rinse in water.
4. Counterstain nuclei in Mayer's carmalum (see p. 28) 10–15 min.
5. Wash in water and mount in an aqueous mountant.

Result

Esterase activity	shades of blue (intense in mast cells, variable in myeloid cells)
Nuclei	red

ALTERNATIVE CHLOROACETATE ESTERASE METHOD

Notes

When preparing stock solution A, mix the two reactants together briskly to allow full nitrogenation until the solution is colourless—usually 1 min; as a guide to the efficacy of the working solution it should be a pale pink colour, if correctly prepared. Formalin-fixed material reacts well but if using blood smears methanol should be avoided (try formalin vapour). The more mature the myeloid cell the weaker the reaction, but myeloblasts may be negative.

Solutions

Stock solution A

Filtered 4% pararosanilin hydrochloride in 2 M hydrochloric acid	3 drops
4% aqueous sodium nitrite	3 drops

Add 60 ml of pH 6.8 veronal-hydrochloric acid buffer and mix.
The final pH of solution should be 6.3 (adjust if necessary).

Stock solution B

Dissolve 20 mg naphthol ASD chloroacetate in 1 ml acetone (or dimethylformamide).

Working solution

Mix solutions A and B and then filter; the resultant solution should be a pale pink colour.

Mayer's haematoxylin (see p. 25)

Technique

1. Frozen or paraffin sections to distilled water.
2. Treat with the working solution for 2 h (at room temperature).
3. Wash in water.
4. Stain the nuclei with haematoxylin for 1–2 min.
5. Wash in tap water for 5–10 min.
6. Dehydrate, clear and mount as desired.

Results

Myeloid blood cells and mast cells	bright red
Nuclei	blue

LACTASE (Indigogenic Method)

Notes

The medium can be used repeatedly. After incubation it is filtered and stored frozen. This can be repeated at least 10 times and is sufficient for 50 biopsies.

Incubation solution

5-bromo-4-chloro-3-indolyl-β-D-fucoside	3 mg

Dissolve in N, N-dimethylformamide	0.3 ml
0.1 M citric acid phosphate buffer, pH 6.0	6 ml
1.650% potassium ferricyanide	0.5 ml
2.11% potassium ferrocyanide	0.5 ml

Mix thoroughly.

Technique

1. Incubate sections in the medium at 37°C for 2 h.
2. Rinse in distilled water.
3. Fix in 10% formalin for 5 min at room temperature.
4. Rinse in distilled water.
5. Counterstain lightly with an alum haematoxylin.
6. Wash, dehydrate, clear and mount as desired.

Results

Enzyme-active sites	blue
Nuclei	reddish blue

β-GALACTOSIDASE

Incubation solution

5-bromo-4-chloro-3-indolyl-β-galactosidase dissolved in 2 drops 2-methoxyethanol	3 mg
McIlvaine buffer pH 4.0	7 ml
2.11% potassium ferrocyanide	0.5 ml
1.65% potassium ferricyanide	0.5 ml
Sodium chloride	47 mg

Technique

1. Cover sections with the medium and incubate at 37°C for 5–18 h.
2. Rinse in water.
3. Counterstain lightly with Mayer's carmalum.
4. Rinse dehydrate, clear and mount as desired.

Result

Enzyme activity	blue
Nuclei	red

DEHYDROGENASES

Dehydrogenases are enzymes that have the ability to remove hydrogen from the substrate and transfer it to another substance. The substance that acts as the hydrogen acceptor is either nicotinamide adenine dinucleotide (NAD), or nicotinamide adenine dinucleotide phosphate (NADP), or a flavoprotein. NAD and

NADP are also known as co-enzymes 1 and 2 respectively (Table 13.4). When they have accepted the hydrogen released by the action of the dehydrogenase they are known as reduced NAD and NADP, signified as NADH and NADPH respectively.

Sometimes the dehydrogenase itself can act as a hydrogen acceptor, and this is reduced by flavoproteins in a subsequent reaction. Because of the ability of dehydrogenases to remove hydrogen from the substrate, they are regarded as oxidative enzymes. Some dehydrogenases can be demonstrated histochemically and, with the reactions they catalyse, are listed in Table 13.4. Dehydrogenases are mitochondrial enzymes and are removed by fixation techniques. The 'diaphorases' are dehydrogenases that catalyse the dehydrogenation of the reduced forms of NAD and NADP, i.e. they catalyse the reactions.

$$\text{NADH} \longrightarrow \text{NAD}^+ + \text{H}$$
$$\text{NADPH} \longrightarrow \text{NADP}^+ + \text{H}$$

RATIONALE OF THE DEMONSTRATION OF DEHYDROGENASES

Dehydrogenase activity is demonstrated histochemically using tetrazolium salts. These salts, which are almost colourless, are water-soluble and able to accept the hydrogen released from the substrate by the enzyme action. Tetrazolium salts that have been reduced in this way produce an insoluble, highly coloured, microcrystalline deposit of a formazan compound. In histochemical reactions the conditions of the method are carefully controlled for the successful production and localization of the formazan deposit. Unfixed frozen sections are incubated in a medium containing the specific substrate, tetrazolium salt, buffer and co-enzyme (if required), plus any activators or chelators necessary.

Types of tetrazolium salts

In the development of enzyme histochemistry many types of tetrazolium salt have been tried in oxidase and dehydrogenase histochemistry. Two main types are used—the monotetrazolium salts and the ditetrazolium salts—and much work has been devoted to these to make them suitable for histochemical procedures. Currently, salts from each of the two groups are in routine use for dehydrogenase methods. Ditetrazolium chloride-nitro-BT (NBT) was introduced into dehydrogenase histochemistry by Nachlas et al (1957) for the demonstration of succinic dehydrogenase. The formazan produced with this salt is highly coloured, microcrystalline and insoluble in lipid; deposits of formazan may be seen in areas of lipid. The salt of the monotetrazolium group is 3(4:5-dimethyl thiazolyl-2): 5-diphenyl tetrazolium bromide (MTT). This monotetrazole was introduced by Pearse (1957). The formazan produced with this salt is immediately chelated to cobalt ions, which are present in the incubating medium. The final formazan deposit is deeply coloured and finely granular, and is soluble in fat deposits. Using this tetrazolium salt, Scarpelli et al (1958), Hess et al (1958) and Pearse (1972) described methods for most dehydrogenase enzymes.

Table 13.4   Dehydrogenase reactions

Dehydrogenase	Reaction catalysed
Succinate dehydrogenase	Succinate -- ► fumarate
Lactate dehydrogenase	Lactate -- ► pyruvate
Malate dehydrogenase	Malate -- ► oxaloacetate
Isocitrate dehydrogenase	Isocitrate -- ► oxalosuccinate
Glutamate dehydrogenase	Glutamate -- ► ketoglutarate
Glucose-6-phosphate dehydrogenase	Glucose-6-phosphate -- ► 6-phosphogluconolactone
Alcohol dehydrogenase	Ethanol -- ► acetaldehyde
NAD diaphorase	NADH -- ► NAD$^+$
NADP diaphorase	NADPH -- ► NADP$^+$

HISTOCHEMICAL METHODS

Succinate dehydrogenase: MTT technique. Succinate dehydrogenase in the section releases hydrogen from the substrate (sodium succinate). The hydrogen reduces the tetrazolium salt to form a formazan that is then chelated with cobalt ions to form a coloured insoluble granular deposit; no co-enzyme is required since the enzyme itself acts as a hydrogen acceptor.

Succinate dehydrogenase: NBT technique. Succinate dehydrogenase in the section releases hydrogen from the succinate that reduces the nitro-BT to form a water-insoluble coloured formazan. Again no co-enzyme is required.

Lactate dehydrogenase: NBT or MTT techniques. Lactate dehydrogenase in the section releases hydrogen from the lactate in the incubating medium. NAD is required as a hydrogen acceptor before the tetrazolium salt can be converted into a formazan.

Other dehydrogenases. Other dehydrogenase methods work on the principles outlined above.

NAD and NADP diaphorases: MTT technique. The NAD and NADP diaphorases oxidize NADH and NADPH to NAD and NADP respectively. The hydrogen passes to the tetrazolium salt which then chelates with the cobalt to form a formazan deposit at the site of activity.

Table 13.5   Co-enzymes

Chemical name	Standard abbreviations
Nicotinamide adenine dinucleotide	NAD
Nicotinamide adenine dinucleotide reduced	NADH
Nicotinamide adenine dinucleotide phosphate	NADP
Nicotinamide adenine dinucleotide phosphate reduced	NADPH

PREPARATION OF SECTIONS AND SOLUTIONS

Sections for the demonstration of dehydrogenases are prepared from fresh unfixed material. Fixation will destroy dehydrogenase activity except a small amount of enzyme firmly bound in the cytoplasm. Sections are incubated unfixed at 37°C for 30 min and then transferred to formalin to stop the reaction and to fix the section. They are then counterstained in 2% methyl green (chloroform-washed) or Mayer's carmalum (see p. 28).

Preparation of tetrazolium stock solution

MTT (1 mg per 1 ml distilled water)	2.5 ml
Tris buffer, pH 7.4	2.5 ml
0.5 M cobalt chloride	0.5 ml
0.5 M magnesium chloride	1.0 ml
Distilled water	2.5 ml

The pH is checked and adjusted to 7.0 if necessary, using either stock Tris buffer or M hydrochloric acid. The stock solution is kept frozen and is stable for many months if stored in this manner. The co-enzymes are added just before use. The pH should be checked and adjusted to 7.0–7.1. Note that in the methods for the diaphorases, the respective co-enzymes are the substrates for the reaction.

PRACTICAL DEMONSTRATION OF DEHYDROGENASES

The method detailed below illustrates the techniques of dehydrogenase histochemistry. The same technique can be applied to the dehydrogenases listed in Table 13.7 by simply applying the specific substrate solutions, with the addition or substitution of the correct co-enzyme if needed.

Solutions

Stock substrate solution (see Table 13.6)
Stock MTT tetrazolium solution
Incubating medium (shown in Table 13.7)

Technique

1. Cover sections with incubating medium at 37°C for 30 min to 1 hr.
2. Transfer sections to 10% neutral buffered formalin for 10–15 min.
3. Wash well in tap water for 2 min.
4. Counterstain in methyl green or carmalum for 5 min.
5. Rinse in tap water.
6. Mount in an aqueous mountant.

Results

Succinate dehydrogenase	black formazan deposit
Nuclei	green or red according to counterstain used

Table 13.6   Preparation of stock substrate solutions with pH adjusted to 7.0

Substrate	Chemical	Conc. (M)	Amount of substance	Vol. water	Neutralization	Final vol.
Succinate	Sodium succinate	2.5	6.75 g	8ml	0.05 ml M HCl approx.	10 ml
Malate	Sodium hydrogenmalate	1	1.55 g	8ml	0.9 ml 40% NaOH	10 ml
Glucose-6-phosphate	Glucose-6-phosphate (disodium salt)	1	0.30 g	0.8ml	0.06 ml M HCl	1.0 ml
Isocitrate	DL-isocitric acid (trisodium salt)	1	0.27 g	0.8ml	0.1 ml 1 M HCl approx.	1.0 ml
Glutamate	L-glutamic acid (sodium salt) Mono.	1	1.87 g	8ml	0.05 ml M HCl	10 ml

Table 13.7   Dehydrogenase working solutions

Enzyme to be demonstrated	Vol. of stock tetrazolium soln. (ml)	Vol. of substrate stock soln (ml)	Vol. of distilled water (ml)	Co-enzyme 2 mg
NAD diaphorase	0.9	Nil	0.1	NADH
NADP .	0.9	Nil	0.1	,NADPH
Succinic dehydrogenase	0.9	0.1	Nil	Nil
Malate dehydrogenase	0.9	0.1	Nil	NAD
Glucose-6-phosphate dehydrogenase	0.9	0.1	Nil	NADP
Isocitrate dehydrogenase	0.9	0.1	Nil	NAD
Glutamic dehydrogenase	0.9	0.1	Nil	NAD

DOPA-OXIDASE

Melanin is produced from tyrosine by the action of an enzyme complex called tyrosinase (syn. DOPA-oxidase). Tyrosinase localized within the cells will oxidize DOPA to form an insoluble pigment. It is possible to demonstrate the sites of tyrosinase activity using a technique suitable for post-fixed cryostat sections. The method was originally designed for blocks of tissue, and both methods are given below. Melanin-producing cells are shown by treating the tissue with dihydroxyphenylalanine (DOPA). The enzyme within the cells will oxidize the DOPA to form insoluble brownish granules. Melanocytes of albino skin contain a relatively inactive form of the enzyme tyrosinase and will not be positive for this reaction.

TISSUE BLOCK METHOD (Bloch 1917, Rodriguez & McGavran 1969)

Notes

Any melanin-producing tissue should act as a suitable positive control. A negative control should always be employed as well, and consists of a duplicate tissue block treated with buffer only.

Solutions

Buffer pH 7.4
   Dissolve 42.8 g sodium cacodylate and 9.6 ml M hydrochloric acid in 1 litre distilled water.
Primary fixative
   10% formalin in the pH 7.4 buffer (v/v) plus 0.44 M sucrose.
Reactant
   0.1% DOPA in the pH 7.4 buffer.

Technique

1. Fix two thin (2 mm) pieces of the test material in the primary fixative for 3 h at 4°C.
2. Rinse in cold (4°C) pH 7.4 buffer for 5 min.
3. Incubate one piece of tissue in the buffered DOPA solution for 16 – 20 h at 37°C. Change the solution for fresh buffered DOPA at least once during this time. The remaining tissue block is treated with buffer only at 37°C during this period.

4. Wash both blocks in distilled water for 5 min. Fix in a conventional 10% formalin solution for 1–2 days.
5. Paraffin process in the usual way. Cut 10 μm sections and mount using an adhesive.
6. Counterstain with Mayer's haematoxylin (see p. 25) in accordance with the standard technique, dehydrate, clear and mount as desired.

Results

Newly-formed melanin will be present in the DOPA-treated block only (compare with the block treated with buffer only).

Nuclei   blue

DOPA-OXIDASE IN SECTIONS TECHNIQUE (Bloch 1917, Laidlaw & Blackberg 1932)

Notes

For this variant of the above reaction, use either fresh frozen sections or frozen sections cut from tissue fixed in formalin for no longer than 2–3 h. It is essential to take through a negative control, in this instance a duplicate section incubated in buffer only.

Solutions

Buffer pH 7.4
Dissolve 42.8 g sodium cacodylate and 9.6 ml M hydrochloric acid in 1 litre distilled water.
Primary fixative
10% formalin in the pH 7.4 buffer (v/v) plus 0.44 M sucrose.
Reactant
0.1% DOPA in the pH 7.4 buffer.

Technique

1. Place frozen sections in distilled water for a few seconds only.
2. Treat with DOPA solution for 30 min at 37°C. A duplicate section should be placed in pH 7.4 buffer only at 37°C and left there for a period corresponding to that received by the test section in DOPA.
3. Change with fresh solution and inspect the section microscopically every 30 min or so. In 2–3 h the solution will turn a reddish colour and in 3–4 h a sepia brown. By this stage the reaction should be complete.
4. Wash in several changes of distilled water. Counterstain with Mayer's haematoxylin solution (see p. 25) for 1–2 min. Blue, wash, dehydrate, clear and mount as desired.

Results

DOPA-oxidase   brown
Nuclei   blue

DOPA-OXIDASE REACTION (from Filipe & Lake 1990)

Note

Presence of a reaction product indicates the capacity of cells to produce melanin and is useful in identifying melanoma cells. Mast cells are also stained by this procedure and are often difficult to distinguish from melanocytes. Diethyl-dithiocarbamate is added to chelate the copper on which DOPA-oxidase is dependent. Cryostat or frozen sections of unfixed tissue or of tissue fixed in cold formalin are suitable.

Incubating solutions

Solution (a):
   0.1 M phosphate buffer, pH 7.4

Solution (b):

Tyrosine	2 mg
DL-DOPA	0.2 mg
0.1 M phosphate buffer, pH 7.4	10 ml

Solution (c):

Tyrosine	2 mg
DL-DOPA	0.2 mg
0.1 M phosphate buffer, pH 7.4	10 ml
Diethyl-dithiocarbamate	4 mg

Method

1. Incubate three 10 μm serial sections in solutions a, b and c for 3 h at 37°C.
2. Rinse all sections in water.
3. Counterstain sections with Mayer's haemalum (see p. 25).
4. Dehydrate, clear and mount as desired.

Results

Pigment formed as a result of the enzymic activity appears brown-black in section b. By comparing with sections a and c this pigment can be distinguished from pre-existing melanin.

REFERENCES

Bancroft J D 1975 Histochemical techniques, 2nd edn. Butterworth, London
Barka T 1960 A simple azo dye method for histochemical demonstration of acid phosphatases. Nature 187: 248
Barnett R J, Seligman A M 1951 Histochemical demonstration of esterases by production of indigo. Science 114: 579
Bloch B 1917 Des problem de pigmentbildung in der haut. Archives of Dermato-Syphiligraphiques 124: 129
Burstone M S 1958 Histochemical demonstration of acid phosphates with naphthol AS-phosphates. Journal of National Cancer Institute 21: 523

Burstone M S 1961 Histochemical demonstration of phosphatases in frozen sections with naphthol AS-phosphates. Journal of Histochemistry and Cytochemistry 9: 146

Davis B J, Ornstein L 1959 High resolution enzyme location with a new diazo reagent hexazonium pararosanilin. Journal of Histochemistry and Cytochemistry 7: 297

Filipe M I, Lake B D (eds) 1990 Histochemistry in Pathology, 2nd ed. Churchill Livingstone, London

Gerebtzoff M A 1959 Cholinesterases. Pergamon, Oxford

Gomori G 1941 Distribution of acid phosphatase in the tissues under normal and pathologic conditions. Archives of Pathology 32: 189

Gomori G 1950 An improved histochemical technique for acid phosphatase. Stain Technology 25: 81

Gomori G 1951 Alkaline phosphatase of cell nuclei. Journal of Laboratory and Clinical Medicine 37: 526

Grogg E, Pearse A G E 1952 Coupling azo dye methods for histochemical demonstration of alkaline phosphatase. Nature, London 170: 578

Hess R, Scarpelli D G, Pearse A G E 1958 Cytochemical localisation of pyridine nucleotide linked dehydrogenases. Nature, London 181: 1531

Holt S J 1954 A new approach to the cytochemical localisation of enzymes. Proceedings of Royal Society Series B 142: 160

Holt S J, Withers R F J 1952 Cytochemical localisation of esterases using indoxyl derivatives. Nature 170: 1012

Laidlaw G F, Blackberg S N 1932 Melanoma studies; DOPA reaction in normal histology. American Journal of Pathology 8: 491

Menton M L, Junge J, Green M H 1944 Coupling azo dye test for alkaline phosphatase in the kidney. Journal of Histochemistry and Cytochemistry 5: 420

Nachlas M M, Seligman A M 1949 The histochemical demonstration of esterase. Journal of the National Cancer Institute 9: 415

Nachlas M M, Tsou K C, Sousa E, Cheng C S, Seligman A M L 1957 Cytochemical demonstration of succinic dehydrogenase by the use of a new p-nitrophenyl substituted ditetrazole. Journal of Histochemistry and Cytochemistry 5: 420

Novikoff A B 1956 Preservation of the fine structure of isolate liver cell particulates with polyvinylpyrollidone sucrose. Journal of Biophysical, Biochemical Cytology 2: 65

Pearse A G E 1953 Histochemistry theoretical and applied. Churchill, London

Pearse A G E 1957 Intracellular localisation of dehydrogenase systems using monotetrazolium salts and metal chelation of their formazans. Journal of Histochemistry and Cytochemistry 5: 515

Pearse A G E 1960 Histochemistry theoretical and applied, 2nd edn. Churchill, London

Pearse A G E 1972 Histochemistry theoretical and applied, 3rd edn. Vol. 2. Churchill Livingstone, Edinburgh

Rodriguez N A, McGavran M H 1969 A modified DOPA reaction for the diagnosis and investigation of pigment cells. American Journal of Clinical Pathology 52: 219

Scarpelli D G, Hess R, Pearse A G E 1958 The cytochemical localisation of oxidative enzymes (1) Diphosphopyridine nucleotide diaphorase and triphosphopyridine nucleotide diaphorase. Journal of Biophysics, Biochemistry and Cytology 4: 747

Stevens A 1983 Personal communication

14. Clinical (exfoliative) cytology

INTRODUCTION

Under the heading of 'cytology' are grouped cells from widely differing environments. The presentation of material is variable due to the different conditions surrounding a given fluid when concentrating the contained cells. For example, where there are few cells in abundant fluid, such as in cerebrospinal fluid or urine, it is useful to be able to filter off the contained cells by passing the fluid through a membrane filter (such as a Millipore filter). These can have a pore size of 5 μm so that only particles of a greater diameter will be retained, i.e. most cells.

Another useful method that has grown in popularity is the use of the cytocentrifuge by which cells in fluid are deposited directly on the slide surface by centrifugal force. Concentration of cells in sputum presents special problems due to the viscous nature of the mucous material. The high viscosity prevents membrane filtration and normal centrifugation methods; mucolytic pretreatments with various enzymes or chemical reagents can be used, with or without ultrasonic disintegration, followed by centrifugation. Many workers prefer to prepare smears of selected material from the untreated sputum specimen. It is important that all specimen preparation is carried out in an approved safety cabinet and that appropriate protective clothing is worn. Tuberculous, or high risk, material needs careful handling and safety measures observed, as prescribed by the *Code of Practice for the prevention of infection in clinical laboratories and post-mortem rooms* (Howie Report). The materials most likely to carry this risk are sputum and serous effusions.

In recent years fine needle aspiration (FNA) techniques have proved of increasing value. Cells from a variety of tissues such as breast, liver thyroid and lymph nodes can be aspirated using fine bore needles. The aspirated material may be put in fixative for subsequent concentration or placed directly on slides for fixation and staining. Other material that may be profitably examined in a clinical cytology laboratory includes seminal fluid (for infertility and vasectomy cases), breast fluids (discharges and cyst contents), gastric brushings and bronchial lavage and brushing.

Choice of fixative is important and most cytological fixatives are based on the use of alcohol. There are three good reasons for this:

1. Alcohol is a protein coagulant, and smears of predominantly protein material remain better attached to the slide during staining. There are problems associated with non-protein fluids such as urine; to help keep these smears on the slide, mix

the centrifuged deposit with carbowax fixative (aqueous wax in alcohol), and use an adhesive on the slide. Other coagulant fixatives have been used, such as mercuric chloride; non-coagulant fixatives such as formalin are not suitable.

2. Alcohol gives good chromatin preservation and delineation.

3. Alcohol in whatever form is easily dispensed to clinics and will store without undue deterioration. It must not be sent through the post and smears should be fixed in carbowax fixative as a routine procedure.

There are several popular alcoholic-type fixatives such as butanol-ethanol, ethanol-acetic and Carnoy's solution. In our experience 95% alcohol (95 parts 74 OP industrial methylated spirit IMS, 5 parts water) or undiluted 74 OP IMS gives perfectly good results.

When smears are made they should be wet-fixed, i.e. the slide should be placed in the fixing solution before the smear dries. If the smear is allowed to dry various artefacts occur; the most common of these are enlarged nuclei exhibiting ill-defined weakly staining chromatin and indistinct cell outlines. It is important also, to fix material as rapidly as possible. This applies particularly to serous effusions, as storage of the specimen even at 4°C will cause some cellular changes. Bulk urine specimens should have an equal volume of alcohol added if a delay in laboratory preparation is anticipated.

The following techniques are in common use in clinical cytology laboratories, but it is important to remember that most histological demonstration techniques can also be used for cytological purposes, including those of immunocytochemistry. The difference is that dye uptake or reagent reaction times will be shorter when dealing with smears. Joint fluid cytology involving crystal identification is discussed on page 416.

The question is sometimes asked 'What is the value of exfoliative cytology in diagnostic pathology?'. The advantages are that earlier indications of a symptomless lesion may be given by exfoliated cells, as in a cervical lesion; there may also be information given over a wider area than is likely with a single surgical biopsy, e.g. sputum examination for carcinoma of the lung. Added to these two important advantages is the accessibility of most exfoliated material and simplicity of technique. Against these advantages must be set the paucity of useful cellular material often gained, and the relatively limited information provided by exfoliated material when compared to an histological preparation. For example, a section of a cervical carcinoma will indicate the degree of invasion, cell differentiation, and so on as an aid to prognosis. Another point to be considered is that, whilst a cytological preparation showing a positive result (such as malignant change or inflammation) is of definite value, a 'negative' result is of considerably less value. For example, a sputum smear showing malignant cells is conclusive whilst a benign smear pattern in a patient suspected of having lung cancer is inconclusive. The failure to demonstrate malignant cells may be due to sampling error or simply failure to expectorate 'positive' material.

In conclusion, providing the aims of exfoliative cytological examination are kept in perspective, it is a facet of laboratory work that has taken its place as a useful member of the pathology community. This chapter is an overview of the demonstration aspects of cytology and should be read in conjunction with Bourne (1990) and Coleman & Chapman (1989).

GENERAL STAINING OF SMEARS

PAPANICOLAOU TECHNIQUE (Papanicolaou 1942)

Notes

This is the standard method for the cytological examination of smears from the female reproductive tract. It produces a variegated colour staining that is helpful, for example, with hormonal studies and the detection of Candida and Trichomonas infestation (immunocytochemistry can be used to advantage, particularly for the latter organism) and partly because the type of picture produced results in less eye fatigue. This latter point is not unimportant when one considers the continuous microscopy involved in screening. Nuclei are popularly stained with Harris's haematoxylin, which seems to give the most precise staining of exfoliated cells. There is considerable division of opinion as to the advisability of incorporating acetic acid in the solution; some workers feel that better results are given by using unacidified Harris's haematoxylin.

Following haematoxylin staining, the smears are stained with 'OG 6'. This solution contains a yellow dye orange G, and stains keratin, for example, in smears of vulval carcinoma. The final stage is where the cytoplasms of the cells are stained with solutions variously termed 'EA 36' or 'EA 50'. Different staining results may be given by solutions from different commercial firms bearing the same EA number, so it is advisable to select the solutions giving the most acceptable results. These EA solutions contain eosin, light green and Bismarck brown. Intermediate (non-cornified) vaginal cells usually stain green and superficial (cornified) cells stain pink. The principle by which this differential staining occurs is not clear; neither is the role of Bismarck brown which increasingly is omitted from the staining solution. The pink or green staining is affected by various conditions, such as inflammation. The distinction between cornified and non-cornified cells is more reliably made using nuclear criteria, i.e. pyknotic nuclei for cornified cells and vesicular nuclei for non-cornified cells.

The staining schedule below is for an automatic staining machine; when staining by hand increase the staining times of the OG and EA stains by 50%. Different sources of stain will vary slightly and the staining times should be adjusted to suit the particular solutions.

Solutions

Harris's haematoxylin
OG 6:

Orange G	0.5 g
Phosphotungstic acid	0.015 g
95% ethanol	100 ml

EA 50:

0.1% light green SF in 95% ethanol	45 ml
0.5% eosin ws yellowish in 95% ethanol	45 ml
0.5% Bismarck brown in 95% ethanol (optional)	45 ml
Phosphotungstic acid	0.2 g
Saturated aqueous lithium carbonate	1 drop

Technique

The following is a 30 min schedule for a staining machine.
1. Treat with 95% alcohol for 1 min.
2. Treat with 70% alcohol for 2 min.
3. Rinse with distilled water for 3 min.
4. Treat with filtered Harris's haematoxylin solution for $2\frac{1}{2}$ min.
5. Rinse in tap water for 1 min.
6. Treat with 1% acid-alcohol for 3 s.
7. Rinse in tap water for 2 min.
8. Treat with ammoniated water (distilled water to which are added a few drops of concentrated ammonia) for 1 min.
9. Rinse in tap water for 3 min.
10. Treat with 70% alcohol for 2 min.
11. Treat with 95% alcohol for 2 min.
12. Stain with OG 6 solution for $1\frac{1}{2}$ min.
13. Treat with 95% alcohol for 2 min.
14. Treat with 95% alcohol for 2 min.
15. Stain with EA 50 solution for $2\frac{1}{2}$ min.
16. Treat with 95% alcohol for 2 min.
17. Treat with absolute alcohol for 1 min.
18. Treat with absolute alcohol for 1 min.
19. Treat with absolute alcohol for 1 min.
20. Treat with xylene for 2 min.
21. Treat with xylene for 2 min.
22. Treat with xylene and mount as desired.

Results

Nuclei	blue
Superficial (cornified) cells	pink
Intermediate (non-cornified) cells	green
Candida (monilia)	red
Trichomonads	grey-green
Parabasal cell cytoplasm	deep green
Red blood cells	orange

HAEMATOXYLIN AND EOSIN TECHNIQUE

Notes

H&E staining of smears follows the same broad pattern as staining of paraffin sections. The principal difference is that smears take up dyes more readily, as discussed earlier, so that staining times are shortened. There is no need to take smears down through xylene before staining. The following technique uses Harris's haematoxylin, which we find gives good results for general smear staining including imprint preparations. It is important that the Harris's haematoxylin be filtered before use.

Solutions

Harris's haematoxylin (see p. 25)

1% hydrochloric acid in 70% alcohol
2% aqueous sodium bicarbonate
0.5% aqueous eosin (ws yellowish)

Technique

1. Alcohol-fixed smears are washed well in water.
2. Stain with haematoxylin for 1 min.
3. Wash in water and differentiate in acid-alcohol until the nuclei are sharply stained and the background is relatively unstained. The length of this step depends on the type of material being stained, the fixative used and, more importantly, the avidity of the particular haematoxylin solution. An average differentiation time is from 2–6 s.
4. Wash in water, blue in the bicarbonate solution for 10–20 s.
5. Wash well in water.
6. Stain with eosin for 10–20 s.
7. Wash in water, dehydrate, clear and mount as desired.

Results

Nuclei	blue
Cytoplasm	pink
Red blood cells	orange

SHORR TECHNIQUE (Shorr 1941)

Notes

This technique gives results similar to the Papanicolaou method. The staining is probably a little brighter although it should be appreciated that nuclear detail is inferior to those techniques that employ an alum haematoxylin step.

Solution

Staining solution:

Biebrich scarlet ws	0.5 g
Orange G	0.25 g
Fast green FCF	0.075 g
Phosphotungstic acid	0.5 g
Phosphomolybdic acid	0.5 g
Acetic acid	1 ml
50% ethanol	100 ml

Technique

1. Stain smears for approximately 1 min.
2. Rinse in 70% alcohol then absolute alcohol for 10 s.
3. Rinse well in xylene and mount as desired.

Results

Nuclei	red
Superficial (cornified) cells	orange-red
Intermediate (non-cornified) cells	green

MODIFIED MAY–GRUNWALD-GIEMSA TECHNIQUE

Notes

Some workers prefer Romanowsky-type stains for examination of FNA, urine and serous fluid smears. Nuclear detail, particularly that of nucleoli, is well-delineated but experience is still needed for accurate cell determination. Used on cervical or vaginal smears the staining effect seems to show *Trichomonas vaginalis* parasites clearly. With serous fluids, adenocarcinoma cells are well picked out, especially if any intracytoplasmic vacuolation is present. For best results smears should always be air dried, followed by fixation in methanol for 5–10 min.

Solutions

May–Grunwald stock solution
Grind 0.3 g of the powered May–Grunwald dye in a little methanol, decant, add more methanol and grind, continue until the dye is in solution and make up to a final volume of 100 ml. Filter.

May–Grunwald working solution
Dilute 20 parts of May–Grunwald solution with 30 parts of pH 6.8 phosphate buffer (see Buffer Tables, Appendix 3).

Giemsa stock solution (see p. 70)

Giemsa working solution
Dilute 10 parts Giemsa with 40 parts of pH 6.8 buffer.

Technique

1. Stain fixed smears in the dilute May–Grunwald solution for 10 min.
2. Rinse in pH 6.8 buffer.
3. Stain in the diluted Giemsa solution for 30 min.
4. Wash and differentiate in pH 6.8 buffer for 5–20 min until the desired colour balance is achieved.
5. Allow smears to dry and mount in a DPX-type mountant.

Results

Nuclei	purple
Cell cytoplasms	blue to mauve
Red blood cells	pink

ACRIDINE ORANGE TECHNIQUE (Von Bertalanffy et al 1956, 1958)

Notes

Fluorescent staining of exfoliated material, particularly that of the female reproductive tract, has enjoyed some popularity owing to the clarity with which the fluorescence of RNA is seen. Rapidly growing cells, such as malignant cells, have an increased cytoplasmic RNA content and this has afforded a means by which malignant cells may be detected. The early popularity of the technique has waned due to the impermanence of the preparations and because interpretation, particularly of squamous carcinoma cells, still requires expertise and experience on a level with other techniques (Lowhagen et al 1966). The technique requires a pH of 6.0 for the differential staining of RNA and DNA. Formalin-fixed material does not stain satisfactorily, neither does material fixed in Bouin's solution; alcohol is the fixative of choice.

Solutions

Acridine orange solution
0.1% aqueous acridine orange. Before use dilute one part stain with 10 parts of pH 6.0 phosphate buffer to give a 0.01% solution.
Buffer
pH 6.0 phosphate buffer (see Buffer Tables, Appendix 3).
Differentiator
0.1 M calcium chloride (11.099 g calcium chloride in 100 ml distilled water).

Technique

1. Alcohol-fixed smears to distilled water.
2. Rinse in 1% acetic acid for a few seconds then two changes of distilled water over 1 min.
3. Stain in the diluted acridine orange solution for 3 min.
4. Rinse in pH 6.0 buffer for 1 min.
5. Differentiate in the 0.1 M calcium chloride solution for $\frac{1}{2}$ min.
6. Wash in phosphate buffer and mount in same.

Results (with fluorescence microscope)

DNA	yellow-green
RNA, some mucins	red

NILE BLUE SULPHATE TECHNIQUE FOR FETAL CELLS (Brosens & Gordon 1965, 1966)

Notes

This technique makes use of the fact that when material containing fetal cells is stained with Nile blue sulphate, the fetal sebaceous cells containing lipid will stain red against the non-lipid cells which stain blue. There are two possible uses for the method; firstly, for detecting leaking fetal membranes near term, vaginal fornix aspiration is done and the fluid stained to detect fetal cells deposited by leaking amniotic fluid; secondly, it sometimes happens that a pregnant patient appears to be past full term according to the menstrual history. It is helpful to the obstetrician to know the precise fetal age before a decision about initiation of parturition can be made. A sample of amniotic fluid is drawn off and the ratio of fetal lipid to non-lipid cells determined using the Nile blue sulphate technique. According to Brosens the stage of pregnancy can be determined as in Table 14.1 (counting at least 200 cell types).

Table 14.1   Pregnancy staging

Fetal lipid-containing cells as % of total cells	Pregnancy development (weeks)
1	Up to 34
1–10	34–38
10–50	38–40
Over 50	Over 40

Most workers have criticized not only the accuracy of such figures but the origin of the fat-containing cells. It seems fairly certain that, whatever type of cell stains red in the method, reliance may only be placed on the cell count at the upper end of the scale. The technique is not permanent and the smear should be examined within an hour or so, as the fat globules tend to disperse. A guide to the identification of the cells if the staining is equivocal, is that the lipid-containing cells are usually anucleate compared to the nucleated non-lipid cells.

Solution

1% aqueous Nile blue sulphate (test for high oxazone content before use, see p. 178). Best results are obtained if the solution is less than 1 month old.

Technique

1. If amniotic fluid is received, centrifuge at low speed (1500 rpm) for 5 min.
2. Decant supernatant and re-suspend the deposit in the remaining fluid.
3. Place one or two loop-fulls on a clean slide, add 1 or 2 drops of filtered Nile blue sulphate and apply a coverslip.

Results

Lipid-containing cells	red
Non-lipid-containing cells	blue

SPERMATOZOA IN SEMINAL FLUID

Notes

The following technique enables the examination of spermatozoa in fixed, stained preparations. Initial fixation is in osmium tetroxide vapour followed by Schaudinn fixation which, being a coagulant fixative, serves to prevent loss of material during staining. Haematoxylin staining of spermatozoon heads is followed by counter-staining with Rose Bengal, a homologue of eosin that gives superior staining of spermatozoon tails.

Solutions

1% osmium tetroxide

Schaudinn's solution:

Saturated aqueous mercuric chloride	2 parts
Absolute alcohol	1 part

Mayer's haematoxylin (see p. 25)
0.5% aqueous Rose Bengal

Technique

1. Make thin smears and wet-fix in osmium tetroxide vapour for 3 min (a Coplin jar painted black containing a few ml of fixative usually suffices).
2. Transfer direct to Schaudinn's solution for 10 min.
3. Wash in water for 5 min.
4. Stain the nuclei with Mayer's haematoxylin solution for 5 min. Wash in water. Differentiate in acid-alcohol and blue. Wash in water.
5. Stain with Rose Bengal solution for 3 min.
6. Wash in water. Dehydrate, clear and mount as desired.

Results

Spermatozoon heads	blue
Spermatozoon tails	bright pink
Background protein	pale pink

SEX CHROMATIN

The sex chromatin mass was first shown to be peculiar to female cells by Barr & Bertram (1949); it can be demonstrated in cells (Moore & Barr 1955) and is popularly known as the 'Barr body'. It is thought to be the genetically inactive X chromosome, the active X chromosome in the female not being seen in interphase nuclei. These Barr bodies are present on the nuclear membrane only (the reason for this is not clear), approximately 1 μm in diameter and typically crescentic in shape. Normal males with XY sex chromosomes do not show the Barr body but those with a cytogenetic abnormality, such as Klinefelter's syndrome with XXY sex chromosomes, will show a sex chromatin mass. Those patients who are XXXY will show two Barr bodies and so on. Similarly, female subjects may show an increase in sex chromatin masses above the normal. The absence of the sex chromatin occurs in disease. A good example of this is Turner's syndrome where the female patient is sex chromatin-negative, i.e. XO, instead of the normal XX.

In the routine laboratory the demonstration of the sex chromatin mass usually revolves around those patients suspected of suffering from Klinefelter's or Turner's syndromes (sex chromatin-positive males and sex chromatin-negative females, respectively). For this purpose the most convenient site for taking smears is from the buccal cavity. To obtain a successful smear there are several points to be observed.

Technique

1. Scrape firmly, otherwise only superficial and less well preserved cells will be gained.
2. Take at least four smears but avoid scraping an area previously scraped.

3. The slides should be covered with an adhesive, e.g. gelatin (see p. 32), to prevent subsequent loss of material during staining.
4. Smears should be wet-fixed; ether-alcohol (equal parts) or 95% alcohol serves equally well for this purpose. Slides should be fixed for at least 30 min but may be safely left in the fixative for several days.
5. Smears should also taken from normal male and female subjects to serve as control material for the particular technique adopted.

Besides the techniques described, either a carefully differentiated Harris's haematoxylin-eosin method or the Feulgen technique may be used. Staining of bacteria with the former method can be suppressed by using a Feulgen-type hydrolysis (Klinger & Ludwig 1957). This will depolymerize the haematoxylin-positive bacterial RNA and thus prevent salt linkage with the component phosphate groups.

CRESYL FAST VIOLET TECHNIQUE (Moore 1962)

Notes

This is a popular technique and simple to do although differentiation of the dye requires experience before good results are obtained.

Solution

1% aqueous cresyl fast (echt) violet

Technique

1. Celloidinize both test and control smears (previously fixed) then harden in water for several minutes.
2. Stain with the cresyl fast violet solution for 15 min.
3. Wash in water and differentiate in 95% alcohol until the chromatin of cell nuclei is clearly seen.
4. Rinse in absolute alcohol, remove celloidin film, clear and mount as desired.

Results

Sex chromatin	purple body lying on the nuclear membrane
Background	pale blue-purple

ACETO-ORCEIN TECHNIQUE (Sanderson & Stewart 1961)

Notes

Highly satisfactory results can be given by this method but, unfortunately, it tends to be inconsistent. This variability is almost certainly due to non-uniformity of dye batches. The technique itself is simple and involves simultaneous fixing and staining with the acetic acid-orcein mixture. Squash preparations are subsequently made and it is important to squash firmly, to be able to render the cells flat and easily seen.

Solution

Staining solution

Dissolve 1 g of synthetic orcein in 45 ml of hot (80–85°C) acetic acid, cool to room temperature and add 55 ml distilled water and filter. Fresh solutions give better results.

Technique

Make a buccal smear on a clean slide and add one or two drops of aceto-orcein solution. Place on a coverslip and make a squash preparation as follows.

Technique for squash preparation

1. Place several sheets of blotting paper on the slide to absorb excess stain and, holding one corner of the coverslip down with one hand, make several firm strokes with the other hand on the blotting paper.
2. Examine microscopically and if satisfactory make a permanent preparation as follows. Freeze the slide on solid carbon dioxide or by using a spray. When frozen, remove the coverslip. Dehydrate in alcohol and clear with two changes of Cellosolve for 5 min.
3. Mount; the method originally called for treatment with Euparal essence for 5 min and mounting in Euparal vert. This is not essential, and routine clearing agents and mountants are satisfactory.

Results

Nuclear chromatin, particularly the sex chromatin body   dark brown
Cytoplasm   light brown

BIEBRICH SCARLET-FAST GREEN TECHNIQUE (Guard 1959, modified)

Notes

In our experience this is undoubtedly the method of choice for sex chromatin demonstration. It is not a short technique in terms of time nor is it particularly simple to do but it has the over-riding advantage of consistency of results even with inexperienced personnel. The principle of the technique is that following short staining in dilute alum haematoxylin (the mechanism of this is obscure), nuclear chromatin is stained red with acidified Biebrich scarlet. Subsequent replacement staining is carried out using acidified fast green until only pyknotic nuclei and the sex chromatin of vesicular nuclei are stained red; other structures are stained green.

In practice this differential staining effect is difficult to achieve consistently and requires freshly prepared Biebrich scarlet solution. We have found it better to overstain with the fast green solution so that the sex chromatin, although also stained green, is a darker colour and stands out against the nuclear membrane. In this way it is possible to obtain consistent, easily achieved results.

Solutions

Mayer's haematoxylin (see p. 25)
   Diluted one part with five parts distilled water.

Biebrich scarlet:

Biebrich scarlet ws	1 g
Phosphotungstic acid	0.3 g
Acetic acid	0.5 ml
50% ethanol	100 ml

Fast green:

Fast green FCF	0.5 g
Phosphomolybdic acid	0.3 g
Phosphotungstic acid	0.3 g
Acetic acid	5 ml
50% ethanol	100 ml

Technique

1. Celloidinize smears, as for cresyl fast violet technique, and take to water.
2. Treat with the diluted Mayer's haematoxylin solution for 15 s.
3. Drain and transfer direct to the Biebrich scarlet solution for 2 min.
4. Rinse in 50% alcohol.
5. Place in a Coplin jar of fast green solution for 3–4 h.
6. Rinse in water. Dehydrate (removing celloidin film), clear and mount as desired.

Results

Nuclear chromatin, particularly the sex chromatin body	dark green
Cell cytoplasm	light green

DEMONSTRATION OF Y CHROMOSOMES

Notes

As a corollary to Barr body X chromosome demonstration in the nuclei of female subjects it is possible to demonstrate the Y chromosome in males, using the following fluorescence technique on buccal smears.

In our limited experience the demonstration and visualization of the Y chromosome by this method is not an easy one. The chromosome appears a small structure (when compared to the female Barr body) and differentiating it from the adjacent chromatin particles requires experience. A good fluorescence microscope is important, preferably of the epi-illumination type. It is essential to stain, in parallel with the test smears, a buccal smear from a normal male and a normal female as a positive and negative control respectively.

Solutions

0.5% aqueous quinacrine hydrochloride (prepare fresh)
1% aqueous potassium chloride

Technique

1. Buccal smears are conventionally fixed in an alcohol-based fixative.
2. Wash in distilled water.
3. Stain with the quinacrine solution for 5 min.
4. Wash in distilled water.
5. Differentiate in the potassium chloride solution for approximately 1 min.
6. Wash in distilled water and 'mount' in same.

Results

Using a BG12 exciter filter and K530 barrier filter with ultraviolet light excitation the Y chromosome appears as a small yellow intranuclear body.

G-BANDING FOR CHROMOSOME IDENTIFICATION (Seabright 1971, modified)

Notes

In order to identify more precisely the different human chromosomes, a technique was devised in which, following partial digestion by the enzyme trypsin, the chromosomes of tissue culture preparations are stained by Giemsa. This so called G-banding technique reveals typical banding of the denatured DNA, in which the heterochromatin areas stain purple in contrast to the relatively unstained euchromatin.

A fluorescent dye, quinacrine, may be used in a similar way to differentiate human chromosomes—a technique termed, appropriately, Q-banding. The former method is more commonly used and is given below. When diluting the Hanks' solution it is important to use de-ionized water for standard results; also, when preparing aliquots of the Trypsin-Hanks' stock solution use aseptic conditions.

Solutions

Trypsin-Hanks' solution
Stock solution:

2.5% trypsin solution	80 ml
1 × Hanks' solution*	22.5 ml

Aliquot in 5 ml amounts and store at -20°C.

Working solution:

Stock solution	5 ml
1 × Hanks' solution*	45 ml

Hanks' solution:

10 × Hanks' solution*	15 ml
De-ionized water	135 ml

5% Giemsa in pH 6.8 buffer

---

*Obtainable from Flow Laboratories Ltd., Irvine, Ayrshire, Scotland.

Technique

1. Test and control slides are washed in Hanks' solution adjusted to pH 6.8 with 0.1 M sodium bicarbonate for 1 min.
2. Treat with the trypsin-Hanks' solution adjusted to pH 6.6 with 0.1 M sodium bicarbonate for 40–60 s.
3. Give slides one quick dip in Hanks' solution adjusted to pH 6.0 with 0.1 M HCl.
4. Stain with Giemsa solution for 4 min.
5. Give slides one quick dip in de-ionized water, blot dry, and remove the last traces of water under a lamp. Examine slides using the oil-immersion (x 100) objective.

Results

Typical chromosomal patterns are shown in purple bands of varying width.

SPUTUM SPECIMENS

INTRODUCTION

A smear technique and a concentration technique are described. The latter method uses hydrochloric acid as a mucolytic agent and has the advantage of allowing subsequent cell concentration. Cell morphology, including that of squamous carcinoma cells, is surprisingly well-preserved. Carnoy's fixative is recommended for sputum, although 95% alcohol gives results almost as good. With the Carnoy fixation red blood cells are lysed, so that haemorrhagic specimens will give a clearer background. Ehrlich's haematoxylin solution should not be used for sputum smears as the component mucins will also stain blue. A suitable H&E method is given below; the Papanicolaou technique is an alternative.

SMEAR TECHNIQUE

Solutions

Carnoy's fixative (see p. 425)
Mayer's haematoxylin solution (see p. 25)
0.5% aqueous eosin ws yellowish

Technique

1. Using a safety cabinet, select suitable material from the sputum specimen displayed in a Petri dish and make smears on two or three slides using either wooden applicator sticks or wire loops.
2. Wet-fix smears in Coplin jars filled with Carnoy's fixative. Leave for a minimum of 20 min but not longer than 24 h.
3. Rinse smears in water for several minutes.
4. Stain with Mayer's haematoxylin solution for 10 min. Wash in water.
5. Differentiate in 1% acid-alcohol for 5–8 s depending on the avidity of the particular haematoxylin batch in use at the time. Wash in water and blue in 2% aqueous sodium bicarbonate. Wash again in water.

6. Treat with the eosin solution for 20–30 s.
7. Wash in water, dehydrate, clear and mount as desired. For thick specimens that do not clear easily, leave in one part alcohol to three parts xylene overnight. Rinse in xylene and mount.

Results

Nuclei	blue
Background	pink

CONCENTRATION TECHNIQUE (Taplin 1966)

Notes

The principle of the technique is that component mucins (particularly sialomucins) are hydrolysed by hydrochloric acid. Thus the sputum viscosity is lowered, enabling concentration by centrifugation. Normally, sputum is treated with acid overnight at a concentration of 8%. If it is necessary on occasion to leave the specimen more than 24 h in acid, then a 4% solution of hydrochloric acid should be employed. When the smears are eventually prepared they may be safely air-dried without, seemingly, producing the usual artefacts. In our hands atypical squamous cells are well-preserved, adenocarcinoma cells less so.

Solutions

8% hydrochloric acid v/v
Scott's tap water substitute:

Sodium bicarbonate	3.5 g
Magnesium sulphate	20 g
Distilled water	1 litre

By using distilled water, moulds occur less often.
Mayer's haematoxylin solution
1% aqueous eosin ws yellowish

Technique

1. Add approximately 15 ml of hydrochloric acid to the specimen in the container. Mix well and leave overnight at room temperature.
2. Pour the now liquid contents into a centrifuge tube and spin at 3000 rpm for 5 min.
3. Pour off supernatant. Add approximately 15 ml of Scott's tap water substitute and re-spin for 5 min at 3000 rpm.
4. Pour off the supernatant and re-suspend the cells in Scott's tap water substitute, using just enough solution to give a 'thin cream' consistency. Make smears on clean slides using wooden applicators. Allow to air dry.
5. Stain with H&E in the same way as for sputum smears (see p. 336) but giving rather less acid-alcohol differentiation.

Results

Cell nuclei	blue
Background	bright pink

SEROUS FLUIDS

CONCENTRATION TECHNIQUE

Notes

This method is useful for highly cellular fluids such as effusions of the peritoneum ('ascitic' fluid) and pleura. Heavy effusions are often the result of non-specific inflammation or infections such as peritonitis or empyema but occasionally are due to serous membrane involvement in a malignant growth. This may be due to direct spread from adjacent organs such as carcinoma of the colon or lung, or to secondary 'seedlings' from tumours elsewhere. For example, ovarian adenocarcinomas frequently involve the peritoneal and pleural membranes, causing a heavy effusion. In addition, a rather uncommon malignant tumour of mesothelial cells lining the serous membranes may occur (mesothelioma). A non-malignant inflammatory effusion will contain a mixed cell population comprising neutrophils, lymphocytes, etc, and varying numbers of mesothelial cells.

Whilst our experience has been mainly concerned with H&E staining of this type of material, there is no reason why the other popular cytological stains (see below) should not be used. The principle of the concentration technique is that the centrifuged deposit of the fluid is mixed with plasma to which thrombin is added. The cells are enmeshed in the resultant clot, which is fixed in formalin and subsequently paraffin processed and sectioned as for a tissue block. An alternative blocking method is to use melted agar that is added to the cell deposit and allowed to set.

Solutions

Plasma
  The source of plasma is a haematology laboratory; at 4°C.
Thrombin
  *Bovine thrombin 20 units/1 ml ampoules.

Technique

1. The serous fluid, which is preferably citrated to prevent spontaneous clotting, is centrifuged for 5–10 min at 3000 rpm.
2. Pour off the supernatant and if the centrifuged deposit is scanty make smears and fix and stain as for sputum smears. If the deposit is reasonably substantial proceed as follows.
3. Add approximately twice the volume of plasma to the centrifuged deposit and remaining fluid. Mix thoroughly and add one drop of thrombin. Mix well. A thrombin clot will form, usually within 1 min. If this does not occur it may be due to an insufficiency of plasma; therefore add a little more plasma and re-mix.

---

*Available from Diagnostic Reagents Ltd., Chinnor Road, Thame, Oxon.

4. When the clot has formed, fill the tube with 10% formalin and allow to fix overnight.
5. Place clot in suitable thin wrapping paper and paraffin process. Cut thin (5 μm) sections at three levels.
6. H & E staining is preferred and is used for paraffin sections (see p. 27).

Results

Cell nuclei	blue
Cytoplasms, plasma clots	pink

DEMONSTRATION OF METACHROMATIC LEUKODYSTROPHY USING URINE SPECIMENS

Notes

We are indebted to Francis (1981) for the following technique in which urine cell deposits are smeared on slides and stained with toluidine blue. In cases of the lipid storage disorder metachromatic leukodystrophy, cells may be discerned containing metachromatic granules.

Staining solution

0.1% toluidine blue in pH 5.0 acetic-acetate buffer (see Appendix 3).

Technique

1. The urine sample is centrifuged and the spun deposit washed in pH 5.0 buffer.
2. Re-centrifuge buffer-urine deposit, make smears on slides coated with an adhesive.
3. Fix the smears in formalin vapour for 30 min. This is done by placing them in a Coplin jar containing a small (0.5–1 ml) amount of concentrated formalin.
4. Allow the smear to dry thoroughly at room temperature (30 min or so).
5. Stain with toluidine blue overnight at room temperature.
6. Rinse slides in pH 5.0 buffer, blot dry and mount in a synthetic mountant.

Results

Positive cells	purple-red stained granules

Other cellular material will stain blue.

IMPRINT (TOUCH) PREPARATIONS

INTRODUCTION

It is possible to obtain a good yield of cells by pressing a glass microscope slide against the cut surface of specimens such as breast lumps and lymph nodes. The more cellular the specimen, the more it lends itself to this type of preparation, but the information gained will be purely of a cellular nature, i.e. it will lack tissue architecture detail that may be important for lymph node pathology. For malignant lesions—particularly carcinomas, either primary or secondary—a diagnosis can often be simply and speedily obtained, as a corollary to an urgent frozen section. The usual range of cytological stains can be performed on these imprint preparations, in particular the standard H&E for smears (see p. 326).

Preparative technique

1. Clean glass slides coated with gelatin (see p. 132) are pressed firmly against the cut surface of the specimen and allowed to dry briefly ($\frac{1}{2}$–1 min).
2. Place in 95% alcohol for 15–30 s (this step is optional but gives improved nuclear staining).
3. Wash in water and stain.

IMMUNOCYTOCHEMISTRY

A wide range of antisera may be employed in the resolution of cytological diagnostic problems; the detailed specific applications are discussed in Chapter 12. There are practical problems which limit the use of immunocytochemistry in this context. Foremost is the fact that in gynaecological cytology, i.e. using cervical smear material, only one or two smears are normally received per patient so that if immunocytochemistry is to be performed retrospectively the Papanicolaou-stained slides will need to be first decolourized. It also means that, at best, only one or two antisera can be deployed.

Fine needle aspirate (FNA) material can be suitable either as smears or tissue fragments, also serous fluids, particularly when a paraffin block has been prepared of the centrifuged deposit (see p. 338). This material is ideal for immunocytochemical investigation and a panel of antisera can identify tumour cells. It follows, of course, that any cytological material can be profitably employed if, besides cell blocks, there are sufficient smears or cytocentrifuge preparations available.

A final word on the appropriate fixation for carrying out immunocytochemistry on cytological material. The ideal situation is when paraffin blocks are prepared using clotted centrifuge deposits fixed in formalin. If this is not possible then imprints or cytocentrifuge preparations are recommended. These should be thoroughly air dried (30 min or so using, if possible, a warm air blower) then fixed for 10–20 min in neat acetone. Conventional alcohol (ethanol or methanol) fixation will give acceptable results with most antisera, but those obtained using acetone will be more sharply delineated with a cleaner background. These remarks apply particularly to peroxidase-based immunocytochemical techniques.

REFERENCES

Barr M L, Bertram E G 1949 A morphological distinction between neurones of the male and female, and the behaviour of the nucleolar satellite during accelerated nucleoprotein synthesis. Nature (London) 163: 676–677

Bourne L D 1990 Non-gynaecological cytology. In: Bancroft J D, Stevens A (eds) Theory and practice of histological techniques, 3rd edn. Churchill Livingstone, London

Brosens I, Gordon H 1965 Cytological diagnosis of ruptured membranes using Nile blue sulphate staining. Journal of Obstetrics and Gynaecology of the British Commonwealth 72: 342

Brosens I, Gordon H 1966 The estimation of maturity by cytological examination of the liquor amnii. Journal of Obstetrics and Gynaecology of the British Commonwealth 73: 88

Coleman D V, Chapman P A 1989 Clinical cytology. Butterworths, London

Francis R J 1981 Personal communication

Guard H R 1959 A new technic for differential staining of the sex chromatin, and the determination of its incidence in exfoliated vaginal epithelial cells. American Journal of Clinical Pathology 32: 145

Klinger H P, Ludwig K S 1957 A universal stain for the sex chromatin body. Stain Technology 2: 235

Lowhagen T, Nasjell M, Granbert I 1966 Acridine orange fluorescence cytology in detection of cervical carcinoma. Acta Cytologica 10: 194–196

Moore K L 1962 The sex chromatin: its discovery and variations in the animal kingdom. Acta Cytologica 6: 1

Moore K L, Barr M L 1955 Smears from the oral mucosa in the detection of chromosomal sex. Lancet 2: 57

Papanicolaou G N 1942 A new procedure for the staining of vaginal smears. Science NY 95: 438

Sanderson A R, Stewart J S 1961 Nuclear sexing with aceto-orcein. British Medical Journal 2: 1065

Seabright M 1971 Rapid banding technique for human chromosomes. Lancet 2: 971

Shorr E 1941 A new technic for staining vaginal smears: III a single differential stain. Science NY 94: 545

Taplin D J 1966 Malignant cells in sputum: a simple method of liquefying sputum. Journal of Medical Laboratory Technology 23: 252–255

von Bertalanffy L, Masin F, Masin M 1956 Use of acridine orange fluorescence technique in exfoliative cytology. Science NY 124: 1024

von Bertalanffy L, Masin F, Masin M 1958 A new and rapid method for diagnosis of vaginal and cervical cancer by fluorescence microscopy. Cancer NY 11: 873

15. Central and peripheral nervous system

INTRODUCTION

This chapter deals with the functional elements that make up the nervous system. There are many special techniques capable of demonstrating nervous tissue entities; the majority are silver impregnations of sections or tissue blocks. It is unfortunate that many methods are not only empirical but capricious. This means, inevitably, that it is a subjective science where consistent success with a method is largely a matter of expertise or experience. Where the rationale of a technique is known it will be given.

A few of the following techniques use celloidin sections, although these are of diminishing popularity, and some expertise is required in dehydrating and clearing the stained section. The following system is one we have found successful and would commend to the novice.

1. Take the stained celloidin section from water, through 70% alcohol to 95% alcohol (95 parts 74 OP spirit and 5 parts water). Flatten the section using camel hair brushes.

2. Place in absolute alcohol (74 OP spirit) and then in a mixture of four parts xylene and one part absolute alcohol to flatten the section by softening the celloidin.

3. Mount on a slide, blot with xylene-soaked blotting paper and then clear in xylene.

4. Brush out any air bubbles under the section whilst wet with xylene. Mount in Canada balsam. If there are any prominent folds in the section, it sometimes helps to cut away the excess celloidin border using a sharp scalpel blade; this should be done when the section is in xylene just before mounting in balsam.

Standard formalin fixation is suitable for most CNS/PNS demonstration techniques, although there are areas, such as myelin and neuroglia, for which specialized fixation is required. Unless otherwise indicated, frozen or celloidin sections give better results than paraffin, particularly with those techniques employing silver impregnation. The reason for this is not clear. However there are silver techniques in which paraffin sections give satisfactory results, and some of these will be described.

Immunocytochemistry has provided a serious challenge to the traditional methods for nervous tissue and will be discussed later in the chapter.

NEURONES AND THEIR PROCESSES (CNS)

As discussed in Chapter 1, when dealing with the normal histology of tissue, neurones may be large, as in the anterior horn of the spinal cord, or small as in the granular layer of the cerebellum. The nucleus is often difficult to see due to the scanty chromatin network, but in the larger neurones has a prominent nucleolus. The cell body contains varying amounts of discrete granular material known as 'Nissl substance' and varying amounts of the pigment lipofuscin which increases in amount with advancing age. From the cell body emerges an axon (axis cylinder) and several dendrites, and in these may be shown delicate fibrils which pass from the cell body into the processes. These fibrils are the 'neurofibrils'.

NISSL SUBSTANCE

Nissl substance is composed of coarse aggregates of RNA, and the component material can be readily demonstrated by most cationic dyes, also by techniques designed for RNA demonstration such as methyl green-pyronin or gallocyanin. Nissl substance also gives a strong yellow primary fluorescence. A selection of the more commonly employed techniques is given below.

Table 15.1   Central and peripheral nervous systems. Demonstration of nerve cells and their processes.

Technique	Recommended use
Bielschowsky: block impregnation	Nerve fibres of CNS
Bielschowsky: frozen sections	Nerve fibres of CNS
Formal-thionin	Nerve fibres of CNS
Golgi–Cox	Some nerve fibres of CNS
von Braunmuhl	Neurofibrils and plaques of CNS
Cresyl fast violet	Nissl substance of CNS
Toluidine blue	Nissl substance of CNS
Glees & Marsland	Nerve fibres of CNS and PNS
Gros–Bielschowsky	Nerve fibres of CNS and PNS
Linder	Nerve fibres of CNS and PNS
Palmgren	Nerve fibres of CNS and PNS
Winklemann & Schmit	Nerve fibres of CNS and PNS
Methylene blue	Nerve endings of PNS
Schofield	Nerve endings of PNS

CRESYL FAST VIOLET FOR NISSL SUBSTANCE (Kawamura & Niimi 1972)

Notes

Although dyes such as thionin, toluidine blue and methyl green-pyronin can be used to demonstrate Nissl substance, undoubtedly cresyl fast violet gives the best results, particularly in the hands of a novice. Gothard's (1898) differentiator gives slightly the better results, but is not mandatory as 96% alcohol can be successfully used; it also has a rather pungent odour. Alcohol or Carnoy fixation gives the best results but formalin-fixed material is adequate. The rationale of the technique is a simple acid-base reaction, where the cationic dyes bond with the anionic RNA of the Nissl substance, plus the DNA and RNA of cell nuclei.

Staining solution

0.1% aqueous cresyl fast violet acidified by 0.7 ml of 10% acetic acid per 100 ml of solution giving a pH of 3.5–3.8.

Technique

1. Sections to water.
2. Stain for 30 min at room temperature.
3. Wash in water. Differentiate in 95% alcohol until the background is relatively clear.
4. Dehydrate, clear and mount as desired.

Results

Nissl substance, nuclei	violet
Background	colourless

TOLUIDINE BLUE TECHNIQUE FOR NISSL SUBSTANCE

Solutions

0.2% aqueous toluidine blue
Gothard's solution:

Pure creosote	50 ml
Cajuput oil	40 ml
Xylene	50 ml
Absolute alcohol	150 ml

Technique

1. Sections to water.
2. Stain with toluidine blue for *either* 6 h at room temperature *or* 30 min at 56°C.
3. Wash in water.
4. Rinse in 90% alcohol.
5. Differentiate in Gothard's solution or 95% alcohol, controlling microscopically until the Nissl substance is clearly seen in the cell bodies of the larger neurones.
6. Dehydrate, clear and mount as desired.

Results

Nucleoli and Nissl substance	dark blue
Nuclei	paler blue

NERVE FIBRES

BIELSCHOWSKY BLOCK IMPREGNATION TECHNIQUE
(Bielschowsky 1904)

Notes

Wherever silver demonstration techniques are concerned the name of Bielschowsky will appear: the father figure of much of argyrophilic fibre demonstration work. In this method the blocks of tissue are impregnated with the sensitizer-ammoniacal silver-reducing solutions and although the method is slow it is, as neurological methods go, a reliable one. When the block is finally sectioned it is always worthwhile cutting a superficial section and then one deeper into the block. In this way both heavily and lightly impregnated areas will be shown. During the impregnation stages the tissue blocks should be allowed to rest on a layer of cotton wool. This will allow for greater solution contact and, therefore, more even impregnation.

Solutions

3% aqueous silver nitrate
Ammoniacal silver
> Add 2 drops of 40% aqueous sodium hydroxide to 5 ml of 20% aqueous silver nitrate. Mix and add successive drops of concentrated ammonia with shaking until the formed precipitate is almost dissolved. Make up to a 40 ml volume with distilled water.

20% formalin in tap water
5% aqueous sodium thiosulphate (hypo)

Technique

1. Place thin (2–3 mm) blocks of formalin-fixed tissue in pyridine for 2 days (this is said to reduce background silver deposition).
2. Wash in running tap water overnight, followed by several changes of distilled water over a day.
3. Treat with the silver nitrate solution for 4–5 days in the dark.
4. Wash well in several changes of distilled water over 2–3 h.
5. Treat with the ammoniacal silver solution for 4–5 h.
6. Wash well in several changes of distilled water for 2–3 h.
7. Reduce in the formalin for 12–16 h.
8. Wash well in water for 1–2 h and paraffin process.
9. Cut conventional sections and deparaffinize in xylene. If the background is clear mount in Canada balsam. If not, tone in 0.2% gold chloride for 2 min. Fix in the hypo solution for 5 min, dehydrate, clear and mount as desired.

Results

Nerve fibres, neurofibrils	black
Neurones, collagen	brown

FORMAL-THIONIN BLOCK IMPREGNATION TECHNIQUE (Min Chueh Chang 1935)

Notes

This is quite a simple and ingenious technique that involves simultaneous fixation and staining of the tissue block. When sectioning the block it is as well not to trim in too far as the dye does not penetrate very deeply. Either fresh or formalin-fixed tissue can be used.

Staining solution

0.4–0.5% thionin in 10% formalin.

Technique

1. If fresh tissue is available, take a thin (2–3 mm) block and treat with formal-thionin for 1 week.
2. If formalin-fixed tissue only is available, take a thin block and wash well in distilled water over 1 day. Treat with formal-thionin for 1 week.
3. Wash in distilled water briefly, then paraffin process (double-embedding may be used, if desired). Dehydration in alcohol should be prolonged, if necessary, until no more thionin diffuses out.
4. Cut sections, deparaffinize and mount as desired.

Results

| Neurones | blue |
| Nerve fibres | red |

GOLGI–COX BLOCK IMPREGNATION TECHNIQUE (Golgi 1878, Cox 1891)

Notes

Although this technique is one of the slowest of the neurological methods it has the unique facility of impregnating only certain of the neurones and their processes. Examination of single nervous entities is therefore eased. Like most of these techniques it is capricious, so it is advisable to take through several blocks and vary the fixation-impregnation period. The rationale of the technique is unknown. Only fresh tissue should be used.

Solutions

Impregnation solution
   Mix 10 ml 5% aqueous potassium dichromate and 10 ml 5% aqueous mercuric chloride.
   To 8 ml of 5% aqueous potassium chlorate add 20 ml distilled water. Add the solutions together and mix.
5% aqueous sodium carbonate or 10% ammonia

Technique

1. Place thin (2–3 mm) blocks of tissue in an ample volume of the fixing-impregnating solution; rest on cotton wool to ensure an even impregnation. Leave for 24 h at 37°C.
2. Change the solution for fresh and leave for a further 24 h at 37°C.
3. Change the solution for fresh, seal the lid of the container with Vaseline petroleum jelly and leave for 1–2 months in a dark place at 37°C.
4. Wash in several changes of distilled water over several hours. Cut thick (50–100 μm) frozen sections.
5. Blacken the impregnation with sodium carbonate or ammonia for 1 h.
6. Wash well in water. Dehydrate, clear and mount. Conventional mounting in balsam will cause fading; it is recommended the section is mounted in thick

balsam and hardened at 40–45°C without a coverslip. Drury &
Wallington (1980) state that it is possible to mount successfully in
synthetic resin with a coverslip.

Results

Some nerve cells and their processes
    (blood vessels may also be impregnated)—   black.

BIELSCHOWSKY TECHNIQUE FOR FROZEN SECTIONS

Notes

The principle of the reaction (which is the same for most silver reactions for
nervous tissue) is that, following 'sensitization' in silver nitrate, the section is
treated with ammoniacal silver. The ammoniacal silver is produced when ammonia
is added to silver nitrate, forming a silver hydroxide precipitate; this is soluble in an
excess of ammonia when a solution of ammoniated silver oxides is formed.
Subsequent treatment with a reducer, such as formalin, will cause a reduced
metallic silver deposit to be selectively laid down. The reason for the silver selectivity (argyrophilia) is unclear. The silver reduction may be followed by toning in
gold chloride that is thought to be a simple metallic substitution of gold for silver.
This is followed by treatment with sodium thiosulphate (hypo) which removes any
un-reduced silver particles, preventing subsequent non-specific blackening by
exposure to light under section storage conditions. This technique is reasonably
reliable but tends to give a darker background than the Bielschowsky block impregnation technique. Formalin-fixed tissue should be used.

Solutions

4% aqueous silver nitrate
Ammoniacal silver
    Add six drops of 40% aqueous sodium hydroxide to 5 ml of 20% aqueous silver
nitrate. Mix and add conc. ammonia drop by drop with mixing, until the formed
precipitate is almost dissolved. Make up to 25 ml volume with distilled water and
filter.
4% formalin in tap water
0.2% aqueous gold chloride
5% aqueous sodium thiosulphate (hypo)

Technique

1. Take 'thin' (15 μm) frozen sections to distilled water and change several
   times over 1 h.
2. Treat with the silver nitrate solution for 4 h in the dark at room temperature.
3. Rinse briefly in distilled water.
4. Treat with the ammoniacal silver solution for 3–10 min (leave until a
   brown colour).
5. Wash briefly in distilled water.
6. Treat with formalin for 10 min.

7. Wash in water. Tone with the gold chloride solution, wash and treat with hypo; both for 1–2 min.
8. Wash, mount on a slide and blot. Dehydrate, clear and mount in Canada balsam.

Results

Nerve fibres, neurofibrils	black
Background	light grey

VON BRAUNMUHL'S TECHNIQUE FOR NEUROFIBRILLARY PLAQUES IN ALZHEIMER'S DISEASE (Von Braunmuhl 1957)

Notes

To demonstrate Alzheimer plaques a variety of silver methods can be used, including the standard Bielschowsky, but this variant seems to give particularly good results (Chalk 1970). It is also a reasonably straightforward type of silver technique; normal neurofibrils and fibres are also demonstrated.

Solutions

2% aqueous silver nitrate
1% aqueous ammonia
20% formalin in tap water
0.25% aqueous gold chloride
5% aqueous sodium thiosulphate (hypo)

Techniques

1. Place 10–30 μm formalin-fixed free-floating frozen sections in distilled water and wash.
2. Place in the silver nitrate solutions for $\frac{1}{2}$–1 h (usually the shorter time), at 56°C.
3. Remove the dish containing the sections from the incubator and leave at room temperature while the following solutions are prepared in separate containers: A—1% ammonia; B—distilled water; C—20% formalin.
4. Treat sections in sequence as follows: A—3s; B—1s; C—3s. Repeat sequence.
5. Wash in distilled water, tone in the gold chloride for $\frac{1}{2}$–1 min, fix in hypo 1–2 min.
6. Mount sections on slides, blot dry, dehydrate, clear and mount in Canada balsam.

Results

Neurofibrils and plaques	black

MYELIN

Myelin sheaths consist of lipids such as cholesterol, phospholipids, cerebrosides and cerebroside sulphate contained in a protein 'neurokeratin' matrix. There are two main groups of methods concerned with demonstrating myelin degeneration: the 'negative' techniques where only normal myelin is stained, and the 'positive' techniques where only the degenerate myelin is stained. There are advantages and disadvantages to the use of each. By demonstrating normal myelin only, degenerated myelin sheaths are shown by absence of staining, and this may not be easy to distinguish if only single fibres are involved. On the other hand, the negative method will demonstrate long-standing degeneration when the products of degeneration, having been removed, would not have reacted with the positive techniques. Techniques which stain degenerate myelin sheaths have an obvious advantage, but they are prone to artefact and show short-term degeneration only (10–60 days). Products of myelin breakdown appear in microglia and can be demonstrated by conventional lipid stains for some weeks after the onset of the disease process. The staining methods are listed in Table 15.2.

NORMAL MYELIN

There are many techniques which demonstrate normal myelin, e.g. PTAH, osmium tetroxide, Sudan black and the iron haematoxylins, but the ones described below give more precise results. Paraffin sections should be cut at 10 μm, as these give better visualization of the myelin sheaths compare to the normal 5 μm sections. Fresh frozen sections can be stained by Sudan dyes or osmium tetroxide for myelin. Due to the greater retention of myelin lipids compared to paraffin sections, the myelin sheaths will appear thicker with a comparatively narrow nerve fibre lumen. Note that besides the 'specialized' techniques for myelin that follow, it is possible to stain with either Weigert's or Heidenhain's iron haematoxylin (see pp. 37 and 86 respectively).

Table 15.2 Demonstration of normal and degenerate myelin

Technique	Normal myelin	Degenerate myelin		
		Early	Later	Long-term
Sudan dyes	yes	no	yes	no
Luxol fast blue	yes	no	no	yes
Loyez	yes	no	no	yes
Weigert-pal	yes	no	no	yes
Iron haematoxylin	yes	no	no	yes
Solochrome cyanine	yes	no	no	yes
Marchi (Swank–Davenport; Busch)	no	yes	no	no

WEIGERT–PAL TECHNIQUE (Weigert 1885, Pal, 1886)

Notes

This is very much a hybrid technique as it employs Weigert's mordant, Pal's differentiator and, usually, Kultschitzky's (1889) haematoxylin. The conventional rationale of the method is mordanting in chrome salts forms a chromium dioxide complex so that normal myelin will subsequently form a lake with haematoxylin. Only long-standing myelin degeneration will show lack of staining. Because the chrome salts act as a fat fixative the resultant myelin sheaths appear more substantial following processing than, say, those demonstrated by Loyez or Luxol fast blue where conventional formalin fixation precedes processing.

With these latter techniques resultant myelin sheaths appear much more slender, presumably due to loss of myelin fats. Paraffin processing can be carried out with this technique but sectioning is difficult; sections become easily detached from the slide so a section adhesive should be used.

Solutions

Weigert primary mordant
   Dissolve 5 g potassium dichromate in 2.5 g fluorochrome (chromic or chromium fluoride) in 100 ml distilled water.
Kultschitzky's haematoxylin:

10% alcoholic haematoxylin (allow to ripen for at least 4 weeks)	10 ml
2% acetic acid	90 ml

Pal's differentiator A
   0.25% aqueous potassium permanganate.
Pal's differentiator B
   Equal parts of 1% aqueous oxalic acid and 1% aqueous potassium sulphite.

Technique

1. Take thin (2–3 mm) pieces of formalin-fixed tissue and treat with the primary mordant 4–7 days.
2. Wash in two changes of alcohol over 30 min. Process through either paraffin or celloidin.
3. Cut 10 μm paraffin or 20 μm celloidin sections and take to water.
4. Stain with the haematoxylin solution overnight at 37°C.
5. Wash in water and blue in any weak alkali such as an aqueous solution of lithium or sodium carbonate.
6. Prepare three containers: one containing the permanganate solution, one distilled water and the other the oxalic-sulphite mixture. The section is differentiated as follows: permanganate 15–20s (agitate); distilled water 1–2s; oxalic-sulphite 4–5 min. This sequence is repeated until the background is reasonably clear and the myelin a blue-black colour.
7. Wash well in distilled water. Counterstain, if desired, in 1% aqueous neutral red solution for 2–3 min. Wash in water.
8. Dehydrate, clear and mount in Canada balsam.

Results

Red blood cells, normal myelin sheaths	blue-black
Nuclei (if counterstained)	red
Background	unstained

LOYEZ TECHNIQUE (Loyez 1910)

Notes

A simple method and one that is applied to routinely fixed, paraffin-processed sections. As mentioned previously, the myelin sheaths stained by this method are considerably more 'anaemic' than those demonstrated by techniques using lipid fixatives. Differentiation may be initiated in either iron alum or 1% acid-alcohol. We prefer the former as it is quicker and gives a clearer background.

Solutions

Haematoxylin:

10% alcoholic haematoxylin	
(ripened and oxidized by standing	
for several weeks)	10 ml
Distilled water	90 ml
Saturated aqueous lithium carbonate	4 ml

Preliminary differentiator
4% aqueous iron alum.
Final differentiator
Dissolve 2 g sodium tetraborate (borax) and 2.5 g potassium ferricyanide in 200 ml distilled water.

Technique

1. Sections to water.
2. Treat with the iron alum solution overnight at room temperature.
3. Wash in water for several minutes.
4. Stain with the haematoxylin solution for either 2–4 h at 56°C, or overnight at room temperature.
5. Wash in water. Differentiate out excess background dye in the iron alum solution. Wash in water. Continue differentiation in the borax-ferricyanide solution until the background is clear. Counterstaining may be carried out in 1% aqueous eosin for 1 min.
6. Wash in water. Dehydrate, clear and mount in Canada balsam.

Results

Red blood cells, normal myelin, nuclei	blue-black
Background	colourless if not counterstained, pink if counterstained

MODIFIED LUXOL FAST BLUE (Kluver & Barrera 1953, Ainge et al 1969)

Notes

Luxol fast blue is one of the copper phthalocyanin dyes (along with alcian blue and methasol fast blue), and has a strong affinity for phospholipids and choline bases; hence its affinity for myelin. It is a popular method because routinely fixed, paraffin-processed sections can be successfully stained a pleasing colour. The following modification has the twin advantages of simplicity and short staining times. Luxol fast blue staining can be followed by oil red O or similar dye, to show degenerate myelin in a contrasting colour.

Staining solution

Luxol fast blue MBS	0.1 g
Methanol	100 ml
1.5 M hydrochloric acid	0.5 ml

Mix and filter (should a precipitate occur following filtration using a standard Whatman No. 1 filter paper, it will be necessary to re-filter through a finer No. 42).
0.05% aqueous lithium carbonate (a saturated solution diluted 1:20 will serve)
1% aqueous neutral red

Technique

1. Paraffin or frozen sections to water.
2. Stain in Luxol fast blue for 1 h at room temperature.
3. Wash in water.
4. Differentiate in lithium carbonate solution for 20 s or so until the background is clear.
5. Wash in water. Counterstain in 1% aqueous neutral red for 5 min.
6. Wash in water. Dehydrate and differentiate the neutral red in alcohol, clear and mount as desired.

Results

Red blood cells, myelin	blue to purple, depending on the amount of counterstain remaining
Nuclei and Nissl substance	red
Background	colourless

SOLOCHROME CYANINE TECHNIQUE (Page 1965, 1970)

Notes

This method is both simple and quick, and has the advantage, unlike Luxol fast blue that also stains collagen, of being equally suitable for PNS or CNS myelin demonstration in paraffin sections. The finished result tends to be rather more delicate than that of the Loyez or Luxol fast blue techniques. Fresh frozen sections can be stained with this technique and should be finally mounted in an aqueous mountant for best results.

Staining solution

Add 0.5 ml conc. sulphuric acid to 0.2 g solochrome cyanine RS in a flask. Stir well with a glass rod until the dye goes into solution. Add 96 ml distilled water and 4 ml 10% aqueous iron alum. Mix and filter; the solution keeps well.
10% aqueous iron alum
1% aqueous neutral red

Technique

1. Paraffin sections to water.

2. Treat with the solochrome cyanine solution for 10–20 min.
3. Wash well in running water.
4. Differentiate in the iron alum solution for 10–30 min until the background and nuclei lose the stain (the myelin will be relatively unaffected).
5. Wash in running water for several minutes.
6. Counterstain with the neutral red solution for 5 min (van Gieson's stain, see p. 36) is an alternative counterstain and will intensify the myelin staining effect).
7. Differentiate the counterstain and dehydrate in alcohol. Clear and mount as desired.

Results

Red blood cells, myelin, muscle	blue
Nuclei, Nissl substance	red
Background	colourless

DEGENERATE MYELIN

Certain methods may be used to demonstrate relatively early degeneration when the period of survival of the patient between occurrence of the lesion and death does not exceed 60–80 days. In such a period the degeneration products may be found in situ. From 75–250 days survival the products will be intracellular (microglial cells). After 250 days there are unlikely to be demonstrable degeneration products.

The original and well-known technique for early myelin degeneration is that of Marchi & Algeri (1885) although this is rather prone to artefacts (the so-called 'pseudo-granulations'), and the Swank & Davenport (1935) variant is considered superior (Fraser 1972). Another technique, the Busch (1898) has given good results in our hands and will also be presented. After 75 days, intracellular degeneration material can be shown with one of the oil-soluble dyes as previously mentioned, either following Luxol fast blue staining for normal myelin, or silver techniques for microglia. The sudanophilic intracellular material is rich in cholesterol esters. Whatever the method chosen, the occurrence of artefact, i.e. false positive material, will be considerably reduced by minimizing trauma to the gross material. In other words, handle the untreated tissue with care.

MARCHI-TYPE TECHNIQUES

SWANK–DAVENPORT TECHNIQUE (Swank & Davenport 1935)

Notes

The rationale of the method is that the tissue is treated with an oxidant, in this case potassium chlorate, in the presence of osmium tetroxide. Normal myelin is readily oxidized and will not subsequently reduce osmium tetroxide. Early degenerate myelin contains oleic acid that is not oxidized and is able to reduce the osmium tetroxide to lower black oxides. Degenerate myelin is shown black against a relatively colourless background. According to Adams (1958) the rationale depends on the hydrophilic normal myelin lipids being permeable and preferentially reducing the potassium chlorate rather than the osmium tetroxide. In degenerate myelin the hydrophobic cholesterol esters are impermeable to potassium chlorate, permitting reduction of the osmium tetroxide that is absorbed.

Solutions

1% potassium chlorate
Impregnating solution:

1% aqueous osmium tetroxide	20 ml
1% aqueous potassium chlorate	60 ml
Conc. formalin	12 ml
Conc. acetic acid	1 ml

Technique

1. Take thin (3 mm) slices of formalin-fixed tissue and leave in aqueous potassium chlorate solution for 10–75 min.
2. Transfer to the impregnating solution for 7–10 days in the dark (turn blocks frequently).
3. Wash in running water for 24 h.
4. Cut either frozen or paraffin sections. If the paraffin process is used, deparaffinize in xylene before mounting in Canada balsam (cut at 10 μm thickness).

Results

Degenerate myelin	black
Background	yellow

BUSCH TECHNIQUE (Busch 1898)

Notes

This method is similar in result to the Swank–Davenport technique but gives a lighter background. The rationale is the same, except in this case the oxidant is sodium iodate.

Solution

Sodium iodate	3 g
Osmium tetroxide	1 g
Distilled water	300 ml

Technique

1. Take thin (3 mm) blocks of formalin-fixed tissue, wash in running water for several hours.
2. Treat with the impregnating solution for 5–7 days in the dark.
3. Wash in running water overnight.
4. Paraffin process and cut 10 μm thick sections. Deparaffinize and mount in Canada balsam.

Results

Myelin	black
Background	almost colourless

NEUROGLIA

Strictly speaking there are only four types of neuroglial cells; these are derived from the neuroectoderm—fibrous astrocytes, protoplasmic astrocytes, oligodendrocytes and ependymal cells. There is a fifth cell that is commonly found in CNS tissue which, although of mesenchymal origin, has similar morphology and is demonstrated by similar techniques. This cell has various names—the Gitter cell, rod cell or, as it is more popularly known, the microglial cell.

Astrocytes possess, as their name implies, many processes and have a supportive and nutritive function. The oligodendrocytes are small cells with few processes and are concerned with myelin formation. The ependymal cells line the ventricles of the brain and choroid plexus, and vary from flattened to cuboidal, from ciliated to non-ciliated in form. Ependymal cells are of little significance from a pathological or demonstration point of view and will not be considered further. The microglial cells are small cells with a typically elongated body having short processes; their function is like the reticulo-endothelial-type connective tissue cells in that they are phagocytic.

In an H&E preparation neuroglial cells are not shown to great advantage as the processes are not seen. It is usually the nuclei that are to be discerned and only the experienced worker can say with any certainty which nucleus belongs to which type of cell. It will be found that the astrocytes have a medium-sized spherical vesicular-type nucleus, the oligodendrocytes have a small semi-pyknotic nucleus (not unlike that of a lymphocyte) whilst microglia have a small vesicular nucleus that is typically kidney-shaped in appearance. For fixation it is safe to use formalin, although for the Cajal and Hortega techniques formal-ammonium-bromide solution is considered to give superior results. The tissue should be fresh for best results.

Besides the techniques to be described, there is the PTAH method that demonstrates the processes rather than the cell bodies, aslo Anderson's Victoria blue technique and many modifications of the Hortega technique. We propose to confine ourselves to those techniques with which we have experienced good results—see Table 15.3. For further details regarding the neuroglia and their demonstration, the reader may like to consult Cox (1973). Astrocytic processes exhibit a weak birefringence that is attributed to the presence of a myosin-like protein.

Table 15.3 Demonstration of glial elements

Technique	Element demonstrated
PTAH	Astrocyte processes
Holzer	Astrocytes and processes
Cajal	Astrocytes and processes
Scharanberg (mod. of Hortega)	Astrocytes and processes
Weil & Davenport	Oligodendroglia and microglia
Marshall (mod. of Weil & Davenport)	Oligodendroglia and microglia
Penfield (mod. of Hortega)	Oligodendroglia and microglia
Naoumenko & Feigin	Microglia

ASTROCYTES

The following techniques are said to demonstrate both types of astrocytes. We find it difficult to distinguish between them, but a useful guide to the identification of protoplasmic astrocytes is the greater branching of their processes compared to fibrous astrocytes.

CAJAL'S GOLD-SUBLIMATE TECHNIQUE (Cajal 1913, 1916)

Notes

This is probably the best-known technique for neuroglia and although it does not give the clarity of 'staining' of some of the Hortega techniques it is reasonably reliable. We prefer to use yellow gold chloride as opposed to brown gold chloride as on occasion we have experienced better results with the former substance. Fixation is best carried out in FAB (formal-ammonium-bromide) or, if already fixed in formalin, the cut sections may be treated with ammonia-hydrobromic acid ('bromuration' treatment).

Solutions

FAB fixative

Formalin	15 ml
Ammonium bromide	2 g
Distilled water	85 ml

1% ammonia
5% aqueous hydrobromic acid
Gold chloride-sublimate
   Add 0.5 g mercuric chloride to 60 ml distilled water and gently warm to dissolve.
   Add 10 ml 1% aqueous yellow gold chloride and mix. Prepare fresh before use.
5% aqueous sodium thiosulphate (hypo)

Technique

1. Fix thin slices of fresh tissue in the FAB fixative for 24 h at 37°C. Cut thin (15–25 μm) frozen sections and place in 1% formalin. Alternatively, cut frozen sections from formalin-fixed tissue and leave in 1% ammonia overnight at room temperature. Transfer direct to hydrobromic acid for 1 h at 37°C. Wash in three short changes of distilled water.
2. Place several sections flat in the gold chloride-sublimate for 4–8 h at room temperature in the dark, removing sections at varying intervals (4 h will often suffice). Impregnation is usually complete when the sections turn a deep purple macroscopically.
3. Rinse in distilled water for several min.
4. Fix in hypo for 5 min. Wash in water.
5. Dehydrate, clear and mount in Canada balsam.

Results

Astrocytes and their processes	purple to black
Neurones and their processes	varying shades of grey to light purple

HOLZER TECHNIQUE (Holzer 1921)

Notes

Good results are given by this method with abnormal astrocytic proliferation (gliosis) in paraffin sections, particularly when demonstrating long-term (8 weeks or more) lesions. Normal CNS sections tend to be unspectacular and show neuroglial fibres poorly. The rationale is obscure although presumably the potassium bromide acts as a 'trapping agent' for the previously applied dye. Helly's fixation gives improved results even when used as a secondary fixative.

Solutions

Alcoholic phosphomolybdic acid solution:

0.5% aqueous phosphomolybdic acid	10 ml
95% alcohol	20 ml

Alcohol-chloroform solution:

Ethanol	2 ml
Chloroform	8 ml

Staining solution
 0.5% crystal violet in alcohol-chloroform solution.
10% aqueous potassium bromide

Differentiator:

Aniline oil	6 ml
Chloroform	9 ml
25% ammonia	1 drop

Technique

1. 10 μm paraffin sections to water.
2. Treat with the alcoholic phosphomolybdic acid solution for 3 min.
3. Drain slide and flood with the alcohol-chloroform solution.
4. Drain slide and stain with the crystal violet solution for 30 s.
5. Rinse quickly in the alcohol-chloroform solution then take through absolute alcohol and 95% alcohol to distilled water.
6. Treat with the potassium bromide solution for 1 min.
7. Wash in distilled water and blot dry.
8. Differentiate in the aniline solution until the neuroglial fibres only are blue-purple.
9. Dehydrate, clear and mount as desired.

Results

Neuroglial fibres (mainly astrocytic)	deep blue-purple
Background	light purple

SCHARANBERG'S 'TRIPLE HORTEGA' (Scharanberg 1954)

Notes

This method is a variant of the Hortega technique for astrocytes and is sometimes known as the 'triple Hortega' due to the impregnation employed. The results given by this technique can be good regarding clarity for neuroglial demonstration and we would rate the results superior to those obtained with the better known Cajal gold-sublimate technique. Either FAB fixation or the bromuration treatment is applied.

Solutions

Sensitizer:

2% aqueous silver nitrate	50 ml
Pyridine	20 drops

Silver carbonate

To 10 ml 10% aqueous silver nitrate add 30 ml of 5% aqueous sodium carbonate. Mix, add conc. ammonia, mixing until the formed precipitate is just dissolved. Make up to a total volume of 70 ml with distilled water.

Ammoniacal silver

Add conc. ammonia to 20% aqueous solution of silver nitrate with frequent mixing, until the formed precipitate is just dissolved.

10% formalin in tap water

5% aqueous sodium thiosulphate(hypo)

Technique

1. 15–20 μm frozen sections to distilled water.
2. Treat with the silver nitrate-pyridine solution for 15 min at 60°C.
3. Drain and transfer direct to the silver carbonate solution to which have been added 20 drops of pyridine. Allow to stand for 15 min at 60°C.
4. Drain and transfer direct to the ammoniacal silver solution for 5 min at room temperature (this stage may sometimes be omitted without affecting the final result).
5. Reduce in the 1% formalin for 2–3 min.
6. Wash in water and tone if desired in 0.2% gold chloride for 2 min.
7. Wash in water and fix in hypo for 5 min.
8. Wash in water and mount the section on a slide. Blot dry.
9. Dehydrate, clear and mount as desired.

Results

Both types of astrocyte and their processes	black
Background	purple-red

OLIGODENDROCYTES AND MICROGLIA

As a rule both types of cell are demonstrated concomitantly by the popular techniques in this group. Oligodendrocyte fibres, in particular, are not easily visualized in normal human material, being best seen in proliferative lesions in animal tissue such as cat. The two techniques presented are similar; one of these, Marshall's, is a variant of the Weil & Davenport method. Each technique has something to offer as will be discussed.

WEIL & DAVENPORT TECHNIQUE (Weil & Davenport 1933)

Notes

Good demonstration of both oligodendrocytes and microglia is given by this technique, with usually a reasonably clear background. It is sometimes possible to demonstrate sparse oligodendrocytic processes in normal human material. Better results are obtained if toning is omitted. Conventional formalin fixation is satisfactory.

Solutions

Ammoniacal silver
   To 2–3 ml concentrated ammonia add 10% aqueous silver nitrate with mixing until the solution becomes slightly opalescent (usually 18 ml or so).
15% formalin
5% aqueous sodium thiosulphate (hypo)

Technique

1. 15 μm frozen or 5 μm paraffin sections to distilled water; give several changes.
2. Treat with the ammoniacal silver solution for 15–20 s.
3. Drain and transfer direct to the formalin and gently agitate until the sections turn a coffee brown colour (usually several minutes).
4. Rinse well in distilled water. Fix in hypo for 5 min and wash in water.
5. Mount on a slide, blot. Dehydrate, clear and mount as desired.

Results

Oligodendrocytes, microglia	black (astrocytes are also impregnated but to a less well-marked degree)
Background	yellow-brown

MARSHALL'S TECHNIQUE (Marshall 1948)

Notes

Whilst oligodendrocytes are also shown by this technique, it is the microglia that are well-demonstrated although the background is usually rather 'dirtier' than that of the preceeding technique. Formalin fixation is suitable and both paraffin and frozen sections can be used. Better results are said to be obtained if the frozen sections are left in 10% ammonia overnight, before carrying out the technique.

Solutions

Ammoniacal silver
   To 2 ml of concentrated ammonia add 5% aqueous silver nitrate until a slight opalescence is obtained.
3% formalin
0.2 aqueous gold chloride
5% sodium thiosulphate (hypo)

Technique

1. 15–20 μm frozen or 5 μm paraffin sections to distilled water; the paraffin sections should be loose (unmounted).
2. Treat with the ammoniacal silver solution for 4–5 s.
3. Transfer sections to the formalin and agitate for approximately 30 s until they are a reddish brown colour.
4. Wash well in distilled water. Tone in the gold chloride, this will help clear the background.
5. Wash in water and fix in hypo for 5 min. Wash in water and mount on a slide.
6. Blot, dehydrate, clear and mount as desired.

Results

Oligodendrocytes, microglia and,
to a lesser degree, astrocytes   black

PENFIELD'S MODIFICATION OF THE HORTEGA TECHNIQUE FOR OLIGODENDROGLIA AND MICROGLIA (Penfield 1928)

Notes

This is one of the classic methods for oligodendroglia and microglia, both cells being demonstrated so that distinction is made on morphological grounds. Formalin ammonium bromide fixation is preferred, although formalin fixation followed by hydrobromic acid treatment of the sections will give acceptable results. The impregnating solution is a silver carbonate one, in contrast to the silver hydroxide solution normally employed in histological silver methods.

Solutions

1% ammonia
5% aqueous hydrobromic acid ('bromurator')
5% aqueous sodium carbonate
Impregnating solution:

10% aqueous silver nitrate	5 ml
5% aqueous sodium carbonate	20 ml

Mix, and add conc. ammonia drop by drop with frequent mixing until the formed precipitate is *almost* re-dissolved. Make up to a 75 ml volume with distilled water and filter.

1% formalin
0.2% aqueous gold chloride
5% aqueous sodium thiosulphate (hypo)

Technique

1. Place free-floating frozen sections in the weak ammonia solution overnight at room temperature.
2. Transfer direct to the hydrobromic acid solution for 1 h at 37°C.
3. Wash sections in three changes of distilled water (several minutes in each).
4. Sensitize in the sodium carbonate solution for 1 h at room temperature.
5. Drain slide and place in the impregnating solution for 3–5 min or until sections are a light brown colour.
6. Reduce in the formalin solution with gentle agitation; the sections should turn a uniform grey colour. This will usually take 1–2 min.
7. Wash in water, and tone if desired in gold chloride for 1–2 min.
8. Wash in water and fix in hypo for 1–2 min.
9. Wash in water, mount sections on slides, blot well, dehydrate, clear and mount as desired.

Results

Oligodendroglia and microglia	black
Background	light grey

NAOUMENKO & FEIGIN TECHNIQUE FOR NEUROGLIA
(Naoumenko & Feigin 1962)

Notes

This is virtually a modification of a Hortega silver technique and demonstrates microglia rather than oligodendroglia. To avoid loss of sections from the slide during the technique they should be mounted using a section adhesive. Either formalin or formalin-ammonium-bromide fixed tissue can be used.

Solutions

Impregnating solution:

20% aqueous silver nitrate	25 ml
5% aqueous sodium carbonate	200 ml

Mix, and add concentrated ammonia drop by drop with constant mixing, until the formed precipitate re-dissolves but the solution remains very faintly turbid. Filter before use.

3% hydrochloric acid
5% aqueous sodium carbonate
0.2% formalin in distilled water
0.2% aqueous gold chloride
5% aqueous sodium thiosulphate (hypo)

Technique

1. 15–20 μm thick paraffin sections to distilled water, washing well in several changes of same.
2. Treat sections with the hydrochloric acid solution for 12 h.
3. Rinse briefly (one quick dip) in each of two jars of distilled water.
4. Place sections in the sodium carbonate solution for 2 h.
5. Place sections in the impregnating solution for 1 min.
6. Drain slide and place in two changes of the dilute formalin solution, agitating until the section is a light brown-grey colour (this takes approximately 10 s in each change).
7. Wash well in distilled water.
8. Tone in gold chloride for 1 min, wash and fix in hypo for 1 min.
9. Wash in water, dehydrate, clear and mount in Canada balsam.

Results

    Microglia   black

PERIPHERAL NERVOUS SYSTEM (PNS)

The demonstration of peripheral nerve fibres, both myelinated and non-myelinated, and nerve endings is something of a specialized art and there are more than a few techniques to be considered. A major point is that techniques that are successful on purely CNS material may well not be successful when dealing with PNS material. This is largely because various other tissues, such as muscle and collagen, may also stain strongly, a complication that does not arise to any extent in CNS tissue.

Formalin fixation, preferably lengthy, is usually satisfactory for most PNS methods although osmium tetroxide-containing fixatives are of use when dealing with myelinated fibres. Prompt fixation in formalin is to be aimed at, except for muscle, which should be allowed to stand for at least 30 min at room temperature before fixing. This will prevent artefacts due to muscular contraction. Besides the techniques to be described there are others such as the solochrome cyanine (see p. 353) and the traditional Ranvier (1889). For futher discussion and details on PNS techniques, see Page (1970, 1971) and Bone (1972).

SCHOFIELD TECHNIQUE FOR NERVE ENDINGS IN MUSCLE AND SKIN (Schofield 1960)

Notes

Although peripheral nerve fibres are also demonstrated, it is the delineation of motor end plates in muscle that is the forte of this technique. Like most silver methods it can be capricious, and it is as well to take through several sections of the same material to enable a subsequent choice to be made. Prolonged formalin fixation gives better results.

Solutions

20% aqueous silver nitrate

10% formalin in tap water.
Ammoniacal silver
   Add concentrated ammonia with mixing to 20% aqueous silver nitrate until the
   formed precipitate is almost dissolved.
5% aqueous sodium thiosulphate (hypo)

Technique

   1. Thick (50–80 μm) formalin-fixed frozen sections to distilled water.
   2. Leave overnight at 37°C in 50% alcohol to which are added 15 drops of
      pyridine per 50 ml volume.
   3. Rinse in two changes of distilled water.
   4. Place in the silver nitrate solution for 15 min at room temperature in the
      dark.
   5. Take up the sections on a glass rod and gently blot dry.
   6. Take sections through three baths of the 10% formalin solution for
      10–15 s in each (change solution for each new section).
   7. Repeat, but use three baths of 2% formalin.
   8. Rinse in two changes of distilled water.
   9. Treat with the ammoniacal silver solution for 30–60 s. Should the
      eventual result be too weak the temperature of the solution may
      profitably be raised to 27°C.
  10. Take up the sections on a glass rod and gently blot dry.
  11. Treat with 1% formalin, agitate for approximately 1 min until the
      sections appear a dark brown colour.
  12. Wash in water, fix in hypo for 5 min.
  13. Wash in water, mount sections on a glass slide. Blot dry, dehydrate,
      clear and mount as desired.

Results

Motor end plates in muscle, nerve endings in skin and nerve fibres	black
Background	yellow-brown

GROS–BIELSCHOWSKY TECHNIQUE FOR CELLOIDIN AND FROZEN SECTIONS

Notes

This popular technique can show inconsistent results and it is important to leave
the sections in the initial silver nitrate solution until they are a light brown in colour.
When transferring sections from the formalin bath to the ammoniacal silver, the
amount of formalin carried over will influence the degree of silver blackening. If the
final impregnation is too weak a repeat section carrying over more of the formalin
may prove successful.

Solutions

20% aqueous silver nitrate
20% formalin in tap water

10% ammonia
1% acetic acid
Ammoniacal silver

   Slowly add concentrated ammonia to 15 ml of 20% aqueous silver nitrate with frequent mixing until the resultant precipitate just dissolves. Add a further 15 drops of concentrated ammonia and mix.

0.2% aqueous gold chloride
5% aqueous sodium thiosulphate (hypo)

Technique

1. Frozen sections to distilled water, washing well in several changes of same.
2. Treat with 20% silver nitrate for 20–60 min in the dark at room temperature.
3. Transfer sections to 20% formalin. Give several changes over 5 min.
4. Transfer sections to the ammoniacal silver solution and observe the silver impregnation microscopically using a low power objective. When the nerve fibres are black against a reasonably clear background (up to 10 min) transfer the sections to 10% ammonia for 5 min to halt impregnation.
5. Wash in 1% acetic for a few minutes, tone in gold chloride for 1–2 min. Wash in water then fix in hypo for 5 min.
6. Dehydrate, clear and mount in Canada balsam.

Results

Nerve fibres, etc.	black
Background	often a grey colour

MODIFIED WINKLEMANN & SCHMIT TECHNIQUE FOR FROZEN SECTIONS (Winklemann & Schmit 1957)

Notes

The main advantages of this technique lie in its simplicity and the fact that it may be used for PNS as well as CNS tissue. Unfortunately, it does tend to produce a rather 'dirty' background. Formalin or Bouin fixation is suitable.

Solutions

20% aqueous silver nitrate
0.2% hydroquinone in 1% aqueous sodium carbonate (prepare fresh)
0.2% aqueous gold chloride
5% aqueous sodium thiosulphate (hypo)

Technique

1. 15–20 μm frozen sections to distilled water. Wash in three changes, each of 10 min.
2. Treat with the silver nitrate solution for 20 min.
3. Take sections through three dishes of distilled water for 1 s in each.
4. Treat with the hydroquinone reducer for 5 min.

5. Wash in water, tone in gold chloride for 2 min.
6. Wash in water, treat with hypo for 5 min. Wash in water, mount on a slide.
7. Dehydrate, clear and mount in Canada balsam.

Results

Nerve fibres, etc.	black
Background	grey

GLEES & MARSLAND TECHNIQUE (Marsland et al 1954)

Notes

Although this method for paraffin sections is prone to be capricious it can give excellent results. It is worthwhile taking through several duplicate sections and positive control sections of CNS material. The sections must be celloidinized using 1% celloidin to give a thick protective coat. This is done not just to keep the sections on the slide but so that, when the celloidin coat is removed at the conclusion of the technique, much of the background silver precipitation will be removed also. Without this precaution, it would be very difficult to pick out tissues such as nerve fibres against the very heavy background that occurs in a successful impregnation. Toning helps suppress a heavy background, but we prefer not to tone if possible as, without it, a clearer distinction can be made between nervous elements and collagen. Both PNS and CNS material can be demonstrated.

Solutions

20% aqueous silver nitrate
10% formalin in tap water
Ammoniacal silver
   To 15 ml of 20% aqueous silver nitrate add 10 ml of ethanol, mix. Add concentrated ammonia, with mixing, until the formed precipitate is almost dissolved (usually 40–45 drops). Finally add two drops of ammonia and mix.
0.2% aqueous gold chloride (optional)
5% aqueous sodium thiosulphate (hypo)

Technique

1. Paraffin sections to alcohol, cover with a thick celloidin film (use a 1% solution in ether-alcohol), and harden in water for up to 5 min.
2. Rinse in several changes of distilled water then place in the 20% silver nitrate solution at 56°C (pre-heated) until the sections turn a light brown colour: this may take from 20 min to 1 h but is essential to the reaction.
3. Rinse in distilled water.
4. Treat with two changes of the formalin for 10 s each.
5. Drain the slide and treat with the ammoniacal silver solution for 30 s.
6. Drain the slide and treat with two changes of the formalin for 1 min each. The sections should turn a black-brown colour. If sufficient impregnation fails to occur rinse the slide well in distilled water and go back to Step 5, repeating the impregnation-reduction step.

7. Wash in water, tone in gold chloride if desired for 2 min.
8. Wash in water, fix in hypo for 5 min.
9. Wash in water, dehydrate in alcohol, remove the celloidin film in ether-alcohol. Clear and mount as desired.

Results

Nerve fibres, etc.	black
Background (ideally)	yellow-brown if untoned

PALMGREN TECHNIQUE FOR PERIPHERAL NERVE FIBRES
(Palmgren 1948)

Notes

This is a popular technique for the demonstration of nerve fibres in paraffin sections. As with most silver methods for nervous system constituents, practice and perseverance are necessary to achieve really good results. To this end, it is advisable to take through several test sections so that slight variations in times of treatment can be achieved and afford a measure of choice of result. In common with the Glees & Marsland technique for nerve fibres in paraffin sections (see p. 366) it is advisable to pre-celloidinize the section thoroughly. This will minimize background silver deposition when the celloidin film is ultimately removed.

Solutions

Acidic formalin:

Formalin	25 ml
Distilled water	75 ml
1% nitric acid	0.2 ml

Silver solution:

Silver nitrate	15 g
Potassium nitrate	10 g
Distilled water	100 ml
5% aqueous glycine	1 ml

Reducer:

Pyrogallic acid	10 g
Distilled water	450 ml
Absolute ethanol	550 ml
1% nitric acid	2 ml

Allow to stand 24 h prior to use.

Toning bath:

Gold chloride	1 g
Distilled water	200 ml
Glacial acetic acid	0.2 ml

Intensifier:

50% ethanol	100 ml
Aniline oil	2 drops

Fixing bath

5% aqueous sodium thiosulphate (hypo).

Technique

1. Celloidinize paraffin sections and take to distilled water.
2. Wash sections in the acidic formalin for at least 5 min.
3. Wash in three changes of distilled water over 5 min.
4. Place in the silver solution for 15 min at room temperature or 4–5 min at 35°C.
5. Drain the slide and place in the reducer that has been heated to 40–45°C, agitate gently and leave for 1 min. The sections should be yellow-brown in colour.
6. Rinse in 50% alcohol for 5–10 s then in three changes of distilled water.
7. Examine microscopically; if there is insufficient impregnation repeat the procedure from the acidic formalin stage, but reduce the time in the silver solution and the temperature of the reducer to 30°C.
8. Tone in the gold chloride solution until the yellow brown colour has faded (several minutes).
9. Drain and place into the intensifier for 15 s.
10. Wash in water, fix in hypo for a few seconds.
11. Wash again in water, dehydrate, clear and mount as desired.

Results

Nerve fibres	black
Background	grey

LINDER'S TECHNIQUE FOR PERIPHERAL NERVES IN PARAFFIN SECTIONS (Linder 1978)

Notes

This is a highly recommended technique for nerve fibres in PNS. Mineralized tissue that has been decalcified in EDTA or formic acid may also be used. When preparing the physical developer working solution, it is important to stir constantly, as otherwise a white precipitate will form.

Solutions

Buffer stock solution:

2.4.6. collidine	6.6 ml
Distilled water	450 ml

Adjust to pH 7.2–7.4 with 10% nitric acid and make up to a total volume of 500 ml with distilled water.

Buffer working solution:

Stock solution	8 ml
Distilled water	92 ml

Impregnating solution:

Distilled water heated to 60°C	84 ml
1% aqueous silver nitrate	4 ml
0.38% aqueous sodium cyanate	4 ml
Buffer stock solution	8 ml

Add, with mixing, the constituents in the order indicated.

Physical developer stock solution:

Sodium sulphite (hydrated)	20 g
Sodium tetraborate	4.75 g
Distilled water	450 ml

Heat the solution to approximately 50°C and add 10 g leaf gelatin.

Physical developer working solution:

Stock solution	95 ml
2% aqueous hydroquinone	5 ml
1% aqueous silve nitrate	2 ml

Technique

1. Paraffin sections to water, celloidinizing en route in the usual way.
2. Place in diluted buffer: soft tissue 10–20 min at 60°C; decalcified tissue overnight at 40–45°C.
3. Drain and transfer slides to the silver impregnating solution: soft tissue 10–30 min at 60°C; decalcified tissue 90 min at 40–45°C.
4. Wash in several changes of distilled water over 3 min.
5. Place sections into the physical developer working solution at approximately 25°C. Leave in the solution until optimal results are achieved by washing with distilled water at intervals and examining microscopically.
6. Wash in distilled water, dehydrate, clear and mount as desired.

Results

Nerve fibres, melanin, carcinoid tumour granules   black

SUDAN BLACK FOR NERVE ENDINGS IN MUSCLE (Cavanagh et al 1964)

Notes

Myelinated nerve fibres of muscle are well-shown by this simple lipid-staining method. Muscle fixed for 2 days in formalin is ideal (allow initial 30 min for muscle fibres to relax before fixing).

Staining solution

Saturated Sudan black B in 70% alcohol. Filter before use.

Technique

1. Thick (80 μm) frozen sections into water.
2. Wash in 70% alcohol for 1 min.
3. Stain with the Sudan black (pre-heated) solution for 30 min at 37°C.
4. Rinse in three changes of 50% alcohol for 2 min each.
5. Wash in water. Mount in an aqueous mountant.

Results

Myelinated axons (also fat globules and red blood cells)	blue-black
Muscle	weak blue-black to colourless

METHYLENE BLUE TECHNIQUE FOR MUSCLE (Coers & Woolf 1959)

Notes

The principle of this technique is one of supravital staining in the presence of oxygen. The staining effect is subsequently fixed by treatment with ammonium molybdate. Both Page (1971) and Bone (1972) have made recommendations regarding the procedure of the technique and their papers should be consulted in the event of any difficulty. Tissues can be left in the ammonium molybdate solution at 40°C for several days, if it is not possible to continue with the technique the following day.

Solutions

0.015% methylene blue in normal saline (supplied in 20 ml ampoules)
8% aqueous ammonium molybdate

Technique

1. The muscle biopsy is laid out on cork so that the fibres are longitudinally placed, and pinned at each end.
2. Using a fine-bore needle inject the dye solution into and along the muscle fibres so that they are thoroughly suffused and until the dye solution runs out of the cut ends of the muscle fibres. Use ample solution.
3. Moisten the tissue with normal saline and lay flat on Kleenex tissue. Oxygenate the tissue by placing in a stream of oxygen for 1 h at a rate of 4 litres per min.
4. Place in the ammonium molybdate solution overnight at 4°C.
5. Wash in several changes of distilled water over 30 min.
6. Dissect out into fine fibres and place as flat as possible on a glass slide. Cover with another glass slide.
7. Squash by placing under a heavy weight (7kg) for 1 h.
8. Place the slides into 70% alcohol for a few minutes, then remove the top slide and complete the dehydration in absolute alcohol. Clear and mount in a DPX-type mountant.

Results

Nerve fibres (sensory and motor) and their endings in muscle and skin	blue
Nuclei	dark blue
Background muscle	weak blue

IMMUNOCYTOCHEMISTRY

As with other facets of histological demonstration technology, neuropathology has felt the impact of immunocytochemistry. This impact has been especially significant in terms of neuroglial cells and their tumours. The most important antiserum in this context is to glial fibrillary acidic protein (GFAP) which has proved popular at the expense of the traditional silver/gold salt techniques for neuroglia. GFAP is found in normal astrocytes, ependyma and immature oligodendrocytes and, pathologically, in gliomas. These include astrocytomas and oligodendrogliomas. Another important, albeit less used, antiserum is to neurofilament protein, which can be demonstrated immunocytochemically in nerve fibres of the CNS and PNS. Diagnostically, it can be used to identify tumours such as the neuroblastoma, medulloblastoma and paraganglioma.

There are other antisera worthy of note in this field. S100 is a marker for Schwann cells and of value for demonstrating both benign and malignant tumours arising from them. Neurone-specific enolase (NSE) and synaptophysin are present in neurons, axons and paraganglia. In terms of CNS/PNS pathology these last two immunocytochemical markers can be used to identify a similar range of tumours to those shown by anti-neurofilament protein.

REFERENCES

Adams C W M 1958 Histochemical mechanisms of the Marchi reaction for degenerating myelin. Journal of Neurochemistry 2: 178

Ainge G, Cook J L, Gisby P R 1969 Rapid staining of myelin in paraffin sections with Luxol Fast Blue MBS. Journal of Medical Laboratory Technology 26: 231–232

Bielschowsky M 1904 Die Silberimprägnation der Neurofibrillen. Journal für Psychologie und Neurologie 3: 169

Bone Q 1972 Some notes on histological methods for peripheral nerves. Medical Laboratory Technology 29: 319–324

Busch J M 1898 Ueber eine Farbungsmethode sekundarer Degenerationen der Nervensystems mit Osmiumsaure. Neurol Zeitbl. 17: 476

Cajal S, Ramon Y 1913 Sobre un nuevo proceder de impregnacion de la neuroglia y sus resultados en los centros nerviosos del Lombre y animales. Travaux du laboratoire de recherches biologiques de l'université de Madrid 11: 219

Cajal S, Ramon Y 1916 El preceder de oro-sublimado para la coloracion de la neuroglia. Travaux du laboratoire de recherches biologiques de l'université de Madrid 14: 155

Cavanagh J B, Passingham R J, Vogt J A 1964 Staining of sensory and motor nerves in muscles with Sudan black B. Journal of Pathology and Bacteriology 88: 89

Chalk B T C 1970 Personal communication

Coers C, Woolf A L 1959 The innervation of the muscle. Blackwell, Oxford

Cox G 1973 Neuroglia and microglia. In: Cook H C (ed) Selected topics. Bailliere Tindall, London

Cox W 1891 Impregnation des centralen Nervensystem mit Quecksilbersalzen. Archiv für mikroskopische Anatomie 37: 16–21

Drury R A B, Wallington E A 1980 Carleton's Histological technique, 5th edn. Oxford University Press, Oxford

Fraser F J 1972 Degenerating myelin: comparative histochemical studies using classical myelin stains and an improved Marchi technique minimising artefacts. Stain Technology 47: 147–154

Golgi C 1878 Rc. 1st Lomb. Sci. Lett. 2nd series 12: 5

Gothard E 1898 Quelques modifications au procede de Nissl, pour la coloration elective des cellules nerveuses. C. R. Seanc. Soc. 69: 530

Holzer W 1921 Uber eine neue Methode der Gliafases Farbung. Zentralblatt für die gesamte Neurologie and psychiatrie 69: 354–460

Kawamura S, Niimi K 1972 Counterstaining of Nanta-Gyaz impregnated sections with Cresyl Violet. Stain Technology 47: 1–6

Kluver H, Barrera A 1953 A method for the combined staining of cells and fibres of the nervous system. Journal of Neuropathology and Experimental Neurology 12: 400

Kultschitzky N 1889 Uber eine neue Methode der Hamatoxylin-Farbung. Anat. Anz. 4: 223

Linder J E 1978 A simple and reliable method for the silver impregnation of soft or mineralized tissues. Journal of Anatomy 127: 534

Loyez M 1910 Coloration des fibres nerveuse par la methode a l'hematoxyline au fer apres inclusion a las celloidine. Compte rendu des seances de la Societe de Biologie 69: 511

Marchi V, Algeri G 1885 Sulle degenerazioni discendenti consecutive a lesioni della corteccia cerebrale. Riv. sper. Freniat. Med. leg. Alien. ment. 11: 492

Marshall A H E 1948 A method for the demonstration of reticulo-endothelial cells in paraffin sections. Journal of Pathology and Bacteriology LX: 3

Marsland T A, Glees P, Erickson L B 1954 Modification of the Glees silver impregnation for paraffin sections. Journal of Neuropathology and Experimental Neurology 13: 587

Min Chueh Chang 1935 Formal-thionin method for fixation and staining of nerve cells and fiber tracts. Anatomical Record 65: 437–441

Naoumenko J, Feigin U 1962 A modification for paraffin sections of silver carbonate impregnation for microglia. Acta Neuropathologica 2: 402–406

Page K M 1965 A stain for myelin using solochrome cyanin. Journal of Medical Laboratory Technology 22: 224

Page K M 1970 Histological methods for peripheral nerves. Part I. Journal of Medical Laboratory Technology 27: 1

Page K M 1971 Histological methods for peripheral nerves. Part II. Medical Laboratory Technology 28: 58

Pal J 1886 Ein Beitrag zur Nervenfarbe Technik. Medizinische Jahrbuechat 1: 619

Palmgren A 1948 A rapid method for selective silver staining of nerve fibres and nerve endings in mounted paraffin sections. Acta Zoologica 29: 377–392

Penfield W 1928 A method of staining oligodendroglia and microglia. American Journal of Pathology 4: 153

Ranvier L A 1889 Traite technique d'histologie, 2nd end. F Savy, Paris

Scharanberg K 1954 Blastomatous oligodendroglia as satellites of nerve cells: study with silver carbonate: American Journal of Pathology 30: 957–969

Schofield G C 1960 Experimental studies on the innervation of the mucous membranes of the gut. Brain 83: 490–514

Swank R L, Davenport H A 1935 Chlorate-osmic formalin method for degeneration myelin. Stain Technology 10: 87–90

von Braunmuhl A 1957 Hdbch. D. Spez. Pathol. Bd. XIII 1 A 337. Springer, Heidelberg

Weigert C 1885 Eine Verbesserung der Haematoxylin-Blutlaungensalzmethode für das Centralnervensystem. Fortschr. Med. 3: 236

Weil A, Davenport H E 1933 Staining of oligodendroglia and microglia in celloidin sections. Archives of Neurology and Psychiatry, Chicago 30: 175

Winklemann R V, Schmit R W 1957 A simple method for nerve axoplasm. Proceedings of the Staff Meetings, Mayo Clinic 32: 217

16. Specialized biopsies

THE RENAL BIOPSY

The development of a simple, safe technique for a needle biopsy of the kidney has resulted in an increase in our understanding of renal disease. The early renal biopsies were fixed in formalin, processed in the normal way, embedded in paraffin wax, cut at 5 μm and stained with haematoxylin and eosin. Latterly, sections were cut at 3 μm, the thinner section enabling greater glomerular detail to be obtained. Changes such as marginal increase in glomerular basement membrane thickening and slight hypercellularity of the glomerular tuft were more easily noticed, whereas they had been obscured in the thicker sections. A further advance in renal biopsy interpretation followed the development of cutting resin sections 1 μm thick. Special stains are used to demonstrate clearly certain components in the renal biopsy.

URGENT BIOPSIES

In cases of acute renal failure of unknown aetiology, the result of a renal biopsy is required within 24 hours. The needle biopsy is treated and processed as below.

1. Upon receipt in the laboratory, place the biopsy in fresh, pre-heated Carnoy's fixative (see p. 425) at 56°C for 45 min to 1 h.
2. Transfer to absolute alcohol and chloroform 1:1 at 56°C for 1 h.
3. Transfer to chloroform at 56°C for 15 min.
4. Transfer to fresh chloroform at 56°C for 30 min.
5. Transfer to paraffin wax for 15 min.
6. Transfer to fresh wax for 30 min.
7. Transfer to fresh wax for 45 min.
8. Embed in fresh wax.

FIXATION

Bouin's fluid is the fixative of choice for paraffin-embedded 3 μm sections, although formalin may be used. Glutaraldehyde is the fixative of choice for toluidine blue-stained 1 μm resin-embedded sections. A useful compromise is paraformaldehyde, which can be used as a fixative for both paraffin and resin embedding. It gives a less than perfect preservation for electron microscopy compared with glutaraldehyde. The methenamine silver 3 μm paraffin section needs longer in silver than the standard time if fixed in paraformaldehyde, but it is a useful fixative when the precise information required from the biopsy material is not known.

STAINING A 3 μm PARAFFIN SECTION FROM A RENAL BIOPSY

There are four prime demonstration techniques for renal biopsies: H&E, PAS, Jones' methenamine silver method and Congo red stain for amyloid. There are others that are used less often; Table 16.1 lists the useful methods and the tissue structures they demonstrate.

Table 16.1 Renal biopsies and useful demonstration methods

Method	Page	Demonstrates
Haematoxylin and eosin	27	General morphology
Martius scarlet-blue (MSB)	125	Fibrin, basement membranes, collagen
Weigert's elastic	55	Elastic fibres
Verhoeff's elastic	59	Elastic fibres
Periodic acid-Schiff	135	Basement membranes, mesangium
Methenamine silver	63	Basement membranes, mesangium
Congo red	113	Amyloid, myeloma casts
Toluidine blue (resin section)	30	Detailed morphology, basement membrane deposits
Methyl green-pyronin	98	Plasma cells, 'immunoblasts'

Haematoxylin and eosin

This is a useful all-round stain but is less so for detecting subtle abnormalities in the glomerulus than the PAS and methenamine silver methods. It is of value for the general assessment of tubules, hypercellularity, interstitium and blood vessels, and should not be neglected.

Periodic acid-Schiff reaction (see p. 135)

This, with the Jones' methenamine silver, is the best method for demonstration of glomerular capillary basement membranes. In capillary basement membrane thickening the severity of the lesion can usually be detected with ease (cf. Jones' methenamine silver). Almost equally important is the fact that the mesangium of the glomerular tuft and, in particular, the acellular mesangial material is well-demonstrated and minor degrees of mesangial increase easily seen. The basement membranes of the tubules are also well-stained, but this is rarely of diagnostic importance.

Jones' methenamine silver stain (see p. 63)

This silver deposition method is a useful stain for renal biopsies. The best results are obtained when the tissue has been fixed in Bouin's fluid. Fixation in formalin or paraformaldehyde will mean the section will require a longer incubation in the methenamine silver method given below. Where fixation has been short the difference is hardly significant, but specimens that have been standing in formalin for a week or two need a longer staining time. Staining is done under microscopic control, examining the section every 30 minutes or so, until the capillary basement membranes and glomerular mesangial material are stained brown. The basement membranes of the tubules stain earlier than those in the glomerular tuft, so are not a suitable 'end-point'.

The methenamine silver method nicely picks out the glomerular capillary basement membrane and the acellular mesangial material component of the mesangium, in a similar manner to the PAS reaction. The method gained its reputation as a capillary basement membrane stain on its ability to demonstrate argyrophilic 'spikes' on the outer surface of the thickened basement membrane in membranous nephropathy. It is possible not to detect a thickened basement membrane on the methenamine silver section, but it can be discerned using a PAS-stained section. So the PAS reaction is the method of choice for glomerular basement membranes in 3 μm sections. The choice of counterstain for use with the silver method is a light haematoxylin and eosin stain, or light green.

Congo red stain for amyloid (see p. 113)

The staining of amyloid is discussed in some detail in Chapter 6. Sometimes amyloid can be detected in an H&E-stained section, but minor degrees of amyloid involvement can normally only be detected by using an amyloid stain. This occurs particularly in cases where the disease involves the walls of vessels in the interstitium. An advantage of the routine Congo red staining of renal biopsies is that the characteristic casts of Bence Jones light chains in the 'myeloma kidney' also stain.

Elastic van Gieson stain (see p. 55)

This is useful in two situations. In an hypertensive kidney the method emphasizes the increase in number of the elastic lamellae in the internal elastic lamina. The van Gieson component of the stain also helps in assessing the muscular and intimal components of the vessel walls in hypertension. It is also useful in biopsies of renal transplants, where breaks in the internal elastic lamina in vessels usually imply a past episode of transplant rejection.

MSB stain (see p. 125)

This trichrome method was developed by Lendrum et al (1962) to demonstrate fibrin and to attempt to differentiate between fibrin of differing ages (see p. 125). Its main application in renal biopsies is in the demonstration of 'fibrinoid' necrosis in arterioles or glomerular tufts in polyarteritis nodosa, scleroderma, lupus nephritis and malignant hypertension. It also demonstrates fibrin plugging of glomerular capillaries in cases of haemolytic-uraemic syndrome. Fibrin can be distinguished on an H&E, but the MSB is useful and aesthetically pleasing.

Methyl green-pyronin (Unna–Pappenheim) (see p. 98)

This stain demonstrates RNA in cell cytoplasm (see p. 98) and is useful in biopsies of renal transplants. A change seen in rejection is the aggregation around blood vessels of large lymphocyte-type cells, many of which have demonstrable RNA in their cytoplasm. The methyl green-pyronin method stains the cytoplasm of these cells red, as it does plasma cell cytoplasm.

PREPARATION OF RENAL BIOPSIES FOR SEMI-THIN RESIN SECTIONING

Notes

In this technique thin 1 μm sections are cut for toluidine blue staining. The tissue can also be used for electron microscopy if required. The biopsy specimen is treated with care and is placed into normal saline and examined under a dissecting microscope. A piece approximately 3 mm long, containing glomeruli, is cut from the specimen and placed in glutaraldehyde. The remainder of the biopsy is processed as for conventional histology.

Solutions

Primary fixative—glutaraldehyde:

2.26% sodium dihydrogen orthophosphate (NaH$_2$PO$_4$.2H$_2$O	83 ml
2.52% sodium hydroxide	17 ml
0.1 M calcium chloride	0.5 ml
Sucrose	3 g
25% glutaraldehyde	3 ml

To the sodium dihydrogen orthophosphate solution add the sodium hydroxide solution, check the pH and adjust to 7.3–7.4 if necessary. Add the calcium chloride solution drop by drop and agitate the solution. Add sufficient of this solution to the sucrose to make a 100 ml total volume. To 22 ml of this solution add the 3 ml quantity of glutaraldehyde to make the working fixative (which should be prepared fresh daily).

Buffer wash:

2.26% sodium dihydrogen orthophosphate (NaH$_2$PO$_4$.2H$_2$O)	83 ml
2.52% sodium hydroxide	17 ml
0.5 M calcium chloride	0.5 ml
Sucrose	5 g

To the sodium dihydrogen orthophosphate solution add the sodium hydroxide solution, check pH and adjust to 7.3–7.4 if necessary. Add the calcium chloride drop by drop, and add the sucrose.

POST-FIXATION

The tissue is post-fixed for 1 hour in 1% osmium tetroxide at room temperature. Although best results are obtained using Millonig's phosphate buffer or cacodylate-buffered osmium, an unbuffered aqueous solution is only slightly inferior when used as a secondary fixative.

RINSING

The osmium tetroxide is decanted, the tissue given two quick changes of distilled water, and then processed through to resin, It must be remembered, however, that post-fixation of some tissues is inadvisable. In tissue which has been treated to demonstrate acid phosphatase activity in nerve cell lipofuscin bodies, post-fixation in osmium tetroxide makes it difficult to distinguish with accuracy between the reaction product of the post-fixative with the lipofuscin granules and the lead phosphate precipitate derived from the enzyme activity (Brunk & Ericsson 1972). Reale & Luciano (1964) have also shown that long periods of post-fixation may extract the end-products of enzyme reactions.

DEHYDRATION METHOD (performed at room temperature)

1. Following a rinse in distilled water, place the tissue in 50% alcohol for 10 min.
2. Transfer to 70% alcohol for 10 min.
3. Transfer to 95% alcohol for 10 min.
4. Transfer to absolute alcohol, previously filtered through anhydrous sodium sulphate, for 30 min.
5. Transfer to a fresh change of absolute alcohol.

ARALDITE EMBEDDING MIXTURE (Glauert & Glauert 1958)

Notes

The amount of accelerator added to the mixture is critical and will affect both the time needed for polymerization and the cutting properties of the cured block. Too much accelerator will produce dark amber-coloured blocks which are brittle and difficult to cut; well-cured blocks are a pale straw colour. Insufficient accelerator will produce blocks which polymerize poorly. The hardness of the final block can also be altered by varying the amount of plasticizer in the mixture. With modern ultramicrotomes most workers prefer a harder block than the ones produced by the original recipe and add only 0.5 ml of dibutyl phthalate.

If a hard specimen is to be processed, the plasticizer is either omitted completely or some of it is replaced by an alternative hardener, methyl nadic anhydride (MNA).

Embedding medium

Araldite CY212	10 ml
Hardener DDSA	10 ml
Accelerator DMP30	0.5 ml
Dibutyl phthalate	1 ml

To ensure thorough mixing of the constituents, the resin and hardener are mixed together and stirred until clear; the dibutyl phthalate is then added and the mixture stirred at 37°C, if necessary, until the plasticizer is dispersed. Finally, the accelerator is added and the final mixture stirred thoroughly before use.

This mixture will polymerize slowly at room temperature, but can be accelerated by using elevated temperatures. The original recipe recommended 2 days at 48°C or overnight at 60°C, but most laboratories allow polymerization to proceed overnight at 60°C.

Technique

1. After dehydration to absolute alcohol, soak the tissue in epoxypropane for 2–5 min changes at room temperature.

2. Decant off the epoxypropane and replace with a 1:1 mixture of epoxypropane and embedding medium for 60 min at room temperature.
3. Decant off this mixture and infiltrate with complete embedding medium for 2–6 h or overnight at room temperature in uncapped vials.
4. Embed in fresh embedding mixture and polymerize overnight at 60°C.

Thorough mixing of the constituents is again important and is easily accomplished with a magnetic stirrer because of the low viscosity.

EMBEDDING METHOD

1. Following the treatment with absolute alcohol place the tissue in 1:2 epoxypropane for 20 min.
2. Give a further change of 1:2 epoxypropane for 20 min.
3. Place in epoxypropane-resin mixture for 1 h.
4. Leave in pure resin overnight in uncapped vials at room temperature.
5. Infiltrate with fresh resin at 60°C, two changes of 30 min each. After each change rotate the vials to ensure contact of the tissue with fresh resin.
6. Embed the tissue in warm resin at 60°C in capsules, and polymerize for 48 h at 60°C.

TOLUIDINE BLUE STAINING OF 1 μm SECTIONS

An advance in renal biopsy interpretation followed the development of 1 μm thick sections. Paraffin wax offers inadequate support to the tissue block for this purpose, so the tissue is embedded in a resin. The tissue is fixed in glutaraldehyde, followed by dehydration in alcohol before embedding in resin. Sections are cut at 1 μm on a suitable microtome, and stained with 0.25% toluidine blue. More information can be obtained from renal biopsies in this way; in particular a far better assessment of basement membrane thickness, marginal mesangial increase and glomerular cellularity can be made. In addition, the various types of deposits in the basement membrane in such conditions as acute post-streptococcal glomerulonephritis, membranous nephropathy and lupus nephritis are seen by this technique. Another advantage of this method is that relevant parts of the same resin-embedded biopsy can then be examined by electron microscopy after trimming.

The toluidine blue method is the most satisfactory way of staining 1 μm resin-embedded sections. Attempts to apply the usual techniques for 3 μm paraffin sections, such as Jones' methenamine silver, are unsatisfactory and, if successful, provide less information.

OTHER STAINING METHODS FOR STRUCTURES IN RENAL TISSUE

JUXTAGLOMERULAR CELLS

Popularly known as 'JG' cells, these are modified smooth muscle cells that are found in the wall of the afferent arteriole where it enters the renal glomerulus. Granules are contained in the cytoplasm of these cells that are thought to secrete renin, a hormone concerned with blood pressure regulation. They were first described in mouse kidney by Ruyter in 1925. The JG granules are not seen in an H&E stain, and their demonstration is now of little diagnostic importance, but their histochemical delineation is of some interest, particularly in research. There is a marked species difference in the size of JG cells and in their histochemical behaviour. Mouse kidney gives the best results whilst those of human tissue are often unsatisfactory. Formalin-containing fixative gives good results, and both paraffin and fixed frozen sections can be used. Fresh, unfixed cryostat sections are not successful (Szokol & Gomba 1971).

One of the more popular techniques is that of Bowie, and this is described in detail. Other techniques, all of which give variable results, are as follows: PAS (see p. 135); aldehyde fuchsin (Harada 1966) (see p. 58); thioflavine T fluorescence (Harada 1969, Szokol & Gomba 1971) (see p. 117); 0.5% crystal violet in 70% alcohol for 1–3 min (Harada 1970).

BOWIE'S NEUTRAL STAIN TECHNIQUE (taken from Cowdry 1952)

Notes

This technique, like those quoted above, is not specific for JG cells but is sufficiently selective to afford reasonably clear-cut demonstration. The preparation of the neutral dye is rather time-consuming and tedious, but the actual technique is reasonably straightforward. As with any technique for JG cells some degree of practical experience with the stain is necessary before really good results are obtained. Fixation in Helly's fluid (see Appendix 1) is recommended, as is the use of rat or mouse kidney tissue.

Solutions

2.5% aqueous potassium dichromate
Bowie's solution
  Dissolve 1 g Biebrich scarlet in 250 ml distilled water and filter. Dissolve 2 g ethyl violet in 500 ml distilled water. Filter a small amount at a time of the latter solution into the Biebrich scarlet solution with constant stirring until a precipitate is formed. The end-point is reached when a small amount of the mixture placed on a No. 1 filter paper shows no colouration other than the precipitate. Filter the mixture and dry the precipitate in the filter paper. Finally, dissolve 0.2 g of the dried precipitate in 20 ml of 95% alcohol and use. There is enough precipitate formed to make 100 ml volume of stain.

Technique

1. Sections to water.
2. Mordant in the potassium dichromate solution overnight at approximately 40°C.
3. Wash well in tap water, then in distilled water.
4. Stain with Bowie's solution, diluted by adding 10–15 drops to 100 ml of 20% alcohol. Leave overnight at room temperature.
5. Drain and blot dry. Remove excess stain by rinsing two or three times in two changes of acetone.
6. Differentiate in equal parts of xylene and clove oil until the section is an overall red or reddish-purple colour, with any elastin picked out as blue-purple fibres.
7. Rinse in xylene and mount as desired.

Results

JG granules, elastin	blue-purple
Renal parenchyma	red to magenta

GOLGI APPARATUS

This intracytoplasmic entity, which was originally described by Golgi in 1898 using tissue from the owl, is of little significance at light microscopy level in diagnostic pathology. To demonstrate the Golgi apparatus, e.g. for normal demonstration purposes, there is a limited range of techniques that may be used. The structure is rich in various lipids and use can be made of this to demonstrate the apparatus with techniques such as osmium tetroxide or Sudan black. There are also silver techniques that can be used with varying degrees of success; two of these are described below. In the standard H&E stain areas of prominent Golgi apparatus appear unstained—the so-called 'negative' staining effect.

Formalin seems to preserve the Golgi apparatus adequately, but special fixation is necessary for optimal demonstration. Equally important, fixation needs to be prompt if reasonable results are to be obtained. Kidney is a suitable tissue for trying out the various techniques as it is rich in this cell organelle.

McDONALD'S MODIFICATION FOR LASCANO'S TECHNIQUE FOR THE GOLGI APPARATUS (Lascano 1959, McDonald 1964)

Notes

Excellent demonstration of the Golgi apparatus is afforded by this technique. The one minor disadvantage is that a full day is required and fresh tissue needs to be available early in the day.

Solutions

Fixative:

Aminoacetic acid (glycine)	1.7 g
Distilled water	85 ml
Formalin	15 ml
Conc. nitric acid	0.5 ml

1.5% aqueous silver nitrate
Reducer
   1.5% hydroquinone in 1.5% formalin.
0.2% aqueous gold chloride
1% aqueous neutral red

Technique

1. Take thin (1.5–2 mm) pieces of fresh tissue and place in a 100 ml volume of the fixative for 2 h with periodic agitation of the solution.
2. Wash in two changes of distilled water for a few seconds.
3. Treat with the silver nitrate solution for 4 h (agitate periodically).

4. Wash in distilled water for a few seconds.
5. Reduce for 1.5–2 h with frequent agitation.
6. Wash in several changes of distilled water for 5–10 min.
7. Paraffin process, cut thin (3–4 μm) sections and take down to water. Tone in the yellow gold chloride solution for 2 min. Wash in water. Counterstain with neutral red for 5 min.
8. Dehydrate, clear and mount as desired.

Results

Golgi apparatus	black
Nuclei	red

DAFANO – CAJAL TECHNIQUE FOR THE GOLGI APPARATUS (Cajal 1912, Da Fano 1919–20)

Notes

The results with this method may be unpredictable, due to variation in fixation or silver impregnation. It is wise to take through more than one block of the tissue to be examined and to vary the times of treatment. Finally, select the block that gives the best results. A rather complex toning solution is usually specified for this technique but we see no obvious advantage in this as against the conventional gold chloride solution.

Solutions

Fixative:

Cobalt nitrate	1 g
Formalin	15 ml
Distilled water	100 ml

1.5% aqueous silver nitrate
Reducer:

Hydroquinone	2 g
Formalin	15 ml
Distilled water	100 ml
Sodium sulphite	0.5 g

0.1% aqueous gold chloride
1% aqueous neutral red

Technique

1. Place thin (1.5–2 mm) slices of fresh tissue in the fixative for 3–8 h (see Notes).
2. Rinse in distilled water for 30 s.
3. Treat with the silver nitrate solution for 36–48 h (change the solution after one day).

4. Rinse in distilled water for 30 s.
5. Reduce for 12–24 h.
6. Wash in water for 5 min.
7. Paraffin process and cut thin (3–4 μm) sections.
8. Either de-paraffinize and mount, or take down to water, tone in 0.1% aqueous yellow gold chloride for 5 min and wash in water. Counterstain with neutral red for 5 min, dehydrate, clear and mount as desired.

Results

Golgi apparatus	black
Mitochondria	brown
Background	grey if toned, yellow-brown if untoned
Nuclei	red

RENAL PATHOLOGY

The kidneys are intra-abdominal retro-peritoneal organs that are found against the lower ribs. As a result they are well-protected from injury, but their situation makes blind closed needle biopsy difficult and biopsies are only performed by experienced operators. Tumours in the kidney are usually malignant, the commonest is the clear cell carcinoma (hypernephroma). This tumour, found in adults usually over the age of 50 years, may metastasize early before the primary lesion has been identified. It is found in the parenchyma of the kidney and has a characteristic clear cell architecture. Tumours in the renal pelvis are commonly transitional cell carcinomas.

The kidney is prone to suffer from infections, termed pyelonephritis, usually from *E.coli*. Infections are more common in women and in patients who have an abnormal urinary tract, either as a result of congenital abnormality, or due to the presence of stones. Renal stones are formed when the urine becomes supersaturated with a solute such as calcium, or when there is a nidus on which stones may form, such as pus in pyelonephritis or fragments of tumours.

Non-malignant lesions of the kidney, presenting as renal failure, may be disease of the tubules, glomeruli or vessels. Tubular disease may be the result of hypotension causing the death of lining cells and is termed acute tubular necrosis. Lesions of the glomeruli are called glomerulonephritis; these are usually immunologically mediated, the result of antibody attack on antigens in the renal basement membrane (type 2 hypersensitivity) or deposited antibodies (type 3 hypersensitivity). This results in thickening of basement membrane, membranous change, or proliferation of cells in the mesangium, termed proliferative change, or in the Bowman's space, termed crescentic change. In children there may be clinical evidence of glomerular disease but no change will be seen on light microscopy—a disease termed minimal change or lipoid nephropathy. Several of the diseases affecting the glomerulus show identical features on routine H&E staining, and the pathologist will require special stains to reach a diagnosis. In addition to the histochemical and immunocytochemical stains discussed above, many histopathologists request electron microscopy. Material stained with conventional EM stains will clearly demonstrate basement membrane material, antigen/antibody complexes, amyloid and other connective tissue components as well as showing ultrastructural features of cells, such as the loss of foot processes, the only abnormality seen in minimal change disease. Access to electron microscopy is therefore essential in the provision of a renal biopsy service.

The kidney may be secondarily involved in many other diseases, as a result of vascular damage for instance in hypertension and diabetes. It may also be involved in autoimmune diseases such as SLE and in diseases such as myeloma which results in tubular damage. The renal glomerulus also shows changes in diabetes and is an important site for the deposition of amyloid.

Besides production of urine, the kidney secretes two major hormones: renin that controls blood pressure through the renin angiotensin system, and erythropoetin which controls the formation of erythrocytes. Patients with renal damage commonly over-secrete renin, becoming hypertensive, and under-secrete erythropoietin, hence becoming anaemic.

LYMPH NODE BIOPSY

THE NORMAL LYMPH NODE

Lymphocytes are distributed throughout the body; they are arranged in aggregations that exhibit various degrees of structural organization such as the tonsils and the Gut-Associated Lymphoid Tissue (GALT). Isolated lymphocytes are found in loose connective tissues and amongst epithelial cells, particularly in the mucosa of the gastrointestinal and respiratory tracts. The vast majority of lymphocytes are located in encapsulated, highly organized structures called lymph nodes, which are interposed along the larger regional vessels of the lymph vascular system. Two principal functions occur within lymph nodes: firstly non-specific 'filtration' of lymph by the phagocytic activity of macrophages, and secondly storage and proliferation of T and B lymphocytes.

T and B lymphocytes occupy different areas within lymph nodes; each area undergoes characteristic histological changes when appropriately stimulated by the presence of antigens. Even in the absence of disease, individuals are exposed to a wide range of antigenic stimulation both from within and outside. The histological appearance of a lymph node at any particular time reflects not only the response to local antigenic stimulation but also the immunological status of the individual. Below is a brief description of the anatomy of a lymph node.

Capsule	
Cortex—B cell area	Lymphoid follicles, germinal centres, small and large cleaved lymphocytes, small and large non-cleaved lymphocytes, tingible body-macrophages, dendritic reticulum cells.
Paracortex—T cell area	Small and large lymphocytes, histiocytes, interdigitating reticulum cells.
Medulla	Plasma cells, lymphocytes, histiocytes
Sinuses	Marginal, intermediary, medullary
Blood vessels	Arteries, veins, capillaries, post-capillary venules

Lymph nodes show distinct compartmentalization of different lymphocyte subsets: B cells form rounded aggregates or follicles in the outer cortex and T cells occupy the paracortex between the follicles. This segregation of the functional populations of lymphocytes is highlighted by immunocytochemistry.

The B cell follicle is a complex structure that is variable in appearance depending on its degree of activity. In the unstimulated state the follicle consists of a rounded mass of small B lymphocytic cells. These have surface IgD and/or IgM immunoglobulin and the cells are admixed with dendritic reticulum cells and T cells. This is termed a primary follicle. More usually the follicles show some degree of stimulation and are called germinal centres, consisting of large aggregates of proliferating B cells. Surrounding the germinal centre is termed the mantle zone where there are small B lymphocytes possessing a similar phenotype to the primary follicle. The germinal centre itself contains an admixture of proliferating and differentiating B cells termed centroblasts and centrocytes, T cells that have a helper cell predominance and specialized antigen-presenting cells called dendritic reticulum cells. The paracortex of the lymph node contains many T cells, the majority showing a peripheral helper phenotype whilst a smaller percentage are suppressor cells. Admixed with the T lymphocytes are specialized paracortical antigen-presenting cells.

THE BIOPSY

Lymph node biopsies are performed on patients in whom there is unexplained enlargement of a node or group of nodes termed lymphadenopathy. A lymph node biopsy usually involves the removal of a complete node by a surgeon, but a closed needle biopsy may be taken from enlarged nodes. The surgeon removes the largest node where possible, as it will show the most advanced changes. Smaller nodes, which may be abnormal, often do not provide adequate diagnostic information. The node should be excised whole as the interpretation of fragments is unreliable and distortion of the tissue prior to fixation is best avoided. Sometimes a single routinely-stained, thin, well-cut section of paraffin-embedded tissue is all that is required to make a diagnosis. However, a great deal more information can often be elicited from the biopsy tissue by additional techniques. The particular circumstances of the case dictate whether or not any additional investigations are likely to be required. The manner in which the biopsied node is handled varies with the laboratory's resources and the expertise available. Imprint preparations can be made from cut surfaces of the fresh tissue; these are air-dried, and fixed later. It is important to process the tissue used to make the imprints for histology, so that both techniques can be compared. Note that the 'dabbing' process can cause distortion, so it is essential to remove tissue for histological examination first.

For routine histology, fixation in 10% neutral buffered formalin is recommended. Whole nodes or large pieces are cut transversely with a sharp blade to allow penetration of fixative. Fixation should be for 24 hours; long periods of fixation are not desirable and may interfere with subsequent staining. Sections of 4 μm or less are used for surgical histology and it is often necessary to produce 2 μm sections, to be able to appreciate the cytology of individual cells. Alternatively, embedding the tissue in resin and sectioning at 1 μm produces excellent thin sections for morphological use. The necessity of a sharp edge for section cutting cannot be over-emphasized. At low power, scores across the field can make interpretation difficult, and at high power, individual cells are damaged beyond recognition.

Routinely, sections are stained with H & E and a silver impregnation method to demonstrate the reticulin fibre framework. Also used in the study of lymph nodes are the methyl green-pyronin method (see p. 98) and periodic acid-Schiff staining method (see p. 135). It is sometimes useful to demonstrate the presence of neutrophil leukocytes in paraffin sections by the naphthol AS-D chloroacetate esterase method (see p. 313). Frequently used techniques for paraffin sections are immunocytochemical methods that are applied in the diagnosis of lymphomas and other tumours.

The lymph node biopsy presents unique problems as the nodes are composed of many cells with little connective tissue to hold them in place. They are surrounded by a capsule inhibiting penetration of chemicals, so the utmost care and skill is required to produce good histological preparations. In no other area of histology is the quality of a section so important. Good histological preparations from lymph node biopsies result when there is full understanding of the factors involved. Well-fixed lymph nodes are difficult to diagnose if the tissue is inadequately processed or poorly sectioned and stained. Conversely, the most competent histologist is unable to prepare good slides from poorly fixed tissue.

TISSUE PREPARATION

The lymphoid tissues show an ordered structure of confusingly similar cells, and there is a need to identify the cell lines positively so the correct diagnosis may be made. The subsequent treatment regime will be determined by the presumptive diagnosis. The investigation of lymphoid tissue requires a multiparameter approach. The H & E-stained paraffin sections form the basis for all diagnoses; the additional information that can be obtained from other techniques improves the prospect of a correct diagnosis. It is necessary to ensure that the material is correctly handled from the onset.

A piece of tissue $1 \times 1 \times 0.3$ cm is selected and snap frozen. The method chosen for freezing should be rapid, causing least distortion by ice crystal artefact. A cardice and alcohol mixture at $50°C$ or isopentane and liquid nitrogen at $-102°C$ is suitable (see p. 290). A further piece of tissue, $1 \times 1 \times 0.3$ cm, is placed into 10% buffered formalin for 24 hours and processed to a resin block. A piece of tissue $2 \times 1 \times 0.3$ cm is also placed into 10% buffered formalin for 24 hours then processed to a paraffin block.

PARAFFIN SECTIONING

The tissue under examination is soft and for that reason it is probably not considered difficult to prepare sections from lymphoid tissue. However distortion can occur and artefacts be produced at every stage of the paraffin process, especially during fixation, section cutting and drying of the section on to the slide. The properly prepared paraffin section is still the foundation of any histological examination, and the most reliable preparation for the demonstration of intracellular immunoglobulin. The other techniques may help in the diagnosis, and occasionally one technique alone will establish the diagnosis. On occasions they will be of no assistance at all. The paraffin section, when properly prepared, is the only technique that, on its own, may enable the experienced pathologist to make a diagnosis.

Fixation

Transporting the biopsy wrapped in dry gauze can produce a drying artefact. The lymph node is bisected with a scalpel and when sliced must not be squeezed or squashed or the cells will show distortion artefact. Distorted cells show elongated nuclei and clumping of cells. Prompt slicing of the node is essential and precedes fixation for two reasons. First, imprint preparations are made from the cut surface of the fresh node. Secondly, the capsule around the node retards penetration of the fixative. Lymph nodes fixed whole show a fixed outer rim and a central area of poor fixation. Thin blocks are essential, a 3 mm thin block ensuring adequate and uniform fixation. As fixation is the most important step in the preparation of tissue sections, inadequately fixed tissue will be ruined. Tissue blocks can be re-processed but nothing can restore them if the initial fixation was inadequate. Poor fixation is responsible for many lymph node sections that are technically too poor to be suitable for diagnosis. Good quality slides can be prepared from lymph nodes with any fixative, if the solution is of proper strength and volume and if the time allotted for fixation is adequate. A 10% buffered formalin solution is used universally for tissue fixation and is satisfactory, overnight or 24 hours being required for adequate fixation. Fixatives containing picric acid should not be used as they cause partial denaturation of DNA with the resultant loss of methyl green staining. The immunocytochemical techniques will require a greater dilution of the primary antiserum following picric acid fixation or a heavy background reaction will occur.

Processing

Frequently check the temperature of the paraffin baths. Over-heating of reagents affects the quality of tissues, but can destroy lymph nodes. It makes them brittle, and when sectioned the tissue often falls out of the ribbon. Microscopic detail is lost due to the cells being coagulated. Lymph node biopsies are embedded in the paraffin wax routinely used in the laboratory. In particular, waxes containing plastic polymer give excellent results.

Sectioning

Too rapid chilling of the paraffin block after embedding or during sectioning causes cracking of the wax, and often the lymph node cracks as well. Sections must be thin, preferably one cell thick. Lymphocytes are small cells so this means 4–5 mm blocks are cut with a slow and even action. Even properly processed lymph node tissue is delicate — attempting to stretch the tissue to its original size on the water bath will cause damage. Any method that distorts the sections when separating them on the water bath should be avoided. The stained slide should show the tissue architecture described previously and the preservation of morphological detail that enables the classification of the cell types to be undertaken. The artefacts appearing in paraffin section are not unique to lymphoid tissue, but do appear more than in other tissue types. Cutting artefacts fall into two categories. They may be gross artefacts such as 'scores' that are caused by a nicked or damaged cutting edge, or alternating thick and thin areas of the section caused by an insecure block. The second category includes those artefacts that are only visible at high magnifications. In a well-prepared section the lymphoid cells appear to be adjacent, evenly spaced and show organization into follicular cuffs and medullary cords. In a poor section the cells appear to pile up on each other, causing spaces to appear in other parts of the tissue. If the section has been marginally better prepared it may yet show splitting of the nuclei, or 'microchattering'. These artefacts are the result of bad technique in section cutting. The block should be cooled and the sections cut with a smooth action that is as slow as possible. There should be little difficulty experienced in cutting a ribbon of sections at a slow cutting rate. The microtomist will observe that the first sections of a ribbon show opaque wax and transparent tissue. As the cutting continues the wax remains opaque, but the tissue in the cut sections also becomes opaque; the best sections are those that are transparent. Under no circumstances should the speed of the cutting stroke be increased so that a ribbon is formed from a dull edge. These sections will show microchatters and piling up of the cells. The artefacts caused by floating out the sections on a water bath are similar to those that can be produced during the drying of the sections on the microscope slide. If the water bath is too warm or the drying temperature too high, then the section will be disrupted with resultant loss of tissue architecture. The water bath should be approximately 10°C below the melting point of the wax. The drying temperature should not exceed 37°C for best results.

IMPRINTS (TOUCH PREPARATIONS, 'DABS')

Imprints are valuable, not only for showing the appearance of the cells in a cytological preparation stained by a Romanowsky method (for comparison with a blood smear), but also for cytochemical studies. An imprint of the cut surface of the tissue is made by touching it against a clean, grease-free microscope slide, taking care not to smudge the preparation. This is repeated on a few slides. When the tissue is removed the imprint should be just moist and will air-dry almost immediately. The cells appear flattened, with the whole of the nucleus visible, and the cytoplasm is spread out enabling granules to be seen. This is different from the picture seen in sectioned material. The enzyme patterns that are characteristic of certain cell types can be identified using the appropriate techniques. The presence of intense chloroacetate esterase activity in a cell line defines the neutrophil myeloid series although mast cells also exhibit this positive reaction. Two or more imprint slides are stained by the May–Grunwald Giemsa method. Other methods of value for staining imprints are:

- Periodic acid-Schiff—for glycogen granules in cells and mucin.
- Oil red O—for intracytoplasmic lipid.
- Acid phosphatase—for histiocytes, T cells and tartrate-stable 'hairy cells' (of 'hairy cell' leukaemia).
- Non-specific esterase —for histiocytes.
- Acid esterase —for T lymphocytes.
- Chloroacetate esterase —for neutrophil granulocytes, their precursors and mast cells.

The enzyme methods are given in Chapter 13 and are the same as those employed for frozen sections.

CRYOSTAT SECTIONS

Enzyme histochemical techniques are of value as cell markers. One cell type may have a unique enzyme profile, not only in normal but also in diseased tissues. The histochemical techniques may be reliably carried out on imprint smears, but only cryostat sections will enable the intercellular relationships to be determined.

Cryostat sections have some disadvantages of resolution and morphological preservation, but the cell relationships are preserved. This alone makes the examination of enzymes in cryostat sections essential.

RESIN SECTIONS

Tissue is processed through to resinous media in the histology department whenever it is necessary to produce thin sections of highly cellular material. The excellent support provided by resins enables sections of 1 μm to be cut. The morphological preservation achieved with this material is excellent and allows critical evaluation of lymphoid tissues.

Table 16.2   Applications of sections

Morphology	Paraffin sections, resin sections
Enzymes	Imprints, cryostat sections, resin sections
Immunocytochemistry	Paraffin sections, cryostat sections, imprints

STAINING (morphological)

Any routine haematoxylin and eosin procedure, properly controlled, is satisfactory for staining lymph nodes. Difficulty arises when slides are over-stained in a regressive type of haematoxylin such as Harris's and not properly differentiated. This can be remedied by using a progressive haematoxylin such as Mayer's that does not overstain and require differentiation in acid-alcohol. Depth of eosin counterstaining has traditionally been based on personal preference. Personal taste and colour perception vary and, unless the nuclear stain is obliterated by the eosin, individual preference should prevail.

STAINING (specialized)

The lymph node is the site of a great diversity of lesions, ranging from purely reactive through inflammatory to neoplastic. In addition, the histiocytic cell elements may be involved in the storage of the abnormal products of the enzyme deficiency-related disorders such as the lipidoses and the mucopolysaccharidoses.

As previously mentioned, reticulin methods may be useful and show, in particular, follicular (as distinct from diffuse) lesions. Other special stains used for lymph nodes are shown below:

- Gram technique: organisms in general.
- ZN technique: mycobacteria.
- Methyl green-pyronin stain: immunoblasts and plasma cells.
- Giemsa stain: protozoa (e.g. toxoplasmosis, Leishmaniasis).
- Grocott hexamine silver: fungi (e.g. histoplasmosis).
- Perls technique: haemosiderin (e.g. haemochromatosis).
- PAS/Schmorl/Sudan black: lipofuscin deposits.
- Masson–Fontana: melanin (secondary melanoma).
- Alcian blue-PAS: mucins or glycogen (secondary adenocarcinoma).

IMMUNOCYTOCHEMISTRY

In recent years, considerable progress has been made in the identification of various lymphoid cell types. The realization that lymphocytes represent heterologous cell populations has stimulated interest for their characterization. New methods based on immunological techniques aiming to identify lymphoid cell types have been developed, immunocytochemistry has been introduced in the study of lymphoid tissue, and immunological methods are routine procedures in diagnosis.

Immunocytochemistry has proved to be a useful adjunct to conventional light microscopy in the diagnosis of lymphoid tumours. There are several areas in which it is particularly valuable. These include the distinction of malignant lymphoma from reactive lymphoid proliferations, the differentiation of Hodgkin's disease from the non-Hodgkin's lymphomas, and the precise categorization of lymphoprolifera-tion disease. Malignant lymphomas are generally accepted to be clonal prolifera-tions of lymphoid cells, and the demonstration of monoclonality provides strong evidence that a lymphoid population is neoplastic. In B cell lymphomas expressing surface or cytoplasmic immunoglobulin it is possible to recognize light chain restriction and prove the clonal origin of the tumour. The situation is more compli-cated in T cell proliferations where no widely available immunocytochemical marker of clonality exists (Maclennan et al 1990).

With the exception of the T cell subsets that are more easily demonstrated using frozen sections or imprints, there are generally reliable antisera that can be used on routinely fixed, paraffin-processed sections of lymph node. These include: leuko-cyte common antigen (LCA) as a general marker for lymphoid cells, L26 for B lymphocytes and UCHLI or CD3 for T lymphocytes. There is some degree of overlap with B and T cell markers, so that the antisera should not be used in isola-tion but form part of a panel.

ELECTRON MICROSCOPY

It is easy and inexpensive to routinely fix small samples of lymph node biopsies in glutaraldehyde at the time of initial processing. The decision on whether to proceed with the embedding for electron microscopic examination can be made after light microscopic examination.

Information on handling lymph nodes has been drawn from Astarita et al, 1979, Berard & Bowling 1975, and Bowling 1979.

LYMPH NODE PATHOLOGY

Lymph nodes are primarily sites of filtration where antigens can be brought into contact with antibody-producing cells. They enlarge as a normal response to infec-tion, when there is proliferation of B and/or T cell zones of the node. They appear as an increase in the size or number of follicles, or an expansion of the paracortex. This is normally accompanied by eradication of the infecting organism and resolu-tion of the changes.

Some organisms, notably mycobacteria, are capable of surviving and proliferating in nodes, and can be identified with the relevant stains: Ziehl–Neelsen for tubercu-losis, a Gram stain for other bacteria. Some infections give characteristic histolog-ical changes but cannot themselves be identified; examples are viruses, notably

Epstein–Barr and HIV. When proliferating in nodes some agents cause areas of necrosis; the classic example is tuberculosis, but toxoplasmosis and other infections can cause similar changes.

The lymph nodes also show reactive changes in non-infectious inflammatory conditions such as the collagen vascular diseases and rheumatoid arthritis. Some of these give characteristic appearances but in others the appearances can mimic infectious or neoplastic disease. Sarcoidosis, a disease of unknown aetiology, affects lymph nodes giving well-formed granulomas; similar granulomas can be seen in lymph nodes draining areas of malignant tumours.

Lymphadenopathy can also occur as a result of the proliferation of a malignant tumour in the node. These can be primary tumours of lymphoid tissue, called lymphomas, or may be metastatic tumours. Lymphomas are divided into Hodgkin's and non-Hodgkin's lymphomas. These two groups may be further subdivided by analysis of the histological appearance of the node and identification of the cell type involved, requiring immunocytochemistry.

Malignant tumours such as carcinomas have the ability to invade surrounding tissues; they frequently invade into lymphatics, and individual cells are carried in the normal lymph flow to the regional nodes. The cells may then grow and divide, forming a metastasis of the primary tumour. Cells from this metastasis may then invade and enter afferent lymphatics, ultimately allowing the tumour to disseminate throughout the body. Identification of lymph node metastases provides useful prognostic information. Occasionally a lymph node will become enlarged by a metastasis before the primary tumour becomes apparent and biopsy of the node is the mechanism by which a pathologist can suggest likely primary sites. Exact identification of the tumour type in metastases may be vital and is facilitated by the use of stains such as:

- Alcian blue-PAS for mucin, demonstrating an adenocarcinoma
- Masson–Fontana for melanin, demonstrating a melanoma.

Immunocytochemistry is becoming increasingly important in this area. Specific antibodies to tissue types such as prostate and thyroid allow identification of primary site. The use of antibody panels (Gamble et al 1993) allows a pathologist to offer a reasonable suggestion as to the primary site of a metastasizing tumour.

THE LIVER BIOPSY

The classification of liver disease is based on morphology; central to this is the liver biopsy, which continues to hold an important place in diagnosis and patient management. Biopsies are received in one of two forms: either as a narrow fragile core of tissue 2 mm across and 10 mm long, removed by needle biopsy (for which several different types of biopsy needle are available) or, alternatively, as a wedge-shaped piece of tissue obtained by open surgery. Specimens obtained by suction are more likely to undergo fragmentation in cases of cirrhosis, but are usually suitable for diagnosis.

The needle biopsy core requires delicate handling, and particular care should be taken during wax embedding to ensure that the core is embedded flat so that full longitudinal sections can be cut. If the orientation is slightly out, valuable pieces of a small specimen may be lost in the trimming of the block. Despite its size a needle biopsy core gives a reasonable picture of the morphology of the liver, although isolated tumours such as a liver cell carcinoma may be missed. Another sampling problem arises when the liver shows severe cirrhosis with thick fibrous bands. The needle tends to ricochet off the hard fibrous tissue and to bore only through the softer parenchymal tissue, producing a non-representative specimen which understates the severity of the fibrosis. A similar situation arises in occasional cases where the liver is packed with metastatic tumour. Here particularly, when the tumour nodules have a strong fibrous stroma as sometimes occurs with secondary carcinoma of the breast, the needle tends to slide in the soft liver parenchyma between tumour nodules.

In many respects the wedge biopsy is better than a needle biopsy. A larger specimen is obtained and the surgeon can select the most abnormal area, so that solitary tumours are less likely to be missed. For reasons of convenience and haemostasis the surgeon usually removes the wedge from the lower margin of the anterior part of the liver, and this produces an important pitfall for the unwary pathologist. At the anterior inferior border of the liver the architecture of the liver's lobular pattern is distorted. The fibrous septa running from the liver capsule to the subcapsular portal triads are thick, split liver lobules, and often run to the central veins. The portal triads themselves may show increased fibrous tissue and bile duct reduplication. These features may suggest cirrhosis to the inexperienced eye. Furthemore, there may be clumps of neutrophils underneath the liver capsule and within the liver parenchyma. In these circumstances the finding is of no significance and is usually seen when the wedge biopsy is performed towards the end of a laparotomy. Fine needle aspiration (FNA) has the advantage that the fluid can be examined cytologically, which is helpful when neoplasms are suspected, and provides fragments of material for immunocytochemistry.

PROCESSING

The needle biopsy may be processed manually or by using a rapid schedule on a tissue processor during a working day. The wedge biopsy would be routinely processed on a tissue processor in the normal way. When a needle biopsy specimen is obtained from the patient it should be expelled gently on to a piece of card, glass or wood to prevent distortion and undue fragmentation of the specimen. Filter paper is less suitable because fibres tend to adhere to the tissue and interfere with sectioning. The tissue should be treated with care and excessive manipulation avoided; for paraffin processing transfer to buffered formalin when possible. Prior to paraffin processing the needle biopsy specimen is wrapped in a suitable material such as thin paper (cigarette paper is ideal).

SECTIONING

The sectioning of a needle biopsy is done with great care. As the biopsy is thin, it is wise to cut serial sections to cover all possible needs (about 12 sections). For a laboratory doing liver needle biopsies as a routine, the following guide may be helpful:

Section no.   *1.* H&E
        2. Reticulin stain
        3. Perls stain for iron

   4. PAS (plus diastase-PAS—optional)
   5. van Gieson
   6. Long ZN, Schmorl, or Sudan black for lipofuscin
   7. Fouchet for bile (optional).

This leaves sections for other stains (e.g. Congo red, elastic stain, MSB) should the need arise.

Frozen sections

Frozen sections for rapid diagnosis of liver disease are rarely indicated, particularly since a needle biopsy specimen can be rapidly processed and a paraffin section obtained within a few hours. Frozen sections of liver biopsies are usually adequate for the diagnosis of obvious lesions such as tumours, abscesses, granulomas or large bile duct obstruction. They are unsuitable for the recognition of more subtle changes, may be misleading, and are little used in surgical pathology (Bancroft & Stevens 1975).

   The only true indication for frozen sectioning is in the diagnosis of lipid and glycogen storage disease. An open wedge biopsy is preferable, as a needle biopsy specimen may present difficulties because of problems with orientation. Sections are cut in a cryostat, using standard freezing and sectioning methods.

STAINING METHODS

   H & E (see p. 27) for general morphology.

   Reticulin silver (see p. 48) to demonstrate the reticulin network and to emphasize any abnormality of the hepatic architecture. It is particularly useful when detecting degrees of cirrhotic change and to pinpoint foci of liver cell necrosis or atrophy, as in infective hepatitis. A reticulin preparation is important for accurate assessment of structural changes; without it, thin layers of connective tissue and hence cirrhosis may be missed. Counterstaining is sometimes used, but is apt to distract rather than help. If it is necessary to distinguish between collagen and reticulin fibres, toning may be omitted.

   Perls iron reaction (see p. 208) demonstrates iron and its distribution, as in haemochromatosis or transfusional siderosis. Lightly counterstained, the method enables not only iron but also other pigments such as bile and lipofuscin to be evaluated as unchanged brown pigments.

   PAS reaction (see p. 135) for detection of glycogen. The diastase-PAS variant displays the globules of α_1-antitrypsin deficiency, and activated macrophages. When glycogen needs to be demonstrated, for instance in a tumour or in storage diseases, either the PAS stain without diastase or Best's carmine may be used.

   Best's carmine (see p. 162) for detection of glycogen.

   van Gieson stain (see p. 36) demonstrates collagen and is useful in the diagnosis of cirrhosis. Collagen staining is advisable whenever there is substantial fatty change. Collagen stains are also employed in the detection of blocked or narrowed vessels in severely congested livers and in non-cirrhotic portal hypertension. An added bonus with van Gieson's stain is that it is a useful and convenient way of demonstrating bile pigments, which it stains green. Specific staining for bile pigments is sometimes necessary; these can be stained bright green by Fouchet's technique (see p. 201)

Elastic Stain (see p. 55) A stain for elastic fibres enables recent blood vessel collapse to be distinguished from old fibrosis, since only the former is positive. Orcein or Victoria blue staining (Tanaka et al 1981) can be used for this purpose; both stain hepatitis B surface antigen and copper-associated protein as well as elastin. They are also helpful in various forms of hepatitis and in cholestatic diseases.

Long Ziehl–Neelsen method (see p. 203). A good stain for the positive identification of lipofuscin and its differentiation from haemosiderin and other pigments.

Rhodanine stain (see p. 214). Demonstrates copper where it is mainly found in primary biliary cirrhosis or in Wilson's disease, although negative staining does not exclude the diagnosis and positive staining does not establish it.

Ziehl–Neelsen method (see p. 245) is used for the demonstration of mycobacteria and the ova of *Schistosoma mansoni*. When relatively large areas of tissue need to be examined for mycobacteria, the fluorescent auramine-rhodamine method (see p. 248) may also be used.

Chromotrope-aniline blue (CAB) stain. This method, given below, demonstrates new collagen formation, especially useful in alcoholic hepatitis and similar lesions, in which pericellular fibrosis is a key diagnostic feature.

A summary of staining methods is given in Table 16.3

Table 16.3 Demonstration methods for liver biopsies

Method	Application	See page
Periodic acid-Schiff	Glycogen and PAS-positive material	135
Best's carmine	Glycogen	162
Bauer–Schiff	Glycogen in frozen sections	163
Perls	Ferric iron	208
Weigert's elastic	Elastic tissue	55
Schmorl	Lipofuscin, melanin	203
Long ZN	Lipofuscin	203
Sudan black	Lipofuscin	202
Reticulin stain	Reticulin network	48
MSB	Fibrin, collagen	125
Congo red	Amyloid	113
Fouchet	Bile pigments	201
Shikata orcein	Copper-associated protein and hepatitis B antigen	258
Rubeanic acid	Copper deposits	214
Rhodanine	Copper deposits	214

OTHER LIVER STRUCTURES AND STAINING METHODS

Mallory bodies (alcoholic hyaline)

Mallory bodies were first described by Mallory, in 1911, who considered them to be peculiar to liver tissue in alcoholic cirrhosis. Whilst there are some reservations about this, it is undoubtedly true that Mallory bodies are usually found in the more active episodes of hepatic cirrhosis due to excessive alcohol intake. Other conditions in which they may be found include primary biliary cirrhosis and Wilson's disease. Another potentially useful marker of alcoholic cirrhosis is the presence of hepatic perisinusoidal deposits of IgA (Kater et al, 1979, Swerdlow et al 1983). Mallory bodies are protein intracytoplasmic hyaline bodies of somewhat irregular shape, and are found in many cells of the affected liver. They are usually peri- or juxtanuclear in position and the electron microscope has shown them to contain both mitochondria and lysosomes. For more detailed information see Horvath et al (1972) and Lyon & Christoffersen (1971). The following is a list of the more popular techniques for demonstrating alcoholic hyaline, but it must be said these may not offer any great advantage over standard H & E preparations. Frozen sections are considered to give better staining results than paraffin.

- H&E—eosinophilic (see p. 27)
- PTAH—blue (see p. 44)
- Congo red–weak red (see p. 113)
- Baker's acid haematein–blue (not extracted by pyridine) (see p. 184)
- Luxol fast blue (see p. 352).

CHROMOTROPE-ANILINE BLUE METHOD FOR COLLAGEN AND MALLORY BODIES (from Scheuer 1988)

Note

This method demonstrates new collagen formation as well as Mallory bodies.

Solutions

CAB solution
  1.5 g aniline blue is dissolved in 2.5 ml conc. HCl and 200 ml distilled water with gentle heat.
  6 g Chromotrope 2R is added. The pH should be 1.0. Filter.
1% aqueous phosphomolybdic acid

Technique

1. Sections to water.
2. Stain nuclei with Weigert's iron haematoxylin (see p. 36). Rinse in distilled water.
3. Immerse in the phosphomolybdic acid for 1–3 min. Rinse well in distilled water.
4. Stain with CAB solution for 8 min. Rinse well in distilled water. Blot dry.
5. Dehydrate quickly, clear and mount as desired.

Results

Collagen is stained blue, Mallory bodies stain blue or sometimes red and giant mitochondria stain red.

VITAMIN C (ascorbic acid)

The following technique is based upon the reduction of acidified silver nitrate in the dark by ascorbic acid. It must be borne in mind that other argentaffin substances such as melanin and inorganic phosphates may also react.

Ascorbic acid is found in the greatest amount in both liver and adrenal cortex.

VITAMIN C DEMONSTRATION (from Giroud & Leblond 1934)

Notes

Tissues should be as fresh as possible and should not be allowed to dry before treatment with the acidified silver nitrate. The pre-silver nitrate treatment with laevulose is to remove any excess chlorides from the tissue which could otherwise give non-specific silver reduction.

The authors recommend that all stages of the technique, from washing with laevulose to the post-hypo washing in water, are carried out in the dark to avoid any non-specific light reduction.

Solutions

5.4% aqueous laevulose (D (-) fructose)
10% aqueous silver nitrate to which are added 2 drops of acetic acid per 1 ml volume
5% aqueous sodium thiosulphate (hypo)
1% aqueous neutral red

Technique

1. Thin (2 mm) pieces of tissue are washed for 2–3 min in ample quantities of laevulose. Wash briefly in distilled water.
2. Treat with acetic-silver nitrate for 30 min.
3. Rinse in several changes of distilled water over 5–10 min.
4. Treat with the hypo for 15–30 min.
5. Wash in water, paraffin process and cut 5 μm sections.
6. Sections are de-paraffinized, taken to water and counterstained with the aqueous neutral red for 2–3 min.
7. Wash in water, dehydrate, clear and mount as desired.

Results

Ascorbic acid	black granules
Nuclei	red

IMMUNOCYTOCHEMISTRY

Among the multitude of immunological methods now available, commonly used ones for liver include staining for α_1-antitrypsin and hepatitis virus markers. The immunocytochemical techniques discussed in Chapter 12 are applied to liver biopsies as appropriate.

ELECTRON MICROSCOPY AND THIN SECTIONS

A small piece of the fresh needle biopsy core is removed with a sharp scalpel blade and fixed in buffered glutaraldehyde for subsequent resin embedding (see p. 337). Information can be obtained from some liver biopsies by the preparation of 1 μm sections of glutaraldehyde-fixed resin-embedded tissues stained by the toluidine blue method. It is of limited value when compared to its use in bone and renal biopsies, for example.

LIVER PATHOLOGY

Liver disease may be focal or diffuse. Focal disease is usually regenerative, hyperplastic or neoplastic, and can be biopsied using an ultrasound guided closed needle biopsy. In the UK neoplastic lesions are usually metastatic but outside the UK primary tumours of hepatocytes, hepatocellular carcinoma, are extremely common, the aetiological agents being Hepatitis B and afeatoxin.

Diffuse disease can be biopsied by blind closed needle biopsy. It may be metabolic, toxic or inflammatory. Metabolic diseases are uncommon inherited diseases, many of which result in deposition of excess substrates in hepatocytes; these interfere with normal liver function and present as signs of liver failure in children.

Toxins commonly affect the liver, as this is the site where detoxification of ingested material occurs. The most widespread hepatotoxin is ethanol; this causes three separate lesions in the liver, which may co-exist, but each does not necessarily precede or follow the other. They are:

- Acute fatty liver which follows a bout of heavy alcohol consumption. Ethanol affects fat metabolism in hepatocytes by increasing production and decreasing secretion. There is excess deposition of lipid in hepatocytes.
- Alcoholic hepatitis in which focal collections of neutrophils surround dead or dying hepatocytes. Elsewhere hepatocytes show areas of condensation of cytoplasm which are strongly eosinophilic and show positive staining with anti-ubiquitin antisera—these are termed Mallory's hyaline.
- Alcoholic cirrhosis, the result of longstanding alcohol abuse. Cirrhosis is a form of liver disease in which fibrous septa grow between portal tracts and between portal tracts and central veins, thus dividing the liver into nodules. Regeneration increases this nodular appearance.

Inflammatory disease of the liver is most commonly the result of viral infection with the hepatitis viruses A, B, C, D, E. The most common of these is hepatitis A, transmitted by the orofaecal route, which has a self-limiting course. The most feared is hepatitis B, transmitted by serous fluid, which may cause chronic disease states and predisposes to hepatocellular carcinoma.

THE MUSCLE BIOPSY

The histopathology of voluntary muscle is differentiated in several ways. **Structurally**, cross striations are demonstrated with the Mallory PTAH or Heiderhain's iron haemotoxylin. The strong acidophilia of muscle sarcoplasm with trichrome techniques and the depth of eosin staining in the routine H & E show its **composition**. **Antigenically**, labelled antisera are employed and finally, **enzymatically** by demonstrating the enzymes that are present to varying degrees in the different muscle fibres.

Which technique is chosen depends to a large extent on the diagnostic information sought. The first three are mainly involved in tumour pathology, whilst the latter is concerned with the various myopathies and it is in this sphere that muscle biopsy is particularly employed. Vascular and neurogenic elements can be similarly studied and methods for nerve fibres, elastic fibres, and fibrinoid necrosis, employed.

Biopsy of voluntary muscle is performed in patients with muscle weakness, tenderness, or atrophy in an attempt to determine the underlying pathology. This area of surgical pathology is one where histochemical techniques are a necessity. The muscle contains constituent fibres that are differentiated into fibre types, the metabolic and contractile properties of which are different. Histochemical methods are able to differentiate between the different fibre types, and this is used in the diagnosis of muscular abnormalities as these will not be apparent in the H&E—Bancroft & Stevens (1975), Johnson (1990).

The histological appearances using enzyme techniques enable the pathologist to distinguish between myopathy, myositis and denervation. A successful muscle biopsy depends on collaboration between the physician, who will indicate which accessible muscle is most likely to show pathological changes, the surgeon, who will excise an adequate specimen from the chosen muscle with care and the laboratory which will optimally prepare the specimen. It is advisable to maintain the muscle at stretch from the outset, so it is helpful if the surgeon ties each end of the biopsy specimen before excision and maintains tension on the silks employed. A useful manoeuvre is for the surgeon to tie the piece of muscle to be removed to either end of a piece of orange stick before excision. This maintains the muscle biopsy at the correct tension and allows neither shrinkage nor over-stretching. Paraffin sections will be used for the tinctorial and immunocytochemical techniques and fresh cryostat sections for the enzyme techniques.

FIXATION

When the main muscle biopsy specimen has been removed, it is pinned on a flat piece of card or cork at its original tension. It is then left in a moist atmosphere on filter paper in a closed petri dish, for 30 minutes before fixation. Fixation is by 10% neutral formalin, formal calcium or formal sublimate for 24 hours, with the biopsy still pinned out on the card. After fixation the biopsy specimen is cut into two pieces with a sharp scalpel blade to produce two histological blocks: one to be cut to provide transverse sections and the other to show the fibres in longitudinal section. Muscle biopsies should always receive adequate fixation and slow careful processing for the most successful results; large pieces of muscle should be double embedded. A small piece of muscle is fixed in glutaraldehyde for possible electron microscopy.

FREEZING OF MUSCLE BIOPSIES

A piece of muscle no larger than $4 \times 4 \times 3$ mm is frozen after being allowed to stand in a moist atmosphere as previously described. This prevents sudden contraction of the muscle on freezing. For freezing, isopentane super-cooled by liquid nitrogen, as this substance has a high rate of thermal conductivity and consequently a rapid rate of freezing. A slower method of freezing will produce the classic freezing artefact and will make interpretation of the stained slides difficult.

SECTIONING FROZEN MUSCLE BLOCKS

The sectioning of a frozen muscle block in the cryostat presents little problem to an experienced histologist providing the temperature is maintained below $-18°C$. It is essential that the frozen specimen is orientated correctly so that the muscle fibres will be cut transversely. Sections should be cut between 8 and 10 μm to give the best results.

ROUTINE STAINING METHODS

The following methods are commonly used for muscle biopsies:

Haematoxylin and eosin (see p. 27). Used for general morphology. In a well-performed H&E, regenerating muscle fibres can be detected because they are slightly more basophilic than normal fibres. The method also demonstrates the nature of any cellular infiltrate or vascular abnormalities.

Elastic van Gieson (see p. 55). This technique demonstrates collagen, and picks up any abnormality of arterial elastica, e.g. in old arteritis, and stains the myelin or peripheral nerve endings. Some pathologists prefer a trichrome stain for these purposes. One advantage of the trichrome method, as opposed to the elastic van Gieson technique, is that it demonstrates the rods in nemaline rod myopathy. Particularly useful in this context is the Gomori one-step trichrome (see p. 43).

Methyl green-pyronin (see p. 98). The method emphasizes any regenerating muscle fibres; these have a high RNA content and are more pyroninophilic than normal fibres. Nemaline rods also stain deep red by this method.

PAS reaction (see p. 135). This technique demonstrates any glycogen in muscle fibres; positive identification of glycogen depends upon the disappearance of PAS positivity after pre-treatment with diastase. Type 2 fibres stain more strongly than the type 1; fresh cryostat sections coated with celloidin (to prevent streaming of the glycogen) should be used.

Table 16.4   Useful histological and histochemical methods for muscle biopsies

Method	Page	Demonstrates
Haematoxylin and eosin	27	General morphology
Elastic van Gieson	55	Elastic fibres
Masson's trichrome	42	Collagen, muscle
MSB	125	Collagen, fibrinoid
Gomori one-step trichrome	43	Nemaline rod myopathy
Congo red	113	Amyloid
Succinate dehydrogenase	317	Types 1 and 2 fibres
PAS with diastase control	135	Glycogen
Methyl green-pyronin	98	Regenerating muscle
ATPase (pH 4.2, 4.6, 9.4)	305	Types 1 and 2 fibres

ENZYME HISTOCHEMICAL METHODS

Many enzyme histochemical methods have been applied to cryostat sections of muscle biopsies. The three given below are probably the most widely used and generally informative.

Succinate dehydrogenase (SDH) (see p. 317). This technique enables type 1 and the different type 2 fibres to be distinguished: type 1 fibres stain darkly and type 2 stain lightly. Other enzymes of the oxidative cycle have similar reactions.

Muscle adenosine triphosphatase (ATPase) (see p. 305). This method enables type 1 and type 2 fibres to be distinguished. Type 1 fibres stain weakly at 9.4 while type 2 react strongly. At pH 4.2, type 1 fibres stain strongly and type 2 are weak or negative. At pH 4.6 it is possible to differentiate between type 2A and 2B, based on this and other enzyme reactions. The type 2 fibres have been further subdivided into types 2A, 2B and 2C (see Table 16.5).

Phosphorylase. This method also enables the two different fibre types to be distinguished, but less clearly than in the two methods mentioned above, since some fibres stain with intermediate intensity. Its value lies in its application to the phosphorylase deficiency myopathy McArdle's disease, which is a glycogen storage disease.

The value of the enzyme methods lies in their ability to distinguish between the two basic types of muscle fibres. Variations in size, number and distribution of the two fibre types have considerable diagnostic importance.

Table 16.5 Enzyme histochemical muscle fibre differentiation

Method	Page	Type 1	2A	2B	2C
ATPase pH 4.2	305	+++	−	−	+
ATPase pH 4.6	305	+++	+	++	++(+)
ATPase pH 9.4	305	+	++	+++	+(+)
NADH	317	+++	++	+	++(+)
Lactic dehydrogenase (LDH)	317	+++	++	+	++(+)
Succinate dehydrogenase (SDH)	317	+++	++	+	++(+)
Phosphorylase	−	+	++	+++	+(+)

ELECTRON MICROSCOPY

Electron microscopy is important in the diagnosis of rare myopathies, and is of confirmatory value in other muscle diseases. Many ultrastructural abnormalities are completely non-specific, however, and the same changes can be seen in a variety of muscle diseases.

PATHOLOGY OF VOLUNTARY MUSCLE

Voluntary muscle disease presents either as pain or fatigue of the affected muscles on exertion; on examination the muscle may be weak or atrophied. Muscle biopsies are usually taken as closed needle biopsies but open biopsies are frequently performed. The tissue must be received fresh, as previously mentioned, so that the various enzyme histochemical techniques can be carried out. The disease may be a primary disorder of the myocytes, an abnormality of innervation or a disease of the vascular supply. Primary abnormalities of myocytes are termed myopathies and fall into the following four groups:

• Muscular dystrophies, e.g. Duchenne. These are a group of inherited muscle disorders presenting as progressive muscle destruction. The time of onset of the disorder and the muscles affected vary with the type of dystrophy. All types show changes on muscle biopsy that, together with the clinical history, allow accurate diagnosis of the type of disease. The genetic basis of each type is known, and thus genetic counselling can be given.

• Inflammatory myopathies. These may be infectious—from bacteria, viruses or parasites—or may be autoimmune, as in the case of polymyositis and dermatomyositis. The changes seen on muscle biopsy consist of fibre necrosis with phagocytosis and an inflammatory infiltrate.

• Toxic and metabolic myopathies. Metabolic myopathies occur as a result of an inborn error of metabolism, such as glycogen storage diseases, toxic myopathies as a result of ingestion of a toxin.

• Congenital myopathies. These are rare congenital abnormalities presenting as neonatal hypotonia; some are familial.

Abnormalities of innervation may arise as a result of damage to upper or lower motor neurones and on biopsy are demonstrated as abnormalities in the ratio and distribution of the muscle fibre types.

Vascular disease affecting muscle causes ischaemia; this may be due to simple occlusion of the vascular supply by atheroma or microvascular angiopathy, or may be vasculitis such as polyarteritis nodosa.

Malignant voluntary muscle tumours are extremely uncommon, occurring predominantly in children. They are termed rhabdomyosarcomas.

THE BONE BIOPSY AND SPECIMENS OF BONE

Bone is a type of connective tissue in which extracellular components are calcified, giving rigidity. It is a store of inorganic ions, notably calcium, and participates in the maintenance of body calcium levels. Bone is always in a state of growth and resorption. It is composed of specialized cells and an organic extracellular matrix containing proteoglycan ground substance and collagen fibres; calcium hydroxyapatite crystals form the mineral component of bone matrix.

Bone salts are a crystalline hydroxyapatite composed largely of hydrated calcium phosphate, but also containing traces of carbonate, citrate and other ions. Mineralization of the osteoid by bone salts takes place shortly after the osteoid has been produced by the osteoblasts.

Bone has a cellular component and there are three important types of cells: the osteoblast, osteoclast and osteocyte:

• Osteoblasts are immature forms of bone cells and are responsible for the formation of the organic component of the matrix of bone osteoid. This substance then undergoes mineralization and the osteoblasts become trapped within the bone and are then termed osteocytes. The fibrous component of bone is mainly collagen, which reacts in a similar manner to collagen found in other sites.

• An osteocyte is generally considered as an osteoblast that has become trapped within the bone that it has helped to produce (see above).

• Osteoclasts are multinucleate cells actively involved in the resorptive process. The osteoclast is a large, sometimes very large, multinucleate giant cell found at sites of bone erosion or resorption. The more active the bone resorption the larger the osteoclasts appear. The mechanism by which osteoclasts erode bone is not fully understood.

Bone is of two main types. Woven bone is immature and shows the woven organization of the fibrous elements. Lamellar bone is formed from woven bone and is the basis of bones. It is seen as a solid mass — either as compact bone or as a spongy form described as cancellous bone. There are, to a greater or lesser extent, two distinct structurally different components, compact bone and loose cancellous bone. Compact bone forms the shafts of long bones and the exterior surfaces of flat bones. It is composed of closely packed cylinders of dense bone with a central canal. It contains concentrically arranged osteocytes with cytoplasmic processes running along narrow channels within the bone (canaliculi) and the Haversian canal system.

Cancellous bone is composed of narrow interconnecting trabeculae of bone, forming a fine network that has both strength and lightness. This type of pattern forms the central area of a bone and is surrounded by the dense compact, or cortical bone. Spongy, trabecular or cancellous bone is found in the marrow cavities of the long bones, the centre of flat bones and the vertebrae. Bone cement lines are particularly well shown if sections are stained overnight in Ehrlich's haematoxylin diluted .1 part to 99 parts distilled water (Germain 1990).

Osteoid is composed largely of proteinaceous collagenous fibres, arranged compactly, with a mixture of proteoglycans. Bone marrow fills the intertrabecular spaces. It contains the primitive stem cells from which the cellular elements of blood are derived. In the young, the bone marrow participates in blood cell formation. Active bone marrow is filled with dividing stem cells and the precursors of mature blood cells. The many maturing erythrocytes produce the red colour of active marrow whilst less active marrow consists of a reticulin framework that supports the developing blood cells. Inactive bone marrow is largely fatty in composition.

FIXATION OF BONE

As with soft tissues, the adequate fixation of bone is important. Many fixatives have been tried with bone but the best results are obtained with 10% neutral formalin. The poor penetration of the fixative is even more of a problem with bone because of the density of the tissue. The average histology block should be fixed for 48 hours and be no thicker than 4 mm to obtain reasonably rapid and good fixation. Some fixatives also contain agents that will decalcify the tissue during fixation; in our experience these produce no better, and often inferior, results to fixation followed by decalcification.

Urgent specimens

Many surgical laboratories receive urgent bone biopsies; for these, fixation requires to be as rapid as possible. To facilitate this, blocks should be only 2–3 mm thick and fixed in formalin at 37°C for 4–6 hours with as little cortical or dense bone as possible.

DECALCIFICATION OR DEMINERALIZATION

The hydroxyapatite crystals are removed from the bone before suitable sections can be produced. The removal of calcium salts is termed decalcification or demineralization. To remove the crystals, the decalcifying agent passes through the organic fraction of the tissue before reaching the inorganic fraction, and in doing so invariably damages these structures. Two types of decalcifying agent can be used, either acids or organic chelating agents. Commercial decalcifying agents have appeared in recent years; they have no advantage over laboratory prepared solutions.

ACIDS

Many different acids have been used for decalcifying bone. The acids are used as simple dilute aqueous solutions or in mixed solutions with other dilute acids or chemicals. Out of the many acids the best results are probably obtained with nitric , formic and trichloracetic.

Nitric acid. This is probably used most often as it decalcifies rapidly and is reliable in that it will complete the decalcification. Unfortunately, if tissue is left too long in nitric acid considerable damage to the tissue will occur; this damage will become apparent after two days or if in concentrations of acid above 8%. Because of its rapid action, nitric acid is ideal for urgent bone biopsies. Nitric acid for routine use should be a 5% solution with a few milligrams of urea added to each 100 ml. After decalcification the tissue is washed well in 70% alcohol before being processed to paraffin wax.

Formic acid. A good routine decalcifying agent, it is slower in its action than nitric acid, but causes less damage to the tissue by over-exposure. As a standard reagent it should be used as a 10% solution in distilled water. Decalcification for a piece of cancellous bone 4 mm thick should be complete in 48 hours, while for dense bone two weeks or longer may be required. It is recommended that the formic acid is changed every two days. The staining results obtained after formic acid are superior to those using nitric acid.

CHELATING AGENTS

Ethylenediamine tetra-acetic acid (EDTA) is the chelating agent used to remove calcium and it produces a much slower rate of decalcification than the acids. The chelation will take place at neutral pH in a 15% solution. Little damage occurs to the tissue although it may be in the EDTA for several months before decalcification is complete. The speed with which the calcium is removed can be accelerated by heating to between 37°C and 42°C, without causing tissue damage. Staining is of an acceptable standard after using this chelating agent and good differential results can be obtained. A recommended solution which combines both an acid and a chelating agent is as follows:

EDTA 0.7 g
Potassium sodium tartrate 0.008 g
Sodium tartrate 0.14 g
Make up to 1 litre with distilled water and add 99.2 ml of conc. HCl. Note that tissue should be left in this solution for no longer than $1\frac{1}{2}$ days.

Detecting the end-point of decalcification

It is important that when decalcification is complete the tissue should be removed from the decalcifying fluid immediately, otherwise difficulty will be encountered with staining. The best way of confirming complete decalcification is to X-ray the specimen; if this facility is not available then a chemical test for the presence of calcium in the decalcifying fluid should be used. Once the fluid is free of calcium, decalcification is complete. This test will not work with EDTA as there are no free calcium ions in the decalcifying fluid. In this instance, experience is used to decide when the specimen is free of calcium if it cannot be X-rayed.

Decalcification damage to tissue

Adequate fixation is necessary to minimize the damaging effects of treatment with acids. In using acids to remove calcium ions, carbon dioxide is produced. The pressure of the gas and its movement through the tissue is believed to be one factor causing the separation of connective tissues seen after decalcification (Brain 1966). Staining is affected by long treatment with acids, e.g. haematoxylin staining may need to be prolonged and eosin staining is non-differential and intense.

Summary

For routine use: (cancellous bone) 5% nitric acid (aqueous, with added urea), 1–2 days, or 10% formic acid (aqueous), 2–4 days. For non-urgent material: EDTA, 2 weeks–3 months. For urgent material: warm (37°C) 5% nitric acid, 5–12 hours.

PROCESSING OF BONE

In handling large pieces of bone consideration is given, after decalcification, to the means by which the material is to be embedded. Most bone specimens cut adequately when embedded in paraffin wax, but sometimes only after double-embedding. Dense cortical bone, particularly a large specimen, will probably give the best results after being embedded in celloidin. Small biopsies of cancellous bone may be processed using an overnight schedule.

Double-embedding paraffin process

This is the most suitable technique for producing good sections of bone. It involves the usual dehydration in alcohol, then alcohol-ether, followed by impregnation of the bone in two changes of 2% celloidin. This is followed by hardening of the celloidin and clearing of the tissue in chloroform; the block is then embedded in paraffin wax. The double-embedding procedure holds the tissue together better, allowing superior sections to be cut. It takes more time than routine paraffin embedding, usually a working week.

Celloidin sections

The embedding and sectioning of bone material in celloidin is time-consuming and tedious compared with paraffin wax; it does, however, produce excellent results with large pieces of bone. It is not recommended for routine surgical use.

Frozen sections

Small pieces of cancellous bone can be successfully frozen and cut in a cryostat. Larger pieces of bone may be cut on freezing microtomes, but this takes practice before good sections can be produced.

UNDECALCIFIED BONE SECTIONS

To investigate the extent of mineralization of bone, it is necessary to examine undecalcified sections of cancellous bone. Firstly, adequate fixation is attained in 10% neutral formalin and the tissue blocks double-embedded or resin-embedded. In our laboratories the undecalcified bone biopsy is embedded in resin as a matter of routine. In osteomalacia there is a failure of mineralization of bone, best seen in the cancellous bone trabeculae; only the central core of the bone is mineralized, the remainder being uncalcified osteoid. This is distinct from osteoporosis, in which although the trabeculae are thin, mineralization is complete, and no unstained outer zone of osteoid can be distinguished.

BONE BIOPSY

Biopsy material of bone for diagnostic purposes is usually obtained by trephine, and will give a tissue sample some 2–3 mm in diameter and approximately 2 cm in length. A well-taken biopsy will be largely composed of cancellous, as opposed to cortical bone, but much depends on the individual skill of the operator. On occasion, a larger (5 mm) diameter biopsy will be taken and is likely to be required in the demonstration of abnormal osteoid seams, as in osteomalacia.

Preparatory technique for trephine (needle) biopsies

The standard fixative is neutral buffered formalin. Other fixatives, such as Zenker or Helly, will give improved cellular detail but difficulties are likely to be encountered when carrying out silver techniques for reticulin fibres. Careful handling of the somewhat fragile needle biopsy is important at all stages of treatment.

Following fixation (preferably overnight) the biopsy is processed into plastic resin or paraffin. Resin blocks do not normally require prior decalcification. For paraffin processing it is recommended that the tissue is first decalcified in a weak organic acid, such as 10% formic acid for 6 h at room temperature. If the needle biopsy is long enough there is, of course, no reason why a small fragment should not be processed into resin and the remainder into paraffin.

The microscopy of bone marrow cells is easier if the sections are cut at 2–3 μm. The one exception is when silver techniques for reticulin fibres are required. These are more easily studied at the conventional paraffin section thickness of 5 μm. It will be found that the cancellous bone with its component marrow tends to lift during staining. The sections are better mounted on acid-alcohol-washed, or adhesive coated slides (see p. 32).

Demonstration techniques for trephine (needle) biopsies

Besides the routine H&E, Giemsa staining (see p. 70) is often performed for the differential demonstration of the marrow cells. Other, optional, techniques include methyl green-pyronin (see p. 98) for plasma cells, and chloroacetate esterase (see p. 313) for cells of the myeloid series. An important technique, also, is the silver staining of reticulin. Normal marrow contains few of these fibres and an increase indicates cell hyperplasia, or certain types of neoplasm. In myelofibrosis, too, there may be complete overgrowth of the bone marrow by reticulin fibres.

Unfortunately, the demonstration of reticulin in decalcified bone tissue is fraught with problems. These include a heavy background, non-specific argyrophilia of cells and their nuclei, beading of reticulin fibres and general inconsistency of fibre demonstration. There is no one simple solution to these problems. A newly prepared ammoniacal silver solution may be found efficacious. It is worth taking through several slides and slightly varying the times of treatment of the ammoniacal silver stage, to provide a measure of choice of stained section.

Immunocytochemistry on these decalcified paraffin bone sections is entirely feasible and will be discussed later.

STAINING AND DEMONSTRATION OF BONE

The staining of bone can be divided into three parts: firstly for general morphology, secondly for the cells of the bone marrow and lastly for metabolic disease. Methods are given for each group and a summary of the staining methods suitable for bone given in Table 16.6.

Table 16.6 Staining methods for use with bone

Method	Page	Application
Haematoxylin and eosin	27	Morphology
van Gieson	36	Connective tissue
Reticulin	48	Myelofibrosis and hyperplastic bone marrow
Periodic acid-Schiff	135	Mucoproteins of woven bone
Schmorl thionin*	405	Lacunae and canaliculi
von Kossa	410	Calcium deposits (undecalcified bone)
Alizarin red S	211	Calcium deposits (undecalcified bone)
Masson's trichrome	42	Connective tissue

* Not recommended for paraffin sections.

PICRO-THIONIN TECHNIQUE (Schmorl 1934)

Notes

The rationale of the technique is that picric acid treatment, following staining with alkaline thionin, causes a precipitate of the dye to form in the canaliculi and lacunae of bone. The method works well with frozen and celloidin sections but gives indifferent results with paraffin. Fixation with mercuric chloride-containing solutions is said to be contraindicated, formalin being the fixative of choice.

Solutions

0.125% aqueous thionin
   Add one drop of concentrated ammonia per 100 ml volume.
Saturated (1.22%) aqueous picric acid

Technique

1. Take sections to distilled water.
2. Filter on the thionin solution for 5–15 min.
3. Rinse in distilled water.
4. Treat with the picric acid solution for $\frac{1}{2}$ min with agitation.

5. Differentiate out the excess blue dye in 70% alcohol for 5–10 min or longer if required.
6. Dehydrate, clear and mount as desired.

Results

Canaliculi, lacunae	dark brown to black
Background bone	yellow to yellow-brown
Nuclei	red-brown

WOLBACH'S GIEMSA STAIN (Lillie, 1965)

Notes

This Romanowsky method works well for bone marrow smears and sections.

Solution

Giemsa stain	1 ml
Methylalcohol	1.25 ml
0.5% aqueous sodium carbonate	0.1 ml
Distilled water	40 ml

Technique

1. Sections to distilled water.
2. Stain in Giemsa solution for 1 h, changing the stain twice.
3. Transfer to a third change of stain and leave overnight.
4. Differentiate in 95% alcohol containing a few drops of 10% colophonium in alcohol.
5. Dehydrate in absolute alcohol, clear in xylene and mount in cedarwood oil.

Results

Nuclei	dark blue
Red blood cells	yellow to pink
Cytoplasm of haemopoietic cells	light blue

LEISHMAN'S STAIN (Leishman 1901, modified)

Solutions

Leishman stain
pH 6.8 buffer
50% methanol in pH 5.0 buffer

Technique

1. Thin paraffin sections to water and leave in pH 6.8 buffer for 30 min.
2. Immerse in Leishman's stain diluted with two parts of pH 6.8 buffer to one part of stain. Leave for 10–15 min.

3. Wash and differentiate in 50% methyl alcohol in pH 5.0 buffer. When the nuclei are purple and the granules of polymorphs are clearly seen, the section is blotted until completely dry, cleared in xylene and mounted in green Euparal or DPX.

Results

Nuclei	purple
Leucocyte granules	red (eosinophils) to dark purple (basophils)
Red blood cells	pink

METABOLIC BONE DISEASE

Except for the Tripp & Mackay method, the sections used are from undecalcified pieces of cancellous bone. The calcium salts are demonstrated to show the bulk of the trabeculae, and the non-mineralized seams are shown by a collagen stain. The production of the undecalcified sections is carried out by embedding in resin or by double-embedding in paraffin wax. The former technique is to be preferred as the harder embedding medium allows for far better sections to be cut. This enables the mineral density to be studied and gives excellent morphological staining of the cells.

HAEMATOXYLIN AND EOSIN STAINING OF METHACRYLATE SECTIONS (Drury & Wallington 1980)

Solutions

Cole's haematoxylin (see p. 26)
1% aqueous eosin

Technique

1. Transfer sections from 70% alcohol to distilled water.
2. Stain in Cole's haematoxylin for 60 min.
3. Wash well in tap water.
4. Stain in 1% aqueous eosin for 30 min.
5. Differentiate in tap water until osteoid is pink and calcified bone a deep purplish brown.
6. Dehydrate sections in 70% followed by 90% alcohol and then absolute alcohol.
7. Transfer sections to Euparal essence.
8. Place section on a slide, apply a strip of smooth hard paper over the section, and remove wrinkles by rolling a glass rod over the paper. Peel off the paper.
9. Mount in Euparal. A small weight applied to the cover glass helps flattening of the sections.

Results

Osteoid tissue	pink
Calcified bone	purplish brown
Nuclei	blue
Erythrocytes	generally remain unstained

MODIFIED VON KOSSA TECHNIQUE (Tripp & Mackay 1972)

Notes

This method makes use of the principle that silver phosphate is formed which does not require decalcification so that sectioning can easily be carried out. By subjecting the tissue block to the von Kossa technique and then decalcifying to remove any unchanged calcium salts, sections of decalcified bone can be cut in the normal way. Van Gieson staining is subsequently applied.

So that non-specific silver nitrate reduction can be avoided, it is important to use either alcohol fixation or conventional formalin fixation followed by thorough washing in distilled water. When decalcifying, avoid using nitric or hydrochloric acids as these tend to dissolve reduced silver salts. It is not possible to establish the end-point of decalcification by X-rays, as the silver impregnation is X-ray opaque.

It is not practicable to reduce the formed silver phosphate in the tissue block using light, and recourse is made to a reducing solution. Even so it will be found that the centres of the thicker trabeculae are not fully blackened. This is not a serious drawback as any osteoid seams are well shown against the blackened perimeters of the trabeculae. Philpotts (1980) suggested using 3% silver nitrate in 80% alcohol at 37°C for 24 h; it is necessary to dissolve the silver nitrate in water before adding the alcohol. The reducing solution is also used at 37°C but only for 24 h. This modification has worked well in our hands.

Solutions

2% aqueous silver nitrate or 3% silver nitrate in 80% ethanol
Reducer:

Sodium hypophosphite	5g
0.1 M sodium hydroxide	0.2 ml
Distilled water	100 ml

van Gieson's solution (see p. 36)
5% aqueous sodium thiosulphate (hypo)

Technique

1. Take thin (2 mm) blocks of bone fixed in alcohol or conventional formalin solutions.
2. If formalin-fixed, wash well in several changes of distilled water. This is best carried out by washing in a large volume of distilled water (with agitation), during the day, changing the distilled water two or three times (a non-enclosed tissue processor can conveniently be adapted for this purpose).
3. Place in the 2% silver nitrate solution in the dark for 2–4 days at room temperature or the modified solution for 24 h at 37°C (according to which is more convenient).
4. Wash in three changes of distilled water for 20 s each.
5. Wash in running water for 4 h.
6. Treat with reducing solution for 2 days at room temperature or for 1 day at 37°C.
7. Wash in running water for 1 h.
8. Treat with the hypo for 24 h.
9. Wash in water for 1 h and decalcify in 5% or 10% formic acid.

10. Wash in water and then paraffin process in the normal manner.
11. Cut (8–10 μm) sections and mount on slides using an adhesive. Heat-dry for a short period.
12. Take the sections to distilled water and stain with van Gieson's solution for 5 min.
13. Drain the slide, dehydrate, clear and mount in a DPX-type mountant.

Results

Mineralized bone	black
Canaliculi and lacunae in the central areas of the non-blackened bone trabeculae	black
Bone marrow	yellow
Osteoid seams	red

GOLDNER'S METHOD (Goldner 1938)

Notes

The technique has proved valuable when applied to resin sections, mainly because of the excellent staining of bone marrow cells. Osteoblast and osteoclast activity are easily assessed.

Solutions

Weigert's haematoxylin (see p. 36)
Ponceau-fuchsin solution:

Ponceau de xylidine	0.75 g
Acid fuchsin	0.25 g
Acetic acid	1 ml

Mix and add to 100 ml distilled water.
Azophloxin solution:

Azophloxin	0.5 g
Acetic acid	0.6 ml

Mix and add to 100 ml distilled water.
Final staining solution:

Ponceau-fuchsin solution	5 –10 ml
Azophloxin solution	2 ml
Acetic acid (0.2%)	88 ml

Light green solution:

Light green	1 g
Acetic acid (0.2%)	1 ml

Mix and add to 500 ml distilled water.
Phosphomolybdic acid/orange G solution:

Phosphomolybdic acid	3g
Orange G	2 g

Dissolve in 500 ml of distilled water, and add a crystal of thymol.

Technique

1. Stand sections in a solution of 90 ml 80% ethanol and 10 ml of 25% ammonia for 1 h.
2. Rinse in water for 15 min.
3. Stain in Weigert's haematoxylin for 1 h.
4. Rinse in water for 10 min.
5. Rinse in distilled water for 5 min.
6. Stain in final ponceau fuchsin/azophloxin solution for 5 min.
7. Rinse in 1% acetic acid for 15s.
8. Stain in phosphomolybdic acid/orange G solution for 20 min.
9. Rinse in 1% acetic acid for 15s.
10. Stain with light green solution for 5 min.
11. Rinse in three changes of 1% acetic acid.
12. Rinse in distilled water, blot dry and mount.

Results

Mineralized bone	green
Osteoid	orange-red
Nuclei	blue-grey
Cartilage	purple

VON KOSSA METHOD FOR CALCIUM SALTS (von Kossa 1901)

Notes

This is the oldest and most widely used method for calcium, in which silver is subsituted for calcium in calcium salts. This silver salt is then reduced to black metallic silver by light or photographic developer. As with any method for calcium, acid fixatives should be avoided, buffered neutral formalin being recommended. The usual post-silver hypo treatment is omitted as partial bleaching of the blackened calcium salts may occur.

Solutions

2% aqueous silver nitrate
van Gieson's stain or 1% aqueous neutral red

Technique

1. Sections to distilled water, two or three changes.
2. Transfer sections to a clear glass container containing the silver nitrate, or place on a slide rack and cover the section with the solution and expose to bright sunlight or a high intensity light source for 60 min. If exposed to sunlight the time may be less; check microscopically.
3. Wash in several changes of distilled water.
4. Wash well in tap water.
5. Counterstain as required, either in van Gieson or neutral red for 5 min.
6. Dehydrate, clear and mount in DPX.

Results

Calcium deposits	black
Background	according to counterstain used.

SOLOCHROME CYANINE

Notes

Solochrome cyanine is used as a differential stain to demonstrate osteoid and its relationship with mineralized bone. It can also be used to show the calcification front and repeating bands within the wider osteoid borders. The solution of Hyman & Poulding (1961) gives the best staining in our hands.

Solution

Solochrome cyanine	1 g
Conc. sulphuric acid	2.5 ml

Mix well to incorporate all the dye in the sludge. Add 500 ml of 0.5% aqueous iron alum (ferric ammonium sulphate). Mix and filter.

Technique

1. Sections to distilled water.
2. Stain in solochrome cyanine solution for 60 min.
3. Differentiate in warm alkaline tap water until the mineralized areas appear blue and other areas light red. Control microscopically as over-differentiation causes all tissues to become blue.
4. Dehydrate, clear and mount as desired.

Results

Mineralized bone	light blue
Calcification front	dark blue
Osteoid	light red-orange
Wide osteoid	light red-orange with pale blue and orange bands
Nuclei	blue

BONE PATHOLOGY

Bone biopsies are carried out either as an open biopsy by an orthopaedic surgeon, or as a needle biopsy taken with a cutting trephine. It is important that the pathology department is aware of the differential disgnosis under consideration as most metabolic bone diseases (described below) cannot be diagnosed on decalcified specimens. The stains used for bone described in this section are largely used for the metabolic bone diseases. These are diseases in which there is an abnormality in the cycle of bone deposition and reabsorption. The three commonest are:

- A failure to calcify the osteoid due to a deficiency in an essential co-factor, vitamin D termed osteomalacia in the adult and rickets in the child.

- A generalized reduction in bone bulk termed osteoporosis. This is seen in postmenopausal women and as a complication of treatment of fractures.
- Abnormal organization of the newly deposited bone, possibly the result of viral infection in Paget's disease.

All of these conditions cause the bone to become weak and present as an increase in the number of fractures. Those occurring in abnormal bone are termed pathological fractures; besides those occurring in metabolic bone diseases such as those described above, pathological fractures also occur in tumours, which may be primary or secondary. Common primary bone tumours arise from osteoblasts and chondroblasts; benign tumours of osteoblasts are termed osteomas or osteoblastomas, benign chondral tumours are chondromas. These tumour types show tissue similar to its mature counterpart. Malignant tumours, osteosarcomas and chondrosarcomas, can be poorly differentiated; osteosarcomas are recognized by the formation of bone, chondrosarcomas by their myxoid matrix. Common secondary malignant tumours in bone are those arising from lung, breast, prostate and kidney.

REFERENCES

Astarita R W, Cramer A D, Taylor C R 1979 Lymph node biopsy diagnosis for the surgical pathologist. American Society of Clinical Pathology
Bancroft J D, Stevens A 1975 Histopathological techiques and their diagnostic uses. Churchill Livingstone, London
Berard C W, Bowling M C 1975 Overcoming technical errors in the histologic preparation of lymph nodes (Profession Educators Series). American Society of Clinical Pathology
Bowling M C 1979 Lymph node specimens: achieving technical excellence. Laboratory Medicine 10: 467–476
Brain E B 1966 The preparation of decalcified sections. Charles C. Thomas, Springfield, Illinois, Ch 3, pp 69–135
Brunk T U, Ericsson J L E 1972 Electron microscopical studies on rat brain neurons. Localisation of acid phosphatase and mode of formation of lipofuscin bodies. Journal of Ultrastructure Research 38: 1
Cajal S, Ramon Y 1912 Travaux du laboratoire de Recherches Biologiques de l' Universite de Madrid 10: 209.
Cowdry E V 1952 Laboratory techniques in biology and medicine, 3rd edn. Williams & Wilkins, Baltimore
Da Fano C 1919 –1920 Method for the demonstration of Golgi's internal apparatus. Journal of Physiology 53: 92
Drury R A B, Wallington E A 1980 Carleton's Histological technique, 5th edn. Oxford University Press, London
Gamble A R, Bell J A, Ronan J E, Pearson D, Ellis I O 1993 Tumour marker immunoreactivity to identify primary site of metastatic cancer. British Medical Journal 306: 295–298
Germain J 1990 Personal communication
Giroud A, Leblond C P 1934 Etude histochemie de la vitamine C dans glande surrenale. Archives Anatomy Microscopy and Morphology Exp. 30: 105
Glauert A M, Glauert R H 1958 Araldite as an embedding medium for electron microscopy. Journal of Biophysical and Biochemical Cytology 4: 191
Goldner J 1938 A modification of the Masson trichrome technique for routine laboratory purposes. American Journal of Pathology 14: 237
Harada K 1966 Fixative stain sequences for selective demonstration of juxtaglomerular cells. Stain Technology 41: 83
Harada K 1969 Staining juxtaglomerular granules with basic fluorescent stains. Stain Technology 44: 293

Harada K 1970 Rapid demonstration of juxtaglomerular granules with alcoholic crystal violet. Stain Technology 45: 71

Horvath E, Kovacs K, Ross R C 1972 Sub-cellular features of alcoholic liver lesions: Alcoholic hyaline. Journal of Pathology 110: 245

Hyman J M, Poulding R H 1961 Solochrome cyanin-iron alum for rapid staining of frozen sections. Journal of Medical Laboratory Technology 18: 107

Johnson M A 1990 Skeletal muscle. Ch. 10 in: Filipe M I, Lake B P (eds) Histochemistry in pathology, 2nd edn. Churchill Livingstone, Edinburgh

Kater L, Jobsis A C, Baart De La Faille-Kuyper E H 1979 Alcoholic hepatic disease. Specificity of IgA deposits in liver. American Journal of Clinical Pathology 71: 51–57

Lascano E F 1959 A new silver method for the Golgi apparatus. Archives of Pathology 68: 499

Leishman W B 1901 Note on a simple and rapid method of producing Romanowsky staining in malarial and other blood films. British Medical Journal 2: 751

Lendrum A C, Fraser D A, Slidders W, Henderson R 1962 Studies on the character and staining of fibrin. Journal of Clinical Pathology 15: 401

Lillie R D 1965 Histopathologic technic and practical histochemistry, 3rd edn. McGraw-Hill, New York

Lyon H, Christoffersen P 1971 Histochemical studies of Mallory bodies. Acta Pathologica Microbiologica Scandinavica 74A: 649

Maclennan K A M, Ellis I O, Robinson G 1990 Immunocytochemistry in diagnostic pathology. In Bancroft JD, Stevens A (eds) Theory and practice of histological techniques, 3rd edn. Churchill Livingstone, London.

McDonald D M 1964 Silver impregnation of the Golgi apparatus with subsequent nitrocellulose embedding. Stain Technology 39: 345

Page K M, Stevens A, Lowe J, Bancroft J D 1990 Bone. In: Bancroft J D, Stevens A (eds) Theory and practice of histological techniques, 3rd edn. Churchill Livingstone, London

Philpotts C J 1980 Personal communication

Reale E, Luciano L 1964 A probable source of errors in electron histochemistry. Journal of Histochemistry and Cytochemistry 12: 713

Scheuer P J 1988 Liver biopsy interpretation, 4th edn. Bailliere Tindall, London.

Schmorl G 1934 Die Pathologisch-Histologischeu Untersuchungsmethoden. Vogel, Berlin, Ch. 14, p. 259

Swerdlow M, Lokendra N, Chowdhury M D, Horn T 1983 Patterns of IgA deposition in liver tissues in alcoholic liver disease. American Journal of Clinical Pathology 77: 259–265

Szokol M, Gomba S Z 1971 Subsequent staining of juxtaglomerular cells in frozen sections. Stain Technology 46: 102

Tanaka K, Mori, W Suwa K 1981 Victoria blue-nuclear fast red stain for HBs antigen detection in paraffin section. Acta Pathologica Japonica 31: 93–98

Tripp E J, Mackay E H 1972 Silver staining of bone prior to decalcification for quantitative determinatiion of osteoid in sections. Stain Technology 47: 129

von Kossa J 1901 Nachweis von Kalk. Beitrage zur pathologischen Anatomie und zur allegemeinen Pathologie 29: 163

17. A miscellany

CORPORA AMYLACEA

These bodies may be found in three main human tissue sites—namely prostate, lungs and brain—but their significance is poorly understood. They contain varying amounts of mucoprotein and the name is derived from 'starch-like bodies', due principally to their reaction with iodine. In veterinary pathology there are similar bodies in bovine mammary glands.

Prostatic corpora amylacea

These varying sized, laminated, round structures are found mainly in the gland lumina, and are almost certainly concretions of the gland secretion.

Pulmonary corpora amylacea

These are mainly found in the alveoli of the lungs. They are laminated bodies of variable size and round in shape; the laminations may not be as marked as those of prostatic corpora amylacea. Unlike corpora amylacea of prostate and CNS, those of lung are only occasionally seen.

Central nervous system corpora amylacea

These occur in brain and spinal cord (particularly the latter) and tend to be smaller in size than the corpora amylacea of prostate and lungs; they are round in shape and non-laminated. Many workers have studied these structures. Chemically they are predominantly composed of an amylopectin-like polysaccharide (Sakai et al 1969) and structurally seem to be composed of fibrillary and granular material forming intra-astrocytic aggregates (Ramsey 1965).

Table 17.1 Staining reactions of corpora amylacea

Method	Prostatic	Pulmonary	CNS
H&E	bright red	red	blue/purple
Iodine	brown	brown	brown
PAS	magenta	weakly positive	magenta
Congo red	red*	red*	—
Azure A	—	—	metachromatic

* Sometimes exhibiting green birefringence.

Crystal identification

In theory it is possible for a wide range of crystals to occur in tissue and fluids; in practice it is limited as regards occurrence and diagnostic necessity. We have chosen the following four crystals as representative of the more important regarding histological demonstration and diagnosis. The reactions are taken from the work of Worsfold (1982) and are summarized in Table 17.2, relating to cytological smears as well as histological sections. In particular, birefringence effects can be studied using alcohol-fixed smears of synovial fluid stained by Giemsa.

Table 17.2   Crystal identification

Technique	Calcium phosphate, carbonate	Calcium oxalate	Calcium pyrophosphate	Urate
H&E	Blue or colourless	Colourless	Blue	Blue
Von Kossa	Positive	Negative	Variably positive	Variably positive
Modified von Kossa	Positive	Positive	Positive	Variably positive
Hexamine silver	Negative	Negative	Variably positive	Positive
Lithium carbonate extraction	Unchanged	Unchanged	Unchanged	Extracted
Polarizing microscopy	Monorefringent	Birefringent	Birefringent	Birefringent

CALCIUM PHOSPHATE/CARBONATE

Included in this group are mineral salts of bone, a complex group of mainly calcium salts collectively termed hydroxyapatite. Calcium deposits in tissue are often associated with necrosis, e.g. caseation necrosis of tuberculosis, atheroma of blood vessels and infarction. Calcium carbonate is often present in both normal and abnormal mineral deposits, but it is the phosphate salt that is of greater significance histochemically.

Non-acid fixatives, such as neutral buffered formalin or alcohol, are preferred. H&E staining is variable: the crystals may appear blue or colourless and any haematoxylin staining is attributed to trace elements of iron in the calcium salts. Other staining methods for calcium include alizarin red, purpurin, nuclear fast red, naphthochrome green B, alcian blue and the fluorescent morin technique. Calcium phosphate and carbonate salts are monorefringent, and in tissue are extremely variable in appearance.

CALCIUM OXALATE

These are rare constituents of tissue and may be found in kidney, heart and thyroid in primary oxalosis, a rare condition caused by an enzyme deficiency in the normal metabolism of glycine residues. Another uncommon cause of calcium oxalate formation in tissue is ethylene glycol (antifreeze) intake; crystals form in renal tubules due to the metabolism of ethylene glycol to oxalic acid. Poisoning involving oxalic acid will also produce calcium oxalate deposits in tissues such as kidney.

For fixation non-acidic fixatives are again preferred. The crystals are not stained by H&E and, using polarizing microscopy, appear as birefringent octahedral clusters. The usual methods for calcium salts are negative, including the von Kossa reaction. The following modified method is recommended for the positive demonstration of calcium oxalate. For further details on the demonstration of oxalate see Chaplin (1977).

MODIFIED VON KOSSA TECHNIQUE (Pizzolato 1964)

Notes

Calcium oxalate crystals are not normally von Kossa-positive but using this modified version positive results may be obtained. Oxidation by hydrogen peroxide converts calcium oxalate to carbonate that is blackened in the usual way by light reduction of silver nitrate. Paraffin sections are easily dislodged from the slide during the method and a section adhesive is advisable. A duplicate section is treated with silver nitrate only, to show any pre-existing calcium carbonate deposits.

Solution

Mix equal volumes of 30% (100 vols) hydrogen peroxide and 5% aqueous silver nitrate.

Technique

1. Sections to distilled water.
2. Drain and add hydrogen peroxide-silver nitrate solution, exposing to an intense light source as per the standard technique (see p. 410) for 15–30 min. If excess bubbling develops, replace with fresh reagent.
3. Wash in distilled water and counterstain as desired, e.g. weak eosin or van Gieson.
4. Dehydrate, clear and mount as desired.

Results

Calcium oxalate (and other calcium salts)	black
Background	according to counterstain used

CALCIUM PYROPHOSPHATE

These crystals occur in joints in the condition known as pseudo-gout, but whereas gout is primarily an affliction of males, both males and females are affected in pyrophosphate crystal synovitis. Synovial tissue fixed in formalin or alcohol can be examined histologically, as well as aspirated fluid from joints. The latter is examined either as wet preparations or by concentrating the crystals and then embedding in fibrin clots for histological processing.

Diagnostically, it is important to distinguish pyrophosphate crystals from urates of gout. In our experience the most reliable means is either to examine the preparations by polarizing microscopy with a quartz first order red compensator or to use lithium carbonate extraction of urates. Pyrophosphates exhibit a *positive* form birefringence whilst urates show a *negative* form birefringence. In an H&E preparation calcium pyrophosphate crystals appear as blue-stained rectangular plates or rhombohedrons. They are variably von Kossa (unmodified) and hexamine silver-positive.

URATES

Crystals of uric acid may occur either as a by-product of excessive purine (DNA) breakdown in renal tubules such as may rarely occur in leukaemia chemotherapy or, more commonly, in gout. Unlike pyrophosphate synovitis, gout tends to affect the smaller joints in the extremities. It is important to distinguish between the two conditions by identifying the component crystals of the affected tissue, although urates and calcium pyrophosphates can uncommonly occur together in crystal synovitis.

Polarizing microscopy using a quartz first order red compensator is a useful procedure, showing the urate crystals to possess a negative form birefringence. Another useful technique is to make use of the fact that only urates are extracted by lithium carbonate treatment prior to hexamine silver demonstration. In H&E preparations, uric acid crystals stain blue and are typically needle-shaped. They are variably von Kossa (un-modified) positive.

LITHIUM CARBONATE EXTRACTION-HEXAMINE SILVER TECHNIQUE FOR URATES (Gomori 1946)

Notes

The rationale of the technique is an argentaffin-type reduction by urates of the hexamine silver. The solution should be pre-heated to the desired temperature and positive control sections taken through to establish its efficacy. For reasons that are not clear, sections containing urates may show a loss of hexamine silver reactivity after long storage. Prior treatment with lithium carbonate solution will selectively extract urates.

Solutions

Hexamine silver (see p. 254)
Saturated aqueous lithium carbonate
5% aqueous sodium thiosulphate (hypo)
0.2% light green in 0.2% acetic acid

Technique

1. Two positive control and two test sections to water.
2. Treat one section of each pair with the lithium carbonate solution for 30 min.
3. Wash all sections well with distilled water, drain, and treat with hexamine silver for 1 h at 45°C.
4. Wash well in distilled water. Treat with hypo for 2–3 min.
5. Wash in water and counterstain in light green solution for 1 min.
6. Wash in water, dehydrate, clear and mount as desired.

Results

Extracted sections	urates only are extracted
Unextracted sections	urates and possibly pyrophosphates are blackened
Background	green

KERATIN

Keratin is a protein rich in sulphur-containing amino acids. It forms structures such as finger nails, hair shafts (hooves and antlers in animals) and the stratum corneum of the thicker skin surfaces. Fixation is not usually important, as most fixatives are satisfactory.

DEMONSTRATION

In addition to the two techniques described below, keratin is stained red by the phloxine-tartrazine method (see p. 71). It is usually Gram-positive (see p. 242) and aldehyde fuchsin-positive (see p. 58). It is also Congo red-positive (see p. 113) and stains brightly with orange G or picric acid. Hair shafts are strongly ZN positive (see p. 245) whilst the Schmorl reaction (see p. 203) is often positive due to the presence of the contained SH groups. In addition, keratin is birefringent with the polarizing microscope and gives a yellow secondary fluorescence with thioflavine T (see p. 118).

AURAMINE-RHODAMINE FLUORESCENT TECHNIQUE FOR KERATIN

Notes

The technique uses the auramine-rhodamine fluorescence method for tubercle bacilli but employs a post-treatment toluidine blue step to quench any background fluorescence. Good results can be obtained but are unfortunately rather variable. Auramine is considered potentially carcinogenic and should be handled with care.

Solutions

Auramine-rhodamine solution
4% aqueous toluidine blue

Technique

1. Section to water and stain with heated auramine-rhodamine, differentiating in acid-alcohol as for the tubercle bacilli technique (see p. 248) (2–3 min).
2. Following acid-alcohol treatment, wash well in tap water.
3. Stain with the toluidine blue solution for 20 s.
4. Wash in water, blot dry. Dehydrate, clear and mount in a DPX-type mountant.

Results

Keratin	yellow fluorescence

PERFORMIC ACID-METHYLENE BLUE/ALCIAN BLUE TECHNIQUE FOR KERATIN (Lake 1974)

Notes

Disulphide groups in the keratin form cysteic acid upon oxidation with performic acid. The contained sulphonate radicals of the cysteic acid will form salt linkages at a low pH with cationic dyes such as methylene blue and alcian blue to give highly selective staining of the keratin. Alcian blue has the advantage of not being extracted by the final dehydrating alcohols.

Solutions

Performic acid solution:

98% formic acid	4 ml
30% (100 volumes) hydrogen peroxide	15.5 ml
Conc. sulphuric acid	0.11 ml

Allow the solution to stand for 2 h before use to allow full formation of performic acid.

0.02% methylene blue (pH 2.5) **or** *0.1% alcian blue*

Dissolve 0.1 g alcian blue in 1 ml conc. sulphuric acid using a glass rod for stirring. Add 9 ml glacial acetic acid and mix.

Technique

1. Sections to distilled water.
2. Treat with the performic acid solution for 30 min.
3. Wash well in distilled water.
4. Stain with the methylene blue solution for 15 min or alcian blue for 1 h.
5. Wash in water and blot dry. Dehydrate quickly, clear and mount in a DPX-type mountant.

Results

Keratin (hair shafts)	blue
Background	colourless

SPERMATOZOA IN TISSUE SECTIONS

Apart from the demonstration of testicular spermatozoa in situ for teaching purposes, it is sometimes useful to be able to distinguish them in sperm granulomas. These are uncommon lesions in which a granulomatous reaction has been provoked by the presence of spermatozoa in testicular tissue, outside their normal location in the seminiferous tubules. Only the spermatozoa heads are stained by the following technique, but they are stained more clearly and selectively than in the ZN technique, which is the usual technique employed.

PUTT'S TECHNIQUE (Putt 1951)

Notes

The post-staining lithium carbonate presumably acts as some sort of trapping agent for the dye. The staining solution does not keep well, and will need to be renewed at intervals of 2–3 months. It is important to counterstain lightly in order not to obscure the spermatozoa.

Solutions

Putt's solution
   New fuchsin 1 g in 10 ml absolute alcohol, and phenol 5 g in 100 ml distilled water. Mix and filter.
Differentiator
   5% acetic acid in absolute alcohol.
Counterstain
   0.2% aqueous methylene blue.

Technique

1. Sections to water.
2. Treat with Putt's solution for 5 min. Place in saturated aqueous lithium carbonate solution for 1 min.
3. Decolourize in the acetic-alcohol solution for 5 min.
4. Wash in two changes of absolute alcohol for 2 min each.
5. Wash in water, and counterstain lightly in the methylene blue solution for 20 s.
6. Wash in water, differentiate well and dehydrate in alcohol; clear and mount as desired.

Results

Spermatozoa heads	dark red
Background	pale blue

IN-SITU HYBRIDIZATION AND POLYMERASE CHAIN REACTION TECHNIQUES

Recent years have produced an exciting new technology by which precise identification of a nucleic acid sequence can be achieved in tissue sections. These techniques are termed in-situ hybridization (ISH) and polymerase chain reaction (PCR). They are complex highly expensive procedures that are carried out in specialized laboratories. The areas of diagnostic interest centre on the detection of viral agents such as the human papillomavirus (HPV), where types 16 and 18 are thought to be implicated in cervical cancer aetiology.

The following is a brief outline of performing the techniques. For a more detailed description the reader is referred to Bos et al (1987), Ehrlich (1989), Warford (1988, 1991) and Syrjanen et al (1990).

IN-SITU HYBRIDIZATION

Although first described in the late 1960s by Pardue & Gall (1969) and John et al (1969), only in recent years has ISH become more widely used as the development and production of the necessary probes accelerated. The principle of the reaction is that test material DNA is hybridized with a labelled nucleic acid probe having a complementary DNA/RNA sequence (base pairing). The label used may be a radioactive isotope (such as ^{32}P and ^{35}S or ^{3}H) or may be a non-isotopic compound like biotin or digoxigenin. In the routine laboratory, the use of non-isotopic detection techniques is obviously to be preferred, although isotopic labelling still has a slight edge of greater sensitivity in certain areas.

The technique consists of an initial denaturation of the double-stranded target DNA into single strands by short high temperature (80°C) treatment. This is followed by hybridization with the appropriate DNA or RNA probe (usually at 37°C) incorporated in a complex solution containing formamide (this solution allows low temperature annealing) and dextran sulphate for concentration of the probe. The final stage is to visualize the annealed probe by either autoradiography or immunocytochemistry. Routinely fixed paraffin-processed material may be employed, but pre-treatment with enzymes such as pepsin or proteinase K is necessary to expose the target DNA for the reaction.

POLYMERASE CHAIN REACTION

This reaction was devised in 1983 by an American research worker in the Cetus Corporation, and is a highly sensitive means by which specific DNA sequences can be amplified. This high degree of sensitivity can be a drawback in that false positivity due to extraneous contamination can occur, for example from the skin.

In outline, the technique comprises a repetitive series of temperature cycles, starting with a high (91°C) temperature stage which denatures the target DNA to a single-strand form. This is followed by a lower (60°C) stage in which the single-stranded DNA is allowed to anneal to the primer. The final stage is the extension of the primer by DNA polymerase at a temperature in the region of 72°C. The solution used in the above reaction contains not only the DNA polymerase, but also the four deoxynucleotide triphosphates that the enzyme adds to the ends of the primers. The polymerase is a heat-stable enzyme obtained from a bacterium *Thermus aquaticus* that is termed Taq polymerase. The primers are single-stranded oligonucleotides that are specifically designed to flank the DNA region of interest.

The net result of the above sequence of a single PCR cycle is a doubling of the target DNA molecules as the newly synthesized DNA strands act as templates for the next round of amplification. Four copies are generated after two cycles, eight after three and so on, ad infinitum. Visualization of the amplified target DNA may be subsequently achieved by agarose gel electrophoresis using a fluorescent dye, ethidium bromide.

REFERENCES

Bos J L, Fearon E R, Hamilton S R, Veerlan-de Vries M, van Boom J H, van der Eb A J, Vogelstein B 1987 Prevalence of *ras* gene mutations in human colorectal cancers. Nature 327: 293

Ehrlich H A 1989 Polymerase chain reaction technology. Stockton Press, New York

Chaplin A J 1977 Histopathological occurrence and characterisation of calcium oxalate: a review. Journal of Clinical Pathology 30: 800–811

Gomori G 1946 A new histochemical test for glycogen and mucin. American Journal of Clinical Pathology 16: 177

John H, Birmsteil M L, Jones K W 1969 RNA-RNA hybrids at the cytological level. Nature
223: 582–587

Lake B 1974 In: Cook H C (ed) Manual of histological demonstration techniques.
Butterworth, London

Pardue M L, Gall J G 1969 Molecular hybridization of radioactive DNA to the DNA of
cytology preparations. Proceedings of the National Academy of Science 24: 600–604

Pizzolato P 1964 Histochemical recognition of calcium oxalate. Journal of Histochemistry
and Cytochemistry 12: 333

Putt F A 1951 A modified Ziehl-Neelsen method for demonstration of leprosy bacilli and
other acid-fast organisms. American Journal of Clinical Pathology 21: 92

Ramsey H J 1965 Ultrastructure of corpora amylacea. Journal of Neuropathology and
Experimental Neurology 24:25

Sakai M, Austin J, Witmer F 1969 Studies of corpora amylacea (1) Isolation and preliminary
characterization by chemical and histochemical techniques. Archives of Neurology 21: 526

Syrjanen S, Saastamoinen J, Chang F, Ji H, Syrjanen K 1990 Colposcopy, punch biopsy, in
situ hybridization and the polymerase chain reaction in searching for genital human
papillomaviruses (HPV) infections in women with normal PAP smears. Journal of Medical
Virology 31: 259–266

Warford A 1988 In situ hybridisation: a new tool in pathology. Medical Laboratory Sciences
45: 381–394

Warford A 1991 In situ hybridisation in perspective. Journal of Clinical Pathology 44:
171–181

Worsfold D 1982 Unpublished data

Appendix 1
Fixative solutions

Acetic alcohol formaldehyde (AAF)
Conc. formalin	10 ml
Glacial acetic acid	5 ml
Absolute alcohol	85 ml

Acetone
Absolute acetone at 4°C

1% Acrolein
Acrolein	1 ml
0.1 M phosphate buffer, pH 7.4	99 ml

(The final pH of this fixative should be checked and adjusted to 7.2–7.6 if necessary).

Alcohol
Alcohol 80–100% at 4°C

Bouin's fixative
Picric acid (saturated aqueous)	75 ml
Conc. formalin	25 ml
Glacial acetic acid	5 ml

Carnoy's fixative
Ethyl alcohol	60 ml
Chloroform	30 ml
Glacial acetic acid	10 ml

Clarke's fixative
Absolute alcohol	75 ml
Glacial acetic acid	25 ml

Flemming's fixative
1% chromic acid	60 ml
2% osmium tetroxide	16 ml
Glacial acetic acid	25 ml

10% Formalin
Conc. formalin	10 ml
Tap or distilled water	90 ml

Formal alcohol
Conc. formalin	10 ml

| Absolute alcohol | 80 ml |
| Tap or distilled water | 10 ml |

Formal ammonium bromide

Conc. formalin	15 ml
Ammonium bromide	2 g
Tap or distilled water	85 ml

10% Formal calcium

Conc. formalin	10 ml
Tap or distilled water	90 ml
Calcium chloride	1.1 g
(or until pH reaches 7.0)	

10% Formal saline

Conc. formalin	100 ml
Sodium chloride	9 g
Tap or distilled water	900 ml

Formal sublimate

| Mercuric chloride (saturated aqueous) | 90 ml |
| Conc. formalin | 10 ml |

Formal sucrose

Conc. formalin	10 ml
Sucrose	7.5 g
0.2 M phosphate buffer, pH 7.4	90 ml

Gendre's fixative

Picric acid (saturated in 95% alcohol)	85 ml
Conc. formalin	10 ml
Glacial acetic acid	5 ml

6% Glutaraldehyde

| Glutaraldehyde (25%) | 24 ml |
| 0.1 M phosphate buffer, pH 7.4 | 76 ml |

On storage, the glutaraldehyde becomes acidic, pH 2.5–3.0. The final pH of the above fixative should be checked and adjusted to 7.0–7.2 if necessary with sodium hydroxide.

Heidenhain's 'Susa'

Tap or distilled water	76 ml
Mercuric chloride	4.5 g
Sodium chloride	0.5 g
Trichloracetic acid	2 g
Glacial acetic acid	4 ml
Conc. formalin	20 ml

Helly's fixative

Tap or distilled water	95 ml
Mercuric chloride	5 g
Potassium dichromate	2.5 g

Sodium sulphate	1 g
Conc. formalin is added before use	5 ml

10% Neutral buffered formalin

Conc. formalin	10 ml
Tap or distilled water	90 ml
Sodium dihydrogen phosphate (anhydrous)	0.35 g
Disodium hydrogen phosphate (anhydrous)	0.65 g

10% Neutral formalin

Conc. formalin	10 ml
Tap or distilled water	90 ml
Calcium carbonate chips to cover bottom of container	

Newcomer's fixative

Isopropanol	50 ml
Propionic acid	25 ml
Petroleum ether	8.3 ml
Acetone	8.3 ml
Dioxane	8.3 ml

Paraformaldehyde fixative

Dissolve paraformaldehyde in distilled water to make a 40% solution by heating in a fume cupboard, stirring constantly until only a faint cloudiness persists. Clarify this solution by adding 10 N NaOH drop by drop until the solution is clear. Cool to room temperature and then to 4°C in a refrigerator. Filter after cooling to 4°C. If the solution is being used only for subsequent paraffin sections, the longevity of the 40% paraformaldehyde can be increased by adding sodium pyrophosphate until the solution is a 0.02 M solution of sodium pyrophosphate in the 40% paraformaldehyde solution.

Regaud's fluid

3% potassium dichromate	80 ml
Conc. formalin	20 ml

(Regaud's fluid does not keep, and the solutions should only be mixed immediately before use.)

Rossman's fluid

100% ethanol saturated with picric acid	90 ml
Neutralized commercial formalin	10 ml

Zenker's fixative

Tap or distilled water	95 ml
Mercuric chloride	5 g
Potassium dichromate	2.5 g
Sodium sulphate	1 g
Glacial acetic acid	5 ml

Appendix 2
Preparation of molar solutions

PREPARATION OF 1 LITRE MOLAR SOLUTION

1. Calculate the gram molecular weight (using atomic weights) of the solute.
2. Weigh out 1 g molecule of the solute.
3. Measure out 1000 ml of distilled water.
4. Dissolve the solute in a small quantity of water.
5. Add the remaining distilled water, to make the solution up to 1 litre volume.

For solutions of different molarity (e.g. 2 M solution = 2 × gram molecular wt in 1000 ml water)

Example: Sodium β-glycerophosphate

- Molecular weight of sodium β-glycerophosphate = 315.13
- Molar solution (M) = 315.13 g in 100 ml distilled water
                    0.1 M = 31.513 g in 1000 ml distilled water
- The chemical is dissolved in a small quantity of the water and the volume made up to a litre.

PREPARATION OF MOLAR SOLUTIONS OF LIQUIDS

1. Calculate the molecular weight of the liquid.
2. Find the liquid's (a) valency, (b) specific gravity, (c) concentration.
3. Using the formula:
   Number of ml of liquid per 1000 ml of distilled water =

$$\frac{\text{molecular weight}}{\text{valency} \times \text{specific gravity} \times \text{concn}}$$

Substitute the values found in (2) in the formula to find the volume of liquid required to make up to a molar solution.

4. Measure out the required volume of liquid and make up to 1000 ml by adding distilled water. For solutions of different molarity adjustments have to be made to the volume of liquid used. For an 0.1 M solution the volume required for a 1 M solution has to be divided by 10, then made up to a litre with distilled water.

Appendix 3
Buffer tables

Notes concerning buffer solutions

The salts and acids used in the preparation of buffers should be at least laboratory reagent grade. When preparing buffers the molecular weight given on the reagent bottle should be checked, as chemicals are available in different states of hydration.

Acetate buffer (Walpole) pH 3.6–5.8

Preparation of stock solutions

   Stock A: 0.2 M acetic acid (mw 60.0) 1.2 ml glacial acetic acid in 100 ml of distilled water.
   Stock B: 0.2 M sodium acetate 1.64 g sodium acetate anhydrous (mw 82.0) or 2.72 g sodium acetate trihydrate (mw 136.0) in 100 ml of distilled water.

Composition of buffer

   x ml of A + y ml of B made up to 100 ml with distilled water.

pH	x	y
3.6	46.3	3.7
3.8	44.0	6.0
4.0	41.0	9.0
4.2	36.8	13.2
4.4	30.6	19.5
4.6	25.5	24.5
4.8	20.0	30.0
5.0	14.8	35.2
5.2	10.5	39.5
5.4	8.8	41.2
5.6	4.8	45.2
5.8	2.5	47.5

Sodium acetate-HCl buffer (Walpole) pH 1.0–5.2

Preparation of solution

Stock A: M *sodium acetate (mw 136.0)* 13.6 g sodium acetate in 100 ml distilled water.

Stock B: M *hydrochloric acid (mw 36.5)* 8.5 ml HCl in 100 ml distilled water.

Composition of buffer

500 ml of A + x ml of B made up to 250 ml with distilled water.

pH	x
1.0	75.0
1.2	65.0
1.5	61.0
1.8	54.0
2.0	52.0
2.3	51.0
2.6	50.0
3.0	49.0
3.3	7.5
3.5	46.3
3.8	42.5
4.0	39.0
4.2	35.0
4.4	30.0
4.8	18.0
5.2	10.0

Phosphate buffer (Sörensen) pH 5.8–8.0

Preparation of stock solutions

Stock A: 0.2 M disodium dihydrogen orthophosphate (mw 156.0) 3.12 g sodium dihydrogen orthophosphate in 100 ml of distilled water.

Stock B: 0.2 M disodium dihydrogen orthophosphate (mw 142.0) 2.83 g dissodium hydrogen orthophosphate in 100 ml of distilled water.

Composition of buffer

x ml of A + y ml of B made up to 100 ml with distilled water.

pH	x	y
5.8	46.0	4.0
6.0	43.8	6.2
6.2	40.7	9.3
6.4	36.7	13.3
6.6	31.2	18.8
6.8	25.5	24.5
7.0	19.5	30.5
7.2	14.0	36.0
7.4	9.5	40.5
7.6	6.5	43.5
7.8	4.2	45.8
8.0	2.6	47.4

Phosphate-citrate buffer (McIlvaine) pH 3.6–7.8

Preparation of solutions

Stock A: 0.2 M sodium dihydrogen orthophosphate (mw 142.0) 2.83 disodium hydrogen orthophosphate in 100 ml distilled water.
Stock B: 0.1 M citric acid (mw 210.0) 2.1 g citric acid in 100 ml distilled water.

Composition of buffer

x ml of A + y ml of B

pH	x	y
3.6	32.2	67.8
3.8	35.5	64.5
4.0	38.5	61.5
4.2	41.4	58.6
4.4	44.1	55.9
4.6	46.7	53.3
4.8	49.3	50.7
5.0	51.5	48.5
5.2	53.6	46.4
5.4	55.7	44.3
5.6	58.0	42.0
5.8	60.4	39.6
6.0	63.1	36.9
6.2	66.1	33.9
6.4	69.2	30.8
6.6	72.7	27.3
6.8	77.2	22.8
7.0	82.3	17.7
7.2	86.9	13.1
7.4	90.8	9.2
7.6	93.6	6.4
7.8	95.7	4.3

Tris-HCl buffer pH 7.2–9.0

Preparation of stock solutions

Stock A: *0.2 M Tris (mw 121.0)* 2.4 g Tris (hydroxymethyl methylamine) in 100 ml of distilled water.

Stock B: *0.2 M HCl (mw 36.5)* 1.7 ml hydrochloric acid in 100 ml of distilled water.

Composition of buffer

25 ml of A + x ml of B, made up to 100 ml with distilled water.

pH	x
7.2	22.1
7.4	20.7
7.6	19.2
7.8	16.3
8.0	13.4
8.2	11.0
8.4	8.3
8.6	6.1
8.8	4.1
9.0	2.5

Tris-maleate buffer pH 5.2–6.8

Preparation of stock solutions

Stock A: *0.2 M Tris acid maleate* 2.42 g Tris (hydroxymethyl methylamine) (mw 121.0), and 2.32 g maleic acid (mw 116) in 100 ml of distilled water.

Stock B: *0.2 M sodium hydroxide (mw 40.0)* 0.8 g sodium hydroxide in 100 ml of distilled water.

Composition of buffer

25 ml of A + x ml of B made up to 100 ml with distilled water.

pH	x
5.2	3.5
5.4	5.4
5.6	7.8
5.8	10.3
6.0	13.0
6.2	15.8
6.4	18.5
6.6	21.3
6.8	22.5

Boric acid-borate buffer (Holmes) pH 7.4–9.0

Preparation of stock solutions

> *Stock A: 0.2 M boric acid (mw 62.0)* 1.24 g boric acid in 100 ml distilled water.
> *Stock B: 0.05 M sodium tetraborate (mw 381.4)* 1.9 g sodium tetraborate in 100 ml distilled water.

Composition of buffer

> *x* ml of A + *y* ml of B.

pH	x	y
7.4	90.0	10.0
7.6	85.0	15.0
7.8	80.0	20.0
8.0	70.0	30.0
8.2	65.0	35.0
8.4	55.0	45.0
8.7	40.0	60.0
9.0	20.0	80.0

Veronal acetate buffer pH 3.6–5.4

Preparation of stock solutions

> *Stock A: veronal acetate stock solution* 1.94 g sodium acetate trihydrate (mw 136) and 2.94 g sodium barbitone (mw 206.0) in 100 ml of distilled water.
> *Stock B: 0.1 M HCl (mw 36.5)* 0.85 ml hydrochloric acid in 100 ml of distilled water.

Composition of buffer

pH	ml of A	ml of B	ml of distilled water
3.6	5.0	14.0	4.0
3.8	5.0	13.0	5.0
4.0	5.0	12.5	5.5
4.2	5.0	12.0	6.0
4.4	5.0	11.0	7.0
4.6	5.0	10.0	8.0
4.8	5.0	9.5	8.5
5.0	5.0	9.0	9.0
5.2	5.0	8.5	9.5
5.4	5.0	8.0	10.0

Veronal-HCl buffer (Michaelis) pH 6.8–9.2

Preparation of stock solutions

Stock A: 0.1 M hydrochloric acid (mw 36.5) 0.85 ml HCl in 100 ml distilled water.
Stock B: sodium veronal (barbitone sodium) 2.9 g in 100 ml distilled water plus
1.9 g sodium acetate (3H$_2$0)

Composition of buffer

x ml of A + *y* ml of B.

pH	x	y
6.8	19.1	20.9
7.0	18.6	21.4
7.2	17.8	22.2
7.4	16.8	23.2
7.6	15.4	24.6
7.8	13.5	26.5
8.0	11.4	28.6
8.2	9.2	30.8
8.4	7.1	32.9
8.6	5.2	34.8
8.8	3.7	36.3
9.0	2.6	37.4
9.2	1.9	38.1

Appendix 4
Suggested control material

α-Fetoprotein	primary carcinoma of liver
Acetylcholinesterase	motor end plates, axons, neurones
Acid phosphatase	prostate, liver, kidney
Adenosine triphosphatase	muscle, liver
Adrenaline	adrenal medulla
Alkaline phosphatase	kidney, small intestine
Aluminium	lung, skin (industrial disease)
Arginine	Paneth cells
Ascorbic acid	liver, adrenal cortex
Basement membranes (basal lamina)	kidney, hair follicles, epididymis
Beryllium	lung (industrial disease)
Bilirubin, biliverdin	biliary cirrhosis, cholelithiasis
Calcitonin (C) cells	thyroid (dog)
Calcium oxalate	oxalosis (kidney, thyroid)
Calcium phosphate/carbonate	bone, teeth, atheroma, necrosis
Calcium pyrophosphate	pyrophosphate synovitis
Cam 5.2	sweat glands of skin, hepatocytes
Carcino-embryonic antigen (CEA)	colon (epithelium—carcinomas of)
Charcot–Leyden crystals	eosinophil granuloma, sputum (asthma)
Chitin	hydatid cysts of liver, lung
Cholesterol	adrenal cortex, atheroma, degenerate myelin
Cholinesterase (non-specific)	C cells of thyroid, SA and AV nodes of heart
Chromaffin tissue	adrenal medulla
Copper	liver (Wilson's disease, primary biliary cirrhosis)
Cysteine	hair follicles
Cystine	stratum corneum, hair shafts
Cytochrome oxidase	liver, muscle, kidney (mitochondria)
Cytokeratin (polyclonal)	epidermis of skin
Degenerate myelin	multiple sclerosis, subacute combined degeneration
Dehydrogenases	liver, kidney, heart (mitochondria)
Desmin	gastrointestinal tract (external muscle coats)

Dopamine	mast cells of rodents
Elastic cartilage	pinna of ear, epiglottis
Elastic fibres	dermis of skin, arteries
EMA	breast
Endocrine cells (argentaffin)	appendix, ileum (epithelium)
Endocrine cells (argyrophil)	stomach (epithelium)
Eosinophils	bone marrow, subacute intestinal inflammation
Factor VIII-related antigen	endothelial cells, megakaryocytes
Fatty acids (free)	fat necrosis
Fibrin	synovitis, peritonitis, pericarditis, acute inflammation
Fibrous astrocytes	CNS white matter, gliosis
Fibrous cartilage	intervertebral discs
Fungi	lungs (*aspergillus*), skin (*Candida*)
Ganglion cells	intestinal plexus of Auerbach
Glucose-6-phosphatase	mitochondria
Glycogen	liver, voluntary muscle, ectocervix, hair follicles
Golgi apparatus	neurones, kidney (lining cells of tubules)
Gram-negative organisms	meningitis, typhoid, colonic abscesses
Gram-positive organisms	gas gangrene, bronchopneumonia, subacute endocarditis
Haematoidin	infarcts, abscesses
Haemosiderin	haemorrhage, haemochromatosis
Haemozoin	malaria (liver)
Herring bodies	pars nervosa of pituitary
Human chorionic gonadotrophin (HCG)	placenta (and tumours of)
Hyaline cartilage	joints
Hyaluronic acid	umbilical cord, skin, early placenta
Intercellular bridges of epidermis	palmar and plantar skin, squamous cell papilloma
Juxtaglomerular (JG) cells	kidney (mouse) (arterioles)
Keratin	hair shafts, palmar and plantar skin
Lipid (for general staining)	corpus luteum of ovary, sebaceous glands of skin
Lipofuscin	ganglion cells, heart, Leydig cells
Lymphoid cells	tonsil
Mallory bodies	liver (active alcoholic cirrhosis)
Mast cells	intermuscular tissue of intestine, breast fibroadenosis
Melanin	negroid skin, naevus tumours

Microglia	CNS grey and white matter, myelin degeneration
Mitochondria	renal tubules, heart, liver
Muramidase (lysozyme)	macrophages (histiocytes), Brunner's glands
Neurosecretory substance	hypothalamus
Neutral fat	subcutaneous tissue, mesentery
Neutral mucin	stomach (epithelium)
Neutrophils	acute inflammations
Nissl substance	anterior horn cells of spinal cord
Non-specific esterase	liver, kidney (tubules)
Noradrenaline	adrenal medulla
6-Nucleotidase	thyroid, liver
Oligodendrocytes	CNS grey and white matter
Osteoid seams	trabecular bone in osteomalacia
Oxytalan fibres	periodontal ligaments
Pacinian corpuscles	subcutaneous tissue (e.g. axilla)
Paneth cells	small intestine (mucosa)
Peroxidase	erythrocytes, granulocytes
Phospholipids	myelin, erythrocytes, mitochondria
Plasma cells	rheumatoid synovitis, nasal polypi, lamina propria of intestine
Plasmalogens	adrenal cortex
Protoplasmic astrocytes	CNS grey matter, gliosis
Purkinje cells	cerebellum
Purkinje fibres	subendocardium of heart
Reinke crystals	Leydig cells and ovarian hilar cells
Reticulin fibres	liver, spleen, lymphoid tissue
RNA (cytoplasmic)	plasma cells, neurones, pancreatic exocrine cells
Russell bodies	rheumatoid synovitis
S100	naevus tumours, peripheral nerves
Serotonin	intestinal argentaffin cells, rodent mast cells
Sex chromatin	buccal scrapings
Sialomucin (sialidase-labile)	submandibular salivary gland
Sialomucin (sialidase-resistant)	colon (epithelium)
Starch granules	glove powder contaminants of surgical specimens
Sterols	adrenal cortex, Leydig cells
Sulphated mucin (connective tissue)	cartilage, walls of large blood vessels
Sulphated mucin (epithelial)	colon (epithelium)
Tryptophan	Paneth cells, pancreas, eosinophils
Tyrosinase	melanocytes of skin

Tyrosine	pancreas (exocrine)
Urates	gouty tophi
Vascular fibrinoid	vasculitis (e.g. polyarteritis nodosa)
Vimentin	endometrial decidual cells
Virus inclusion bodies	viral warts, herpes simplex, cytomegalovirus

Appendix 5
Index of common dyes

Dye name	Generic name	3rd ed. CI No.
Acridine orange	Basic orange 14	46005
Alcian blue 8GX	Ingrain blue 1	74240
Alizarin red S	Mordant red 3	58005
Aniline blue (water sol) (soluble blue 3M or 2R, water blue)	Acid blue 22	42755
Auramine O	Basic yellow 2	41000
Azophloxine	Acid red 1	18050
Azur A (McNeal)		52005
Biebrich scarlet	Acid red 66	26905
Brilliant crystal scarlet 6R	Acid red 44	16250
Bismarck brown Y	Basic brown 1	21000
Carmine	Natural red 4	75470
Carminic acid		75470
Celestine blue B	Mordant blue 14	51050
Chromotrope 2R	Acid red 29	16570
Congo red	Direct red 28	22120
Crystal ponceau 6R (Brilliant crystal scarlet 6R, ponceau 6R)	Acid red 44	16250
Crystal violet	Basic violet 3	42555
Eosin, yellowish (water & alcohol sol, eosin Y)	Acid red 87	45380
Eosin bluish (eosin B, erythrosin B)	Acid red 51	45430
Fast garnet GBC salt	Azoic diazo component 4	37210
Fast green FCF	Food green 3	42053
Fast red B salt	Azoic diazo component 5	37125
Fast red TR salt	Azoic diazo component 11	37085
Fluorescein	Acid yellow 73	45350
Fuchsin acid	Acid violet 19	42685
Fuchsin basic	Basic violet 14	42510
Fuchsin new	Basic violet 2	42520
Gallocyanin	Mordant blue 10	51030
Haematein		75290
Haematoxylin	Natural black 1	75290
Janus green B	-	11050
Light green SF	Acid green 5	42095
Luxol fast blue	Solvent blue 38	–
Malachite green	Basic green 4	42000
Martius yellow	Acid yellow 36	10315
Metanil yellow	Acid yellow 36	13065
Methyl blue	Acid blue 93	42780
Methyl green	Basic blue 20	42585
Methyl violet 2B	Basic violet 1	42535

Dye name	Generic name	3rd ed. CI No.
Methylene blue	Basic blue 9	52015
Neutral red	Basic red 5	50040
Nile blue sulphate	Basic blue 12	51180
Oil red O	Solvent red 27	26125
Orange G	Acid orange 10	16230
Patent blue	Acid blue 1	42045
Phloxine	Acid red 92	45410
Phosphine	Basic orange 15	46045
Picric acid	–	10305
Ponceau 2R (ponceau de xylidene)	Acid red 26	16150
Pyronin Y (pyronin G)		45005
Rhodamine B	Basic violet 10	45170
Safranin O	Basic red 2	50240
Solochrome cyanine RS (eriochrome cyanine R)	Mordant blue 3	43820
Scarlet R (Sudan IV)	Solvent red 24	26105
Sudan black B	Solvent black 3	26150
Tartrazine	Food yellow 4	19140
Thioflavine T	Basic yellow 1	49005
Thionin	–	52000
Toluidine blue	Basic blue 17	52040
Victoria blue B	Basic blue 26	44045

Index